Early Breast Cancer

Histopathology, Diagnosis and Treatment

Edited by J. Zander and J. Baltzer

With 217 Figures and 154 Tables

Springer-Verlag
Berlin Heidelberg New York Tokyo

Prof. Dr. J. Zander
Prof. Dr. J. Baltzer

I. Frauenklinik der Universität München, Maistraße 11,
D-8000 München 2, Federal Republik of Germany

ISBN 3-540-15059-5 Springer-Verlag Berlin Heidelberg New York Tokyo
ISBN 0-387-15059-5 Springer-Verlag New York Heidelberg Berlin Tokyo

Library of Congress Cataloging in Publication Data. Main entry under title: Early brest cancer.
Includes bibliographies and index. 1. Breast–Cancer. I. Zander, Josef, 1918-. II. Baltzer, J. (Jörg),
1941-. [DNLM: 1. Breast Neoplasms. WP 870 E114] RC280.B8E228 1985 616.99'449 85-2649
ISBN 0-387-15059-5 (U.S.)

© Springer-Verlag Berlin Heidelberg 1985
Printed in Germany

Printing: Beltz Offsetdruckerei, Hemsbach/Bergst. Binding: J. Schäffer OHG, 6718 Grünstadt.
2125/3140-5 4 3 2 1 0

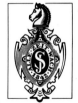

Preface

March 23 and 24, 1983 saw the first international symposium held under the auspices of the Wilhelm Vaillant Foundation for the Advancement of Prophylactic Medicine in the I. Frauenklinik der Ludwig Maximilians Universität München. This symposium was concerned with Advances in Early Detection and Treatment of Breast Cancer and brought together pathologists, gynecologists, and radiologists from Denmark, England, France, Italy, Sweden, Switzerland, the German Democratic Republic, and the Federal Republic of Germany.

The first session dealt with problems concerned with the biology, pathogenesis, and histopathology of early carcinoma of the breast, with special reference to the clinical aspects. The second session was taken up with topical developments in the early diagnosis of breast carcinoma and indicated the present limitations of early diagnosis. In the third session the latest results of the experiences by groups working on the treatment of early carcinoma of the breast in France, the United Kingdom, Italy, the United States of America, and the Federal Republic of Germany were discussed. The main emphasis lay on conservative treatment methods with complete or partial preservation of the breast. These vary quite widely. Some of the conclusions presented on the basis of long-term clinical studies must be regarded as significant breakthroughs, and at the stage these have reached they must no longer be overlooked.

The symposium has highlighted numerous unsolved problems and made it clear that conflicting opinions abound. It has also paved the way for further endeavors directed at conservative treatment of early breast cancer to save women from the fate of having a mutilated body.

The idea of publishing this volume was conceived subsequent to the symposium. It does not contain the text of the papers actually presented, but versions specifically prepared for this book.

The editors are greatly indepted to all the authors, who have made great efforts in the preparation of this publication. Prompt submission of their manuscripts has made it possible for the book to appear while the subject matter is still topical.

Thanks are also due to Springer-Verlag, and especially to Dr. Heinz Götze, for accepting this project and for the scrupulous care his staff has taken, as always in processing the material for publications.

Finally, the editors are indebted to the Wilhelm Vaillant Foundation for the Advancement of Prophylactic Medicine, and in particular to Prof. W. Vaillant. It was the Foundations's generous support that made it possible for the symposium to take place and, indirectly, for this book to be published.

We hope the book will stimulate the basic and clinical research sectors to devote even greater effort than hitherto to the diagnosis and treatment of early carcinoma of the breast, and also that it will promote international cooperation in this very urgent area. We also hope that the clinical practitioner will gain a cleare understanding of when treatment of early breast carcinoma with preservation of the breast is currently justified, and of what problems are still involved. One of our urgent priorities for the near future must be to draw up criteria for conservative treatment in early carcinoma of the breast.

Munich, December 1984   Josef Zander, FACOG (Hon) FACS
                                           Jörg Baltzer

Table of Contents

Histopathology

Diagnosis

Treatment

Author Index

The page numbers indicate the articles to which each author has contributed.

What is Early Breast Cancer?

Edwin R. Fisher

Institute of Pathology, Shadyside Hospital, Pittsburgh, PA 15232, USA
Department of Pathology, University of Pittsburgh, Pittsburgh, PA 15232, USA

It is most unfortunate that many still view the progression of cancer in general, and breast cancer in particular, from what now appears to be an anachronistic perspective. This so-called conventional view assumes that cancer grows with time and subsequently spreads to regional lymph nodes, and that after another time interval spread from these structures occurs, resulting in disseminated disease. Because of this algorithm a concept of early cancer has evolved, for it can be readily, and one might add quite simplistically, recognized that interruption of this cycle prior to spread to regional lymph nodes or dissemination from these ought to result in cure. The cancer is regarded as having been removed at an early or favorable stage. According to this, breast cancer is not only exclusively a temporal phenomenon, but a surgical disease whose outcome depends upon the surgeons' or radiotherapists' ability to eradicate all of the sources of dissemination. Yet, what is overlooked by proponents of this conventional concept is that despite refinements of surgical and radiotherapeutic technics to eliminate local disease and efforts to diagnose the disease early, the survival rate for breast cancer has not significantly improved over a span of at least five decades. Indeed, therapeutic measures are now being explored in which lesser operative procedures are being performed. This new attitude has not been provoked solely for cosmetic reasons, but has knowingly or unknowingly arisen from studies revealing a new or alternative hypothesis concerning the biology of breast cancers and, one migt add, other cancers as well.

It cannot be denied that a primary tumor takes time to grow, as we shall note, but relating spread regionally and subsequently systemically to time is, according to more modern tenets and experiences, not only entirely misleading but also inaccurate. If a breast cancer is found to be large when removed, this does not indicate that it was present for a longer time than another whose measurements are smaller. Such an erroneous conclusion fails to recognize that both may have encompassed identical periods but that the larger was more rapid in its growth than the smaller. This simple scenario clearly reflects one of many aspects of the heterogeneity of breast cancers. Further, it should also be recognized that an individual breast cancer, like other cancers, may also be comprised of heterogeneous cell populations or phenotypes. Some may be metastasizing, others may not. Some may exhibit rapid growth characteristics, others may not. Some may be responsive to various chemotherapeutic modalities, whereas others may not, etc. Despite this lack of uniformity, there are certain general principles that apply to the growth of cancers, including those of the breast, which further provokes skepticism concerning clinical designations of "early" or "late." It is well appreciated that most breast cancers cannot be palpated until they have

Early Breast Cancer
Edited by J. Zander and J. Baltzer
© Springer-Verlag Berlin Heidelberg 1985

achieved a size of 1 cm, or 1 billion cells. Many kinetic studies have indicated that this requires 30 population doubles. When it is recognized that a doubling time might encompass 30–200 or more days it becomes apparent that a tumor that is regarded as clinically early is in truth biologically late, requiring only 10–20 more doubles before causing the death of the host. A small 0.5-cm breast cancer detected by mammography, although regarded as early clinically, has already passed through 27 doubles, and is again biologically a late tumor.

The most important consideration, of course, is the time when a tumor, if it does contain metastasizing phenotypes, exhibits such a phenomenon. Most evidence suggests that when metastases occur they do so within the first 10–20 doubling times, that is to say at a stage which is undetectable by prevailing methodologies (Bauer et al. 1980). It has been estimated that 50% of women with breast cancers measuring 1 cm already have systemic disease. It is difficult to rationalize the experiences noted in some women with untreated breast cancer with the concept of early breast cancer or the pejorative effects of delay in diagnosis and treatment. It has been noted that 35% of the women with untreated breast cancer survive for 5 years, and 68% who presented with localized disease and were untreated survived at least this long (MacKay and Sellars 1965). Certainly the results obtained with protocol 4 of the NSABP refutes the significance of delay in diagnosis and surgical treatment on survival. No difference in disease-free survival was observed in this cohort of patients when they were grouped according to duration of symptoms, i.e., 0–3, 3–6, 6–9 and > 9 months (Fisher ER et al. 1977). Further, one subset of patients with clinically negative nodes was subjected to total mastectomy only, without dissection of the ipsilateral axilla (Fisher B et al. 1977). It is estimated that 40% of the patients in this subset most probably had positive nodes, since the patients were prospectively randomized and this estimate represents the error in clinical as opposed to pathological staging of negative-node patients (Fisher et al. 1975a). Yet, surprisingly, only 16% have evidenced axillary recurrence within 10 years after mastectomy, and the treatment failure rate in the tenth postoperative year for this subset is no different statistically than that for other subsets who were subjected to either radical mastectomy or irradiation following total mastectomy. In keeping with this observation is the recognition of comparable survival rates in patients with occult micronodal metastases and those lacking such a phenomenon (Fisher et al. 1978). These considerations indicate one of the most salient shortcomings of the conventional concept of tumor biology − the failure to recognize the significance of host response and tumor characteristics in its equation. Certainly our own experimental studies, which have revealed a large number of host and other factors that influence the development of hepatic metastases (Fisher and Fisher 1967a), indicate that this is indeed a most significant oversight. Another defect in the conventional concept of cancer progression is the pivotal role attributed to the regional lymph nodes in that scheme. Apparently this view evolved from studies performed by Virchow (1863) and by others, in which it was demonstrated that these structures were barriers to such materials as India ink, red blood cells, etc. However, again, our own experimental studies have clearly demonstrated that the situation with regard to tumor cells may be, and indeed is, different from that observed with the particulates noted. Experiments have been performed which clearly indicate that tumor cells may traverse lymph nodes either through the efferent lymph channel or through lymphaticovenous communications, and that this event, like passage through interstitial spaces, occurs with alarming alacrity (Fisher and Fisher 1966, 1967b, c). Thus, the lymph nodes do not represent barriers to tumor cells. Their removal, in our view, is performed for proper staging of the neoplastic disease rather than for removal of tumor per se and prevention of subsequent metastases.

It appears, therefore, that the long-held conventional view concerning the biology of cancer, with its implications concerning what is early or late cancer, is not substantiated by either experimental or clinical observations. This has led to an alternate hypothesis (Fisher B 1980), which emphasizes that the positive regional lymph node is not an instigator of cell dissemination but an indicator of a host-tumor interrelationship that permits the development of metastases. Regional lymph nodes are of biological rather than mechanical importance and they do not represent effective barriers to tumor cells. The blood vascular system is an important pathway of tumor dissemination. It is, however, closely interrelated to the lymphatic system. Complex, and to date often unclear, host-tumor relationships are operative, which probably affect every facet of the disease. Operable breast cancer, in a large proportion of instances, is already a systemic disease. Because of this it is unlikely that variations in loco-regional treatment will affect survival rates – experience, as noted above, has made this historically evident.

This alternative hypothesis is not intended to convey a cavalier attitude toward the prompt diagnosis of breast cancer, but hopefully will provide a better understanding of its natural history. Certainly it is good medical practice to treat disease promptly. Yet, it must not be done under the illusion that this promptness invariably plays a decisive role in the outcome. Theoretically, the elimination of tumor burden is highly desirable if combative host factors or chemotherapeutic agents are to achieve their maximum efficiency. Yet, it remains to be demonstrated whether this will exert a beneficial effect even in the adjuvant setting for all patients or just for certain subsets, in accordance with the heterogeneity of breast cancers. Lastly, until survival rates can be demonstrated to be substantially improved in prospective, randomized clinical trials with the removal of tumors regarded clinically as early, it appears that the main benefit of recognition of small tumors may lie in the resulting possibility of more cosmetic operative intervention rather than in biologic reasons.

These considerations also appear relevant to the use of the term "minimal cancer" (Gallagher and Martin 1971), an expression that connotes curability as well as earliness. By definition, minimal cancer includes lobular carcinoma in situ, intraductal cancers, and invasive cancers measuring no greater than 0.5 cm. There is no biologic reason why in situ cancers should not be curable, and it is the author's opinion that relatively few cancers ≤ 0.5 cm will be encountered with the detection methods currently available. Further, there are other cancers that exhibit a favorable clinical course and do not qualify to be regarded as minimal cancer. Mucinous, tubular, and papillary forms of breast cancer are frequently larger than 0.5 cm, yet have a favorable prognosis. Because of these inconsistencies I refrain from using the general term and regard precise designations or descriptions of a particular lesion to be more meaningful.

The above indicates that the identifying features of what constitutes an early cancer have not been well defined, at least in the present state of the art. On the other hand, there are certain mammary changes that have long been suspected of being precursor lesions. Although these too defy a precise connotation of time, we are more certain that they are both morphologically and biologically early. It has long been held that most, if not all, cancers appear at least structurally to evolve from a sequence of changes designated by pathologists as hyperplasia, atypical hyperplasia, and carcinoma in situ. Although this seriation of events appears to be fairly well established in cervical cancer, where access to biopsies is relatively simple, extension of this data to other sites, such as the breast, appears more intuitive than real. This does not disclaim the existence of such a pattern but it should be realized that such a progression may be nonobligate or discontinuous (see below). Nevertheless, it must be emphasized that it is the proliferative form of fibrocystic disease or the mammary alteration characterized by ductal hyperplasia, vis-à-vis papillomatosis, epitheliosis, and multiple papillomas, that represents one form of precancerous change (Fisher 1981). Our own electron-microscopic studies (Fisher 1976) of such lesions, including those designated as atypical hyperplasia, because the delineation between hyperplasia and intraductal cancer might be regarded as equivocal, revealed that the banal type of hyperplasia was comprised of normal ductal epithelial cells, whereas the atypical form contained many, but not all cells, possessing features indistinguishable from those found in overt invasive carcinomas. More objective evidence concerning the relationship between banal hyperplasia and carcinoma was obtained from experimental studies performed with 3-methylcholanthrene (MCA) in syngeneic rats. In this model the mammary ductal epithelium sequentially progresses through phases of banal and atypical hyperplasia and finally cancer. Karyotypic abnormalities, including marker forms, were noted in ductal cells from all phases of this process, with fewest occurring in cells from banal hyperplasia and most in the cancers (Fisher et al. 1975b). Electron microscopy, as in the human material, disclosed a commonality of features in cells comprising atypical hyperplasia and cancer. Varying incidences of aneuploidy were also observed with cultured cells from human hyperplastic lesions and cancer (Fisher and Paulson 1978). Studies by Gullino and associates (1976, 1977), using a different model system, complement these findings. They observed an angiogenic response in the rabbit iris with 30% − not all − of xenografted fragments of hyperplastic nodules of the mouse mammary gland and human hyperplastic nodules. All cancer transplants produced neovascularization, whereas normal breast fragments and those from other forms of fibrocystic disease or gynecomastia failed to do so. The findings from both studies constitute compelling evidence that at least the proliferative form of fibrocystic disease is not only a precursor lesion of mammary carcinoma, but perhaps one of its earliest morphological expressions. The failure to find karyotypic aberrations in all samples of proliferative fibrocystic disease, or as in the case of Gullino and associates, angiogenesis following xenografting to the anterior chamber of the rabbit eye, does not militate against such an interpretation. The inconsistency of aberrant chromosomal forms in proliferative fibrocystic disease, as opposed to their consistent appearance in overt cancer cells, suggests that the former disorder may lack the clonal nature of overt cancer, even though both disorders show karyotypic instability. Further, as has long been recognized, hyperplasia of the breast may be induced by other experimental modalities, notably hormones, which do not result in the evolution of cancer. Indeed, lesions indistinguishable from those of early hyperplasia in the methylcholanthrene (MCA) model occur after the administration of estradiol or progesterone. Yet, hyperplastic lesions were not noted to develop into lesions of advanced hyperplasia or cancer (Fisher et al. 1975c). The lesions could not be grafted to suitable hosts and, more importantly, when induced only by hormones they lacked the karyotypic abnormalities found in the ductal cells of the early hyperplasia produced by MCA. Thus, not all hyperplastic lesions evolve into cancer. The arrest of such evolution appears to occur prior to the development of the advanced or atypical stage (lesions which possess only subtle light- and electron-micro-scopic and karyotypic differences from those designated as cancer). These experiments indicate that the evolutionary process is complicated and certainly nonobligate. Unfortunately, there are no simple methods available that allow the identification of those hyperplastic lesions representing the high-risk forms of hyperplasia.

Black and Kwon (1980) have also noted similar morphological characteristics, which they considered to reflect temporal and immunological factors in so-called precancerous lesions and in situ and invasive cancers. Their observations also suggested that oral contraceptives favored the transition from the precursor stage to invasive cancer only in women with a familial history (grandmothers and aunts) of breast cancer. Thus, the evolution of breast cancer from the precursor lesion is not only nonobligate or discontinuous, but apparently under the influence of a variety of other factors.

It is apparent from the preceding paragraphs that the proliferative or hyperplastic form of fibrocystic disease is most significant as a precursor lesion for breast cancer. This is not to imply that it represents a unique form of fibrocystic disease. Indeed, in most if not all instances, it is accompanied by nonproliferative alterations characterized by simple cysts and duct ectasia, stromal hyalinization or so-called fibrous mazoplasia, apocrine metaplasia, and sclerosing or blunt duct adenosis. It has been our practice to regard only papillomas, papillomatosis, multiple papillomas, and lobular hyperplasia as manifestations of proliferative fibrocystic disease, vis-à-vis risk lesions.

Evidence is now accumulating to suggest that another lesion may be a precursor for some cancers of the breast. The alteration is represented by a central sclerotic core often containing elastic fibers and tubules radiating into the surrounding breast parenchyma (Fig. 1). Ducts within the latter frequently exhibit ectasia and/or hyperplastic epithelial changes (Fig. 2). Descriptions of this lesion have appeared sporadically in the literature under a variety of appelations, which emphasize its varying characteristics. Some of these designations are rosette-like lesion (Semb 1928), sclerosing papillar proliferation − a benign lesion often mistaken for carcinoma (Fenoglio and Lattes 1974), *strahlige Narben* (Hamperl 1975), benign sclerosing proliferation (Tremblay 1977), infiltrating epitheliosis (Azzopardi 1979), *lesioni focali sclero-elastotiche mammaries simulanti il carcinoma infiltrante* (Eusebi et al. 1976), radial scar (Linell et al. 1980), nonencapsulated sclerosing lesion (NESL) (Fisher et al. 1979), and indurative mastopathy − a benign sclerosing lesion with elastosis which may simulate carcinoma (Richert et al. 1981). All signify the benignity of the lesion, although Hamperl (1975), like ourselves (Fisher et al. 1979) and more recently Linell and associates (1980), have suggested the possibility that it may be a precursor form of tubular and perhaps other histological types of breast cancer. Indeed, Linell and associates (1980) indicated that 50% of the cancers they studied in 555 mastectomy specimens could be traced to an origin in a radial scar, their translation of Hamperl's *strahlige Narben*. Our own interest in the nature of this lesion has been sustained not only because of the potential significance of the findings of Linell and his associates (1980), but also by frequent consultative inquiries concerning its distinction from tubular cancer. It became quite apparent that interpretation of the radial scar was as frequently worrisome to pathologists as was the differential diagnosis of intraductal hyperplasia from intraductal cancer. This was not totally unexpected, since our previous study (Fisher et al. 1979) of the nonencapsulated sclerosing lesion (NESL) revealed a striking commonality of histological features between its tubular elements and those of overt tubular cancers. The consultative material and our own personally studied cases contained some examples whose morphological appearance strongly suggested that the tubular cancer did indeed arise from such a banal lesion. Cancers arising in the NESL exhibited a profusion of peripheral elements and, more importantly from a diagnostic standpoint, contained "naked" tubular elements within adjacent fatty tissue without the surrounding mantle or apposition to collagen that accompanies such structures in the adipose tissue of the banal NESL (Figs. 3 and 4).

These considerations prompted us to review the pathological material from 1,569 patients with invasive stage I and II operable breast cancer entered in the National Surgical Adjuvant Breast Project (NSABP), protocol 4 (Fisher et al. 1983). All these cases had been studied previously according to a designated protocol allowing for the assessment of 36 pathological and 6 clinical features.

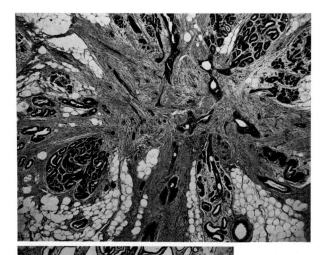

Fig. 1. Banal nonencapsulated sclerosing lesion (NESL) disclosing ductal elements within a radial "scar". × 22.5

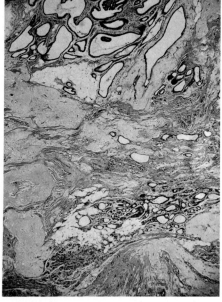

Fig. 2. This NESL or radial scar exhibits duct ectasia and rare papilloma formation at its periphery. The core contains ducts and/or blood vessels obliterated by elastosis (appearing gray). × 10

Examination disclosed that there were actually five types of "scar cancer," which constituted 38% of all cases of invasive cancer. It should be emphasized that the term "scar" is used with full awareness that the hyaline core might not be a scar in the classic sense but simply a stromal reaction to the epithelial neoplastic elements. Yet, it is our opinion that if this latter view is correct it is a unique form of such a stromal reaction. It should also be emphasized that the scar is in no manner related to a reparative process following prior breast biopsy. As noted by Linell and associates (1980), scar cancers of the breast may be analogous to comparable cancers of the lung. In both instances the core often contains elastic fibers, which is unusual in a reparative scar. Adjacent bronchioles and bronchoalveolar units in scar cancers of the lung may exhibit hyperplasia; this is often prominent in the ducts surrounding the banal scar and in cancers which appear to arise from it in the breast. In both sites both well-differentiated and less-differentiated cancers may occur. Lastly, scar cancers of the lung are considered to arise in areas of pulmonary

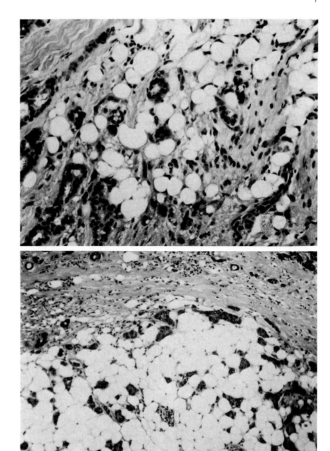

Fig. 3. The ductal elements in breast adipose tissue in this instance appear to be apposed to or surrounded by collagen. This appearance is not considered to be representative of true fat invasion. × 125

Fig. 4. Presence of tubular elements lying free or unassociated with collagen within adipose tissue of breast represents true fat invasion. × 90

hypoxia, e.g., tuberculous scars, infarcts, interstitial fibrosis (Raeburn and Spencer 1953; Spencer 1977; Themel and Luders 1955). Although a hypoxic influence is difficult to establish in the mammary situation, it is of interest to note that obliterative arterial vascular changes may be identified and indeed represent a salient feature of scar cancers. Interestingly, Hamperl (1975) suggested that ductal obliteration might be pathogenetically significant for radial scars of the breast. Apparently all previous investigators overlooked these large blood vessel changes, which are characterized by elastotic change of their wall with or without fibrosis. The intima of affected vessels is often thickened, resulting in luminal obliteration resembling atherosclerosis of the fibrous intimal type (Figs. 5–7). As noted above, we are uncertain as to the possible pathogenetic significance of these vascular changes, but they do appear unique to the scar cancers of the breast.

The type 1 scar cancer is represented by the classic NESL core comprised of radiating, relatively acellular, hyaline-containing isolated tubules or ducts. Some ducts in the core may demonstrate intraductal carcinoma (Figs. 8 and 9). The type 2 scar exhibits the same topographical features as noted in type 1. However, the core exhibits either edema or dense acellular connective tissue without tubular elements (Fig. 10), an appearance suggesting end-stage scar. In type 3 the central core contains overt carcinomatous elements

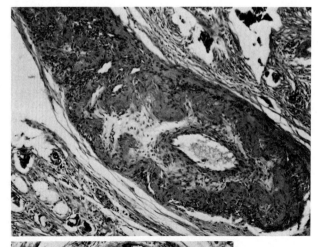

Fig. 5. Alteration of large vessel observed in scar cancer characterized by elastotic and fibrous change in the subintimal zone. × 90

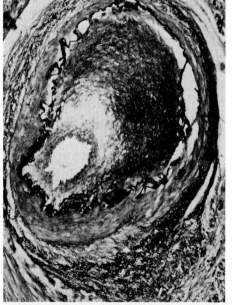

Fig. 6. Artery in scar cancer stained by orcein elastica method, revealing atherosclerotic change of fibrous intimal type. × 90

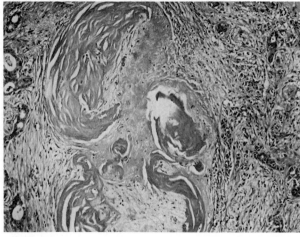

Fig. 7. End-stage vascular or ductal obliteration not uncommonly found in scar cancers. Identifying features are no longer evident. × 90

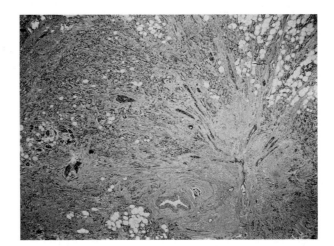

Fig. 8. Tubular cancer containing central core of the NESL or radial scar characteristic of type 1 scar cancer. × 22.5

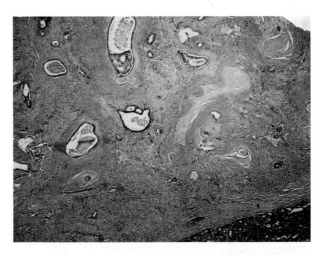

Fig. 9. The core of this type 1 scar cancer contains some ducts with features of intraductal cancer. × 15

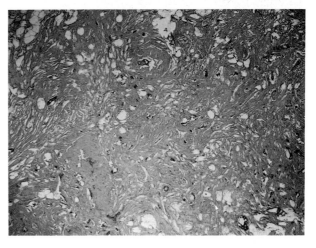

Fig. 10. The core of this type 2 scar cancer exhibits some edema and sparse, small tubular elements. × 22.5

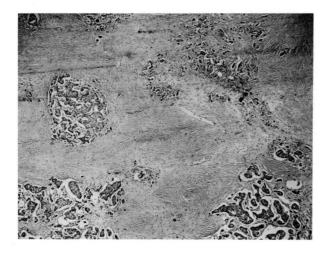

Fig. 11. The central core of this type 3 scar cancer is somewhat less radially situated than with types 1 and 2. Overt carcinomatous elements of nontubular type are present. × 125

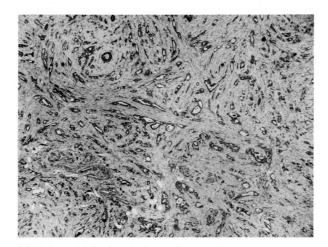

Fig. 12. Type 4 scar is characterized by an interweaving pattern of connective tissue about the neoplastic tubular elements. × 125

of nontubular type, or cancer in which the tubular component is minimal (Fig. 11). An interweaving stromal pattern was observed in type 4 scar cancers (Fig. 12). The scars of type 5 were more frequently circumferential than radial, and were obviously multifocal (Fig. 13). This form was encountered exclusively in some lobular invasive carcinomas, although in a rare example of the latter type 1 scar formation was observed. Although tubular cancers and the combination forms are most frequently found in types 1, 2, and 4 scar cancers, others, such as papillary and lobular invasive cancers, may also be noted, as mentioned above.

Admittedly, the type 1, 2, and 3, and even perhaps the type 4 scar cancers may be variants of the same histogenetic process. Yet, analyses have revealed that these have distinctive histologic characteristics. This has prompted us to regard them as entities, at least tentatively.

The most significant practical feature of the scar cancers is the recognition of a statistically better disease-free survival rate in patients with types 1 and 4 scar cancers (9% of all invasive breast cancers) 6 years following mastectomy than in those without scar cancers or

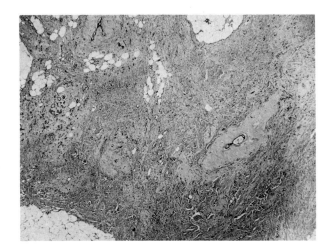

Fig. 13. Type 5 scar cancer, as depicted in this example of tubulolobular invasive cancer, is characterized by multifocal, more globoid, "scars." × 22.5

types 2, 3, 5 (Fisher et al. 1983). Extension of our analyses into the 10th post-mastectomy year however, has revealed that recognition of types 1, 2, and 4 scar cancers (16% of all invasive breast cancers) may be of predicitive value in assessing whether patients surviving 5 years will also survive into the 10th year (Fisher et al., in press). There is also a strong statistical trend to indicate the delineation of these types of scar cancers may allow for the discrimination of disease-free survival regardless of nodal status into the 10th year. Thus, recognition of scar cancers, and particularly of their various types, has prognostic value.

The evidence for regarding the nonencapsulated sclerosing lesion or radial scar as a precursor form for some breast cancers (at least 7% for type 1 scar is compelling. Although we are uncertain about the significance of vascular changes in the pathogenesis of the banal scar or scar cancers, its presence in these situations is highly provocative. Lastly, it becomes apparent that hyperplastic intraductal change and the NESL or radial scar most probably represent the earliest morphological expressions of breast cancer. However, experience has revealed that such "academic" forms of breast cancer can be satisfactorily managed by local conservative extirpation.

References

Azzopardi JG (ed) (1978) Problems in breast pathology. Saunders, London, pp 186–325

Bauer W, Igot JP, Le Gal Y (1980) Chronologie du cancer mammaire utilisant un modele de croissance de Gompertz. Ann Anat Pathol 25: 39–56

Black MM, Kwon S (1980) Precancerous mastopathy; structural and biologic considerations. Pathol Res Pract 166: 491–514

Eusebi V, Gassigli A, Grosso F (1976) Lesioni focali sclero-elastotiche mammarie simulanti il carcinoma infiltrante. Pathologica 68: 507–518

Fenoglio C, Lattes R (1974) Sclerosing papillar proliferations in the female breast. A benign lesion often mistaken for carcinoma. Cancer 33: 691–700

Fisher B (1980) Laboratory and clinical research in breast-cancer – a personal adventure: The David A. Karnofsky memorial lecture. Cancer Res 40: 3863–3874

Fisher B, Fisher ER (1966) Transmigration of lymph nodes by tumor cells. Science 152: 1397–1398

Fisher B, Fisher ER (1967a) Host-tumor relationship in the development and growth of hepatic metastases. In: Wissler RW, Dao TL, Wood SW Jr (eds) Endogenous factors influencing host-tumor balance. International symposium sponsored by the Argonne Cancer Research Hospital, University of Chicago 1966. University of Chicago Press, Chicago, pp 149−166

Fisher B, Fisher ER (1967b) Barrier function of lymph node to tumor cells and erythrocytes. I. Normal nodes. Cancer 20: 1907−1913

Fisher B, Fisher ER (1967c) Barrier function of lymph node to tumor cells and erythrocytes. II. Effect of x-ray, inflammation, sensitization and tumor growth. Cancer 20: 1914−1919

Fisher B, Montague E, Redmond C, Barton B, Borland D, Fisher ER, Deutsch M, Schwarz G, Margolese R, Donegan W, Volk H, Konvolinka C, Gardner B, Cohn I, Lesnick G, Cruz A, Lawrence W, Nealon T, Butcher H, Lawton R (1977) Comparison of radical mastectomy with alternative treatments for primary breast cancer: a first report of results from a prospective randomized clinical trial. Cancer 39: 2827−2839

Fisher ER (1976) Ultrastructure of human breast and its disorders. Am J Clin Pathol 66: 291−374

Fisher ER (1981) Relationship of fibrocystic disease to cancer of the breast. In: Hoogstraten B (ed) Breast cancer CRC, Boca Raton Fl, pp 120−135

Fisher ER, Paulson JD (1978) Karyotypic abnormalities in precursor lesions of human cancer of the breast. Am J Clin Pathol 69: 284−288

Fisher ER, Gregorio RM, Fisher B (1975a) The pathology of invasive breast cancer. A syllabus derived from the findings of the National Surgical Adjuvant Breast Project (protocol 4). Cancer 36: 1−85

Fisher ER, Shoemaker RH, Sabnis A (1975b) Relationship of hyperplasia to cancer in 3-methyl-cholanthrene-induced mammary tumorogenesis. Lab Invest 33: 33−42

Fischer ER, Shoemaker RH, Palekar AS (1975c) Identification of premalignant hyperplasia in methyl-cholanthrene-induced mammary tumorogenesis. Lab Invest 33: 466−450

Fisher ER, Redmond C, Fisher B (1977) A perspective concerning the relationship of duration of symptoms to treatment failure in patients with breast cancer. Cancer 40: 3160−3167

Fisher ER, Swamidoss S, Lee CH, Rockette H, Redmond C, Fisher B (1978b) Detection and significance of occult axillary metastases in patients with invasive breast cancer. Cancer 42: 2025−2031

Fisher ER, Palekar AS, Kotwal N, Lipana NA (1979) A non-encapsulated sclerosing lesion of the breast. Am J Clin Pathol 71: 240−246

Fisher ER, Palekar AS, Rockette H, Redmond C, Fisher B (1981) Pathologic findings from the National Surgical Adjuvant Breast Project (protocol 4) V. Significance of axillary nodal micro and macrometastases. Cancer 42: 2032−2038

Fisher ER, Palekar AS, Sass R, Fisher B (1983) Scar cancers: Pathologic findings from the National Surgical Adjuvant Breast Project (protocol 4). IX. Breast Cancer Res Treat 3: 39−59

Fisher ER, Sass R, Fisher B (in press) Pathologic findings from the National Surgical Adjuvant Breast Project (protocol 4). X. Discriminants for tenth year treatment failure. Cancer

Gallager HS, Martin JE (1971) An orientation to the concept of minimal breast cancer. Cancer 28: 1505−1507

Gimbrone MA Jr, Gullino PM (1976) Neovascularization induced by intraocular xenografts of normal, preneoplastic mouse mammary tissue. JNCI 56: 305−318

Gullino PM (1977) Natural history of breast cancer. Progression from hyperplasia. Cancer 39: 2697−2703

Hamperl H (1975) Strahlige Narben und obliterierende Mastopathie. Beiträge zur pathologischen Histologie der Mamma. XI. Virchows Arch [Pathol Anat] 369: 55−568

Linell F, Ljungsberg O, Andersson I (1980) Breast carcinoma. Aspects of early stages, progression and related problems. Acta Pathol Microbiol Scand [A] (Suppl 272)

Mackay EN, Sellars AH (1965) Breast cancer at the Ontario Cancer Clinics, a statistical review 1938−1956. Medical Statistics Branch, Ontario Dept Health, Ontario

Raeburn C, Spencer H (1953) Study of origin and development of lung cancer. Thorax 8: 1−10

Richert RR, Kalisher L, Hutter RVP (1981) Indurative mastopathy: A benign sclerosing lesion of breast with elastosis which may simulate carcinoma. Cancer 47: 561−571

Semb C (1928) Fibroadenomatosis cystica mammae. Acta Chir Scand [Suppl] 10: 1−484

Spencer H (ed) (1977) Pathology of the lung, 3rd edn. Saunders, Philadelphia, p 814

Themel KG, Luders CJ (1955) Die Bedeutung tuberkuloser Narben für die Entstehung des peripheren Lungenkarzinoms. Dtsch Med Wochenschr 80: 1360−1363

Tremblay G, Buell RH, Seemayer ThA (1977) Elastosis in benign sclerosing ductal proliferation of the female breast. Am J Surg Pathol 1: 155−159

Virchow R (1863) Cellular pathology. (Translated by Frank Chance) Lippincott, Philadelphia

Pathogenesis of Early Breast Cancer

H. Stephen Gallager

The University of Texas System Cancer Center, MD Anderson Hospital,
Houston, TX 77030, USA

Introduction

In 1961, Dr. John Martin and I undertook a collaborative histopathological and radiologic study of breast cancer. We were stimulated to this by the then current upsurge of interest in mammography. We hoped by our study to clarify the relationships between mammographic and histopathological findings in breast cancer. To this end we adopted a subserial whole-organ section technique, a modification of that used by Cheatle many years earlier. Women suspected of having breast cancer were routinely submitted to preoperative mammography. Diagnoses of carcinoma were established by trephine-needle biopsy only, thus leaving tumors essentially intact within the breasts. Each mastectomy specimen was first examined grossly, and the axillary lymph nodes were removed and processed in the usual manner. The breast itself was divided into three large vertical blocks. Each of these was fixed, processed, and embedded in paraffin. Giant sections 12−15 μm thick were cut at 1-mm intervals through each block. Thus, each breast yielded a set of 80−200 large sections that could be arranged in order to provide a three-dimensional representation of the breast. Lesions could be directly compared with mammographic images and point-for-point correlations established.

During the ensuing 12 years, we examined 209 breasts from 201 patients by this technique (Gallager and Martin 1969a, b). All but a few of the specimens contained invasive carcinomas ranging from 2 cm to 5 cm in diameter. In 12 of the specimens there were invasive carcinomas less than 2 cm in diameter. Three showed intraductal carcinoma only and two contained no malignant lesions.

The major objective of this investigation was to establish correlations between pathological and radiographic appearances in breast cancer and thereby to contribute to an improvement in the sensitivity and specificity of mammography. This objective was in large measure achieved (Gallager and Martin 1970). Of more fundamental importance, however, was the information we gained relating to the manner in which breast carcinoma arises and progresses. In this presentation I shall describe some of these findings and the conclusions we drew from them. Additionally, I shall review several more recent studies of breast cancer pathogenesis and present a schema that attempts to show relationships among the several mechanisms that have been proposed.

Early Breast Cancer
Edited by J. Zander and J. Baltzer
© Springer-Verlag Berlin Heidelberg 1985

Findings of the Whole-Organ Study

It was an early observation that invasive breast masses vary in their intrinsic structures. Two distinct types make up more than 85% of all masses. The more common of these (48% of cases) we have designated the multinodular mass. It is typified by a fairly well-circumscribed margin that is multiply scalloped in cross section. Neoplastic cells are concentrated at the periphery of the mass, while the center is largely fibrotic and contains relatively few cells. The fibrotic area is often geographically patterned, following the major contours of the periphery of the mass. Slightly less common was the stellate mass, which has a central solid core and long tentaculate projections extending in many directions. The central region is diffusely fibrotic, with carcinoma cells evenly scattered through a background of mixed fibrous and elastic tissue. The tentacles consist of ducts containing intraductal carcinoma. Each duct is surrounded by a thick sleeve of acellular connective tissue. Stellate carcinomas tend to occur at an older age and have a more favorable average nuclear grade; they are associated with a survival rate about 15% higher than that of the multinodular carcinomas.

The incidence of multicentricity was remarkably high in this material. Multicentricity was defined for the purposes of this study simply as multiple sites of carcinoma not demonstrably connected with one another. Multiple sites of invasive carcinoma were found in 37% of cases, and foci of intraductal carcinoma not associated with an invasive mass were identified in an additional 37%. In about two-thirds of the cases of multicentric invasion there were either small satellite nodules adjacent to a major invasive mass or multiple invasive nodules of similar size clustered near a single locus. In the remaining cases secondary invasive nodules, usually small, were found in locations remote from an index mass. Almost all the secondary masses occurred in the courses of ducts containing intraductal carcinoma.

Proliferative changes in duct epithelium were almost universally present in breasts containing invasive carcinomas and involved ducts of all sizes, although involvement of third-order and smaller ducts was most frequent. Within most breasts the epithelial changes constituted a broad spectrum ranging from simple hyperplasia through hyperplasia with atypia to frank intraductal carcinoma. In many cases equivocal foci were found in which it was impossible to decide whether the alteration represented atypical hyperplasia or noninvasive carcinoma. By the use of mapping techniques it was possible to demonstrate that proliferative changes may be either continuous or discontinuous within a single duct system. We have observed ducts in which intraductal carcinoma extended from the subareolar region continuously into deep portions of the breast. We have also seen ducts in which considerable stretches of normal epithelium intervened between areas of intraductal carcinoma. Microscopic invasive nodules, when they were present, invariably were found surrounding or immediately adjacent to ducts containing intraductal carcinoma. Both papillary and nonpapillary patterns of proliferation were observed.

Lobular epithelial hyperplasia was found regularly, but less frequently than was ductal hyperplasia. When present, lobular epithelial hyperplasia was similar to ductal hyperplasia in that it ranged through a wide spectrum, extending from simple increase in size and number of lobules to frank lobular carcinoma in situ. In no specimen was atypical lobular hyperplasia or in situ lobular carcinoma found without significant ductal abnormality.

Ducts containing intraductal carcinoma were frequently found to be surrounded by a layer of mixed collagenous and elastic tissue. The thickness of this layer tended to be greater in intraductal carcinoma that was associated with invasive masses of stellate pattern than in that seen with multinodular carcinomas. It was noticeably thicker in the few cases of comedocarcinoma included in the series. A similar mixture of acellular connective tissue was found in the fibrotic portions of invasive masses and also in areas of focally thickened dermis overlying invasive masses.

Conclusions of the Whole-Organ Study

Basing our reasoning on these data, we have hypothesized (Gallager 1974) that the common forms of invasive ductal carcinoma of breast arise from the epithelium of mammary ducts. Hyperplasia of ductal epithelium is regarded as a preneoplastic lesion in the sense that it is a regularly occurring precursor of invasive carcinoma. Ductal hyperplasia is a lesion of high incidence, however, and it seems obvious that outcomes other than the development of carcinoma must be possible. For this reason, we have designated ductal hyperplasia as a nonobligate form of preneoplasia.

We believe that intraductal carcinoma is the result of neoplastic transformation of the cells of epithelial hyperplasia. Once the intraepithelial carcinomatous process is initiated, it extends to adjacent epithelium within the duct of origin but remains confined within its basement membrane for a relatively long period. Multifocality of the transformation is considered to be a common phenomenon.

The differences in the patterns of invasive masses are believed to be related to differences in rates of cell multiplication. The multinodular mass is the result of a relatively rapidly growing neoplastic cell population. Invasion occurs in an explosive fashion from multiple foci, often in close proximity to one another. As the invasive nodules continue to increase in size they coalesce, producing the characteristic multinodular outline. Fibrosis within multiple nodules occurs following necrosis of tumor cells, accounting for the patterned fibrotic central region of the conglomerate mass. Stellate carcinoma arises as a result of a slower proliferation, invasion occurring as a gradual transmigration of cells through the focally destroyed basement membrane. The resulting mass with its diffuse fibrosis forms a caricature of a duct branching pattern altered by fibrous tissue contraction. It seems likely that invasive comedocarcinoma arises when the neoplastic cell population is an exceedingly indolent one.

Many of these ideas have been incorporated in a graphic representation of our understanding of the natural history of breast cancer (Gallager 1980). In this model the early stages, up to the point of initial invasion, form a linear array. The sequence of events within this period is predictable, and the probability of regional or systemic spread is low. After significant mass formation has occurred the course becomes more random. This formulation supports the importance of early diagnosis and the effectiveness of simple treatment for those carcinomas that fall within our definition of minimal breast cancer (Gallager and Martin 1971).

Discussion

Several studies in recent years tend to corroborate our concept. Ozzello has reported ultrastructural investigations of hyperplastic ducts and intraductal carcinoma and has arrived at similar conclusions (Ozzello 1971). Page et al. carried out a long-term follow-up study of patients who had had breast biopsies for benign disease and found that those with ductal hyperplasia had a risk of subsequent breast carcinoma double that expected (Dupont et al. 1980). Patients with atypical lobular hyperplasia had an even higher risk of

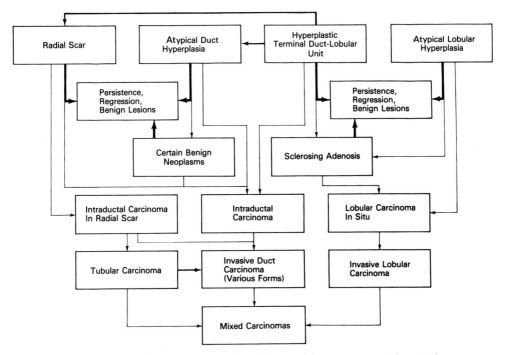

Fig. 1. Proposed schema integrating diverse hypotheses of breast cancer pathogenesis

carcinoma. There have been four follow-up studies of patients with minimal breast cancer (Wanebo et al. 1974; Frazier et al. 1977; Peters et al. 1977; Nevin et al. 1980). All these confirm that this group is characterized by a low rate of axillary node metastasis, a high disease-free survival rate, and a relatively high incidence of bilaterality.

Other possible pathways for the development of breast carcinoma have also been suggested. Wellings and his colleagues have presented evidence that lobules and terminal lobular ducts represent the primary site of involvement (Wellings et al. 1975). These structures are dilated by epithelial hyperplasia, usually with metaplasia, to an epithelial type more like that of mammary ducts. Progression to intraductal carcinoma may take place against this background. Hyperplastic lesions grading into both ductal and lobular preinvasive carcinoma have been observed in the terminal ducts and lobules of the mammary tree. Wellings' group considers it possible that ductal and lobular carcinomas arise in the same location from identical reserve cells. This viewpoint has been supported by a study of breast tissue removed from patients whose breast patterns had been evaluated according to the mammographic technique of Wolfe (Wellings and Wolfe 1978). It was found that the presence of a P2 or DY mammographic pattern had strong correlation with the presence of the type of lesions regarded by Wellings as preneoplastic.

Linell et al. have called attention to the significance of the radial scar, a sclerotic stellate formation that has been referred to by a variety of names (Linell et al. 1980). These authors present compelling evidence for the development of tubular carcinoma within such lesions, and have demonstrated lesions in which transitional stages can be recognized as well as fully developed tubular carcinomas in which remnants of radial scars can be recognized. They further propose that tubular carcinoma is not a stable lesion but is capable of progression to a solid form of invasive carcinoma that except for its background is indistinguishable from invasive duct carcinomas of other origins. My own studies of tubular carcinoma tend to support at least one part of this hypothesis. It is unusual to find a pure tubular carcinoma greater than 1 cm in diameter. Larger lesions that are partly tubular usually also contain focal areas of solid growth.

These several viewpoints are not necessarily discordant. The concept of progression from epithelial hyperplasia to atypical epithelial hyperplasia, noninvasive carcinoma, and invasive carcinoma is integral to all of them. The points of disagreement relate to the location of the epithelium most frequently involved and the specific process through which the lesion passes in its development. It seems possible that all the hypotheses are correct and that, as Linell has implied, there are multiple pathways of histogenesis capable of terminating in invasive carcinoma. The diagram in Fig. 1 is an attempt to express the possible relationships among the various proposals. For example, similarities in the two lesions suggest that at least some radial scars may be variants or derivatives of Wellings' hyperplastic terminal duct lobular unit. The differences in findings among these various studies may be due to differences in methdology, variations in study population, or a combination of these. It is interesting, for example, that the radial scar is apparently a fairly commonly encountered abnormality in Europe, but it is rare in the United States. The population that provided the specimens we studied consisted largely of rural women and contained high percentages of blacks and Latin Americans. Wellings' study group, by contrast, was largely white and urban.

Conclusion

There is now strong evidence that epithelial hyperplasia in the breast, whatever its source, is a nonobligate preneoplastic lesion. There are also sufficient data to conclude, at least tentatively, that evolution of epithelial hyperplasia may involve a variety of pathogenetic pathways. In all the proposed processes, progression to malignant neoplasia and invasive carcinoma appears to be the exception rather than the rule. While it is reasonable to suppose that greater degrees of cytologic atypia are associated with stronger probabilities of neoplastic evolution, the state of our knowledge does not yet permit accurate prognosis in individual cases. No generalizations can yet be made as to which preneoplastic lesions are sufficiently ominous to warrant mastectomy or other treatment as a means of preventing breast cancer.

References

Dupont WD, Rogers LW, Vander Zwaage R, Page DL (1980) The epidemiologic study of anatomic markers for increased risk in mammary cancer. Pathol Res Pract 166: 471–480

Frazier TG, Copeland EM, Gallager HS, Paulus DD, White EC (1977) Prognosis and treatment in minimal breast cancer. Am J Surg 139: 357–359

Gallager HS (1974) Never understandings of the pathology of breast cancer. In: Castro JR (ed) Current concepts in breast cancer and tumor immunology. Medical Examination, Flushing, NY, pp 27–41

Gallager HS (1980) The developmental pathology of breast cancer. Cancer 46: 905–907

Gallager HS, Martin JE (1969a) The study of mammary carcinoma by correlated mammography and subserial whole organ sectioning: Early observations. Cancer 23: 855–873

Gallager HS, Martin JE (1969b) Early phases in the development of breast cancer. Cancer 243: 1170–1178

Gallager HS, Martin JE (1970) The pathology of early breast cancer. In: Breast cancer early and late. Year Book Medical, Chicago, pp 37–50

Gallager HS, Martin JE (1971) An introduction to the concept of minimal breast cancer. Cancer 28: 1505–1507

Linell F, Ljungberg O, Anderssen I (1980) Breast carcinoma: aspects of early stages, progression and related problems. Acta Pathol Microbiol Scand [A] [Suppl] 272: 1–233

Nevin JE, Pinzon G, Moran TJ, Baggerly JT (1980) Minimal breast cancer. Am J Surg 139: 357–359

Ozzello L (1971) Ultrastructure of the human mammary gland. Pathol Annu 6: 1–60

Peters TG, Donegan WL, Burg EA (1977) Minimal breast cancer: a clinical appraisal. Ann Surg 186: 704–710

Wanebo HJ, Huvos AG, Urban JA (1974) Treatment of minimal breast cancer. Cancer 33: 349–357

Wellings SR, Wolfe JN (1975) Correlative studies of the histological and radiographic appearance of the breast parenchyme. Radiology 129: 299–306

Wellings SR, Jensen HM, Marcum RG (1975) An atlas of subgross pathology of the human breast with special reference to possible precancerous lesions. JNCI 55: 231–273

Histological Study on Multicentricity of Breast Carcinoma by Means of Whole-Organ Sections

H. Kalbfleisch and C. Thomas

Department of Pathology, Philipps-University,
Robert-Koch-Str. 5, 3550 Marburg, Federal Republic of Germany

Introduction

The improved preoperative diagnosis of breast tumors in recent years has led to increasingly frequent detection of smaller or "earlier" cancers, raising the question of restricting surgical treatment. The implications of this are close cooperation between the clinician and the pathologist, and increased refinement of the histopathological techniques. In addition to the diagnosis of malignancy, the pathologist has to work out prognostically relevant parameters based on the histological type of the tumor, its size and infiltration of the surrounding tissue, metastases, and multicentricity. For this purpose whole-organ or large-area sections yield the best results concerning exact determination of the extent of the tumor (Lüttges 1982), its contour, and the reaction of the surrounding, as well as its location within the breast. Even the finest radial branches of carcinomatous tissue, lymph vessel invasion, infiltration of the dermis, fascia, or muscle, or multiple tumorous foci are discernible without effort. Conventional sampling of recognizable lesions and random blocks are not adequate for these purposes.

In this study primary mastectomy specimens were examined by means of whole-organ sections especially when multiple-site carcinoma was suspected, and secondary mastectomy specimens were used to check for residual carcinoma at the site of previous local tumor excision. The advantages of large-area sections are compared with diagnosis from conventional slides.

Materials and Methods

From November 1978 to December 1982 all the 432 mastectomy specimens, representing 426 patients with breast cancer, were examined by the large-block technique. In this series 193 patients had undergone right, 234 left, and 6 bilateral mastectomy. In 5 cases the side was not recorded. In the majority of cases the amputation was performed in the Department of Gynecology at Marburg University and the preoperative histopathological diagnosis was carried out by the Department of Pathology at Marburg University. Some specimens were submitted from other hospitals, and the primary histopathological diagnosis was done by other pathology departments in some cases. Primary mastectomy was performed after carcinoma was established by "triple diagnosis," i.e., diagnosis of breast cancer by means of clinical, mammographic and cytological methods. As we have strong reservations about performing mastectomy on the basis of cytolgcial evidence alone without histological confirmation of malignancy, in our Pathology Department we have introduced

Early Breast Cancer
Edited by J. Zander and J. Baltzer
© Springer-Verlag Berlin Heidelberg 1985

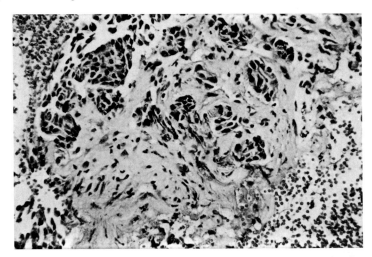

Fig. 1. Microhistology of tissue fragments obtained by fine-needle puncture of the breast, showing aggregates of invasive tumor cells. H & E, × 300

microhistological processing of minute tissue fragments collected by fine-needle puncture (Köhler et al. 1977). Serial sections of paraffin-embedded material yield more comprehensive information than cytological examination of smear preparations alone, mostly making the diagnosis of invasive carcinoma possible without difficulty (Fig. 1). Secondary mastectomy was done after excisional biopsy with histopathological diagnosis of carcinoma in patients in whom clear triple diagnosis was not achieved. A simple or total mastectomy was performed, with axillary revision in most cases. After radiographic examination the whole-breast preparation was serially sliced at 10-mm intervals at right angles to the skin. The cut surfaces were inspected macroscopically and small pieces of tissue were cut off for conventional histological examination. Each tissue slice was radiographed and completely embedded in paraffin blocks in toto. Tissue preparation was done with a "Paraffinator" (rapid embedding device) to save time. The number of slices depended on the size of the mammary gland. Axillary fat was prepared separately; the lymph nodes were isolated and histological slides were prepared. The size of the tumor was measured during the macroscopic examination. This measurement was confirmed in the radiographs and the whole-organ sections. In the large-area sections the site of the main tumor, its connection to the surrounding tissue, multiple foci of the carcinoma, dysplastic lesions of the mammary gland and, in cases of secondary mastectomy, the evidence of residual carcinoma were ascertained (Fig. 2). The pathological findings were registered in a breast carcinoma schedule. The term "main tumor" is used in this report to describe the clinical preoperatively known tumor for which the surgical intervention was necessary, as against occult secondary nidus or multiple cancerous foci. The term "residual carcinoma" indicates all remaining carcinomatous tissue in secondary mastectomy specimens when the object of surgery was excision of the total carcinoma in the first step of the operation, i.e., excisional biopsy for the purpose of histological confirmation of the cancer diagnosis. In 264 cases a primary, in 164 a secondary, and in 4 a subcutaneous mastectomy was performed. The mean age of the patients was 55.6 years, with a range of 30–91 years. The age distribution of our patients is shown in Table 1.

Results

Size of Carcinoma

The size of the main tumor (taken as the largest diameter) was between 0.4 and 10.2 cm. There were 9 minimal cancers and 175 cases with a tumor size of 2 cm or less or tumor stage

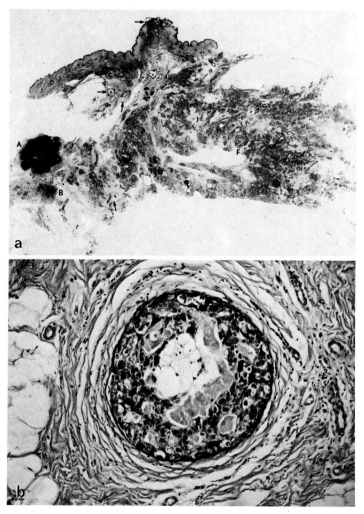

Fig. 2. (a) Whole-organ section of the breast; section through the nipple and the main tumor mass (two tumor foci; *A, B*). *Arrows* indicate intraductal carcinoma **(b)** and nipple involvement **(c)**. In middle and on right fibrocystic disease with ductal papillomatosis, adenosis and atypical hyperplasia. *F*, smal fibroadenoma; H & E, × 1. **(b)** higher magnification of focus of intraductal carcinoma; H & E, × 120.

I. In 34 cases the exact tumor size could not be determined due to multiple tumor foci. In 45 additional cases in whom the preliminary histopathological examinations had been conducted in other pathology departments the size of the main tumor was unknown. The performance of primary, secondary, or subcutaneous mastectomy related to the size of the main tumor is presented in Table 2.

Secondary mastectomy was performed in a higher percentage of women with smaller tumors or with multicentric carcinoma, whereas primary mastectomy was done more often in older patients, as already seen in Table 1.

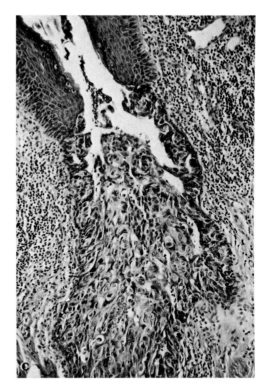

Fig. 2. c Higher magnification of the nipple region, showing section through the lactiferous duct within the nipple with intraductal carcinoma. H & E, × 120

Table 1. Age distribution of patients undergoing primary, secondary, and subcutaneous mastectomy

Age years	Total patients	Mastectomy		
		Primary	Secondary	Subcutaneous
30–39	28	10	17	1
40–49	66	31	35[a]	–
50–59	110	67[b]	41[a]	2[a]
60–69	120	74	46	–
70–79	83	62	21[a]	–
80–89	17	16	1	–
90	2	2	–	–
Total	426	262	161	3

[a] Bilateral mastectomy in one patient; [b] Bilateral mastectomy in two patients

Histology of the Main Tumor

The histological tumor types were classified according to the WHO nomenclature (1981) (see Table 3). With the exception of medullary and mucinous carcinoma there are no significant differences in the histological type of the main tumor between primary and secondary mastectomy. Both medullary and mucinous carcinomas were treated mainly by primary mastectomy. Conversely, noninvasive ductal and lobular carcinoma were found more often in the secondary mastectomy specimens.

Table 2. Size of the main tumor removed at primary, secondary, and subcutaneous mastectomy

Size of main tumor	Total	Mastectomy		
		Primary	Secondary	Subcutaneous
0.5 cm or less	9	1	8	–
1.0 cm or less	29	12	17	–
2.0 cm or less	146	95	50	1
2.0–5.0 cm	144	123	21	–
More than 5 cm	25	23	2	–
Multiple sites	34	10	21	3
Unknown	45	–	45	–
Total	432	264	164	4

Table 3. Histological tumor types according to the WHO classification in cases of primary, secondary, or subcutaneous mastectomy

Tumor type	Total	Mastectomy		
		Primary	Secondary	Subcutaneous
Noninvasive				
Intraductal carcinoma	4	–	4	–
Lobular carcinoma in situ	5	1	2	2
Invasive				
Invasive ductal carcinoma	295	201	94	–
With predominant intraductal component	19	6	13	–
Invasive lobular carcinoma	27	12	15	–
Mucinous carcinoma	12	11	1	–
Medullary carcinoma	12	10	2	–
Papillary carcinoma	5	4	1	–
Tubular carcinoma	19	9	8	2
Adenoid cystic carcinoma	4	3	1	–
Apocrine carcinoma	1	1	–	–
Carcinoma with metaplasia				
Squamous type	1	1	–	–
Cartilagineous type	1	1	–	–
Paget's disease	7	5	2	–
Unknown	20	–	20	–
Total	432	264	164	4

Staging of the Carcinoma

Postoperative histopathological staging of the main tumor according to the TNM criteria (1979) revealed the following distribution (cf. Table 4).

Primary mastectomy was performed mainly in advanced tumor cases. In 33 cases invasion of the dermis or the pectoral muscle was found and in 16 cases infiltration of the chest wall

Table 4. Postsurgical histopathologic staging of the main tumor according to the TNM categories in primary, secondary, or subcutaneous mastectomy

pT	Total no. of cases	Mastectomy		
		Primary	Secondary	Subcutaneous
pT is	9	1	6	2
pT I	175	104	70	1
pT II	142	121	21	–
pT III	17	15	2	–
pT IV	16	15	1	–
pT X	73	8	64	1
Total	432	264	164	4

Table 5. Regional lymph node status, postsurgical staging according to the TNM categories in primary, secondary, or subcutaneous mastectomy

pN	Total no. of cases	Mastectomy		
		Primary	Secondary	Subcutaneous
0	200	110	89	1
1a	18	12	6	–
1ba	38	22	16	–
1bb	15	12	3	–
1bc	71	48	22	1
2	33	22	10	1
3	2	1	1	–
x	55	37	17	1
Total	432	264	164	4

or ulceration of the skin. In 7 cases histological examination revealed Paget's disease of the nipple. In five patients with dissolute carcinoma all the large-area sections from the whole breast showed carcinomatous dissemination. In this study 175 cases were allocated to stage pT I, 142 to pT II, 17 to pT III, and 16 to stage pT IV.

Regional lymph nodes were available in 377 specimens for histopathological evaluation, i.e., in 87% of all cases; 200 of these (53%) revealed no tumor metastases. Micrometastases were found in 18 cases and macrometastases in 159 cases. The distribution according the TNM criteria (1979) is given in Table 5.

Multicentric and Multifocal Carcinoma

The term "multicentricity" or "multicentric carcinoma" describes multiple foci of noninvasive or invasive mammary carcinoma located in different mammary quadrants. A carcinoma is described as multifocal if more than one nidus of cancer tissue is found within

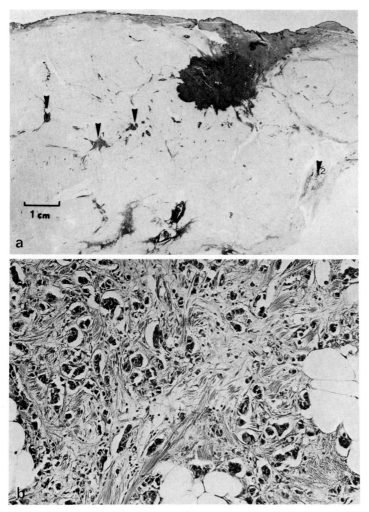

Fig. 3. (a) Whole-organ section of a breast with multicentric carcinoma. Besides the rather well-circumscribed main tumor there are also multiple intraductal and invasive ductal carcinomas (*arrows*); H & E, × 1, **b** higher magnification of nidus of infiltrating carcinoma shown in the whole-organ section (*1* in **a**); H & E, × 120

the main tumor-bearing mammary quadrant and if the additional foci are separated by a tumor-free tissue region 2 cm wide.

Solitary carcinoma was ascertained in the whole-organ sections of 154 specimens, i.e., 36%, while in 255 cases or 59% multiple foci of cancer were found. According to our definition, multifocal tumors appeared in 110 cases or 26% and multicentric tumors in 145 or 34% (Fig. 3). In 23 cases the tumor could not be classified because no residual carcinoma was detectable in secondary mastectomy specimens with previous external diagnosis (14 cases) or only minute cancerous foci were found at the margins of the wound cavity of the previous excisional diagnostic biopsy (9 cases). These findings present difficulties in distinction between branches of a stellate main tumor or separate satellite foci or multifocal carcinoma. (For details see Table 6.)

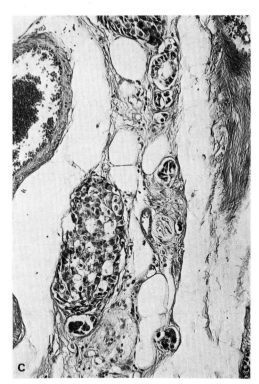

Fig. 3. c Higher magnification of another part of the same multicentric carcinoma (*2* in **a**). H & E, × 120

Table 6. Multicentricity of breast cancer and size of the main tumor

Size of the main tumor	Total cases	Carcinoma			
		Solitary	Multi-centric	Multi-focal	Indefinite
0.5 cm or less	9	4	2	3	–
1.0 cm or less	29	17	6	6	–
2.0 cm or less	146	79 (54.1)	25 (17.1)	42 (28.8)	–
2.0–5.0 cm	144	52 (36.1)	55 (38.2)	37 (25.7)	–
More than 5 cm	25	2 (8)	20 (80)	3 (12)	–
Multiple sites	34	–	25	9	–
Unknown	45	–	12	10	23[a]
Total (%)	432	154 (35.6)	145 (33.6)	110 (25.5)	23[a] (5.3)

[a] Includes 9 cases with residual carcinoma

Residual Carcinoma

In cases of secondary mastectomy with complete removal of the clinically diagnosed tumor within the margins of evidently noncancerous tissue, we searched for residual carcinoma macroscopically as usual and also microscopically, both in conventional slides and in the whole-organ sections. In the 164 specimens taken at secondary mastectomy we found 112

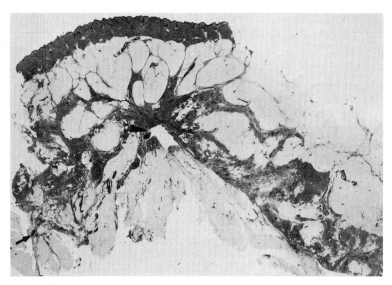

Fig. 4. This secondary mastectomy specimen contains a minute invasive carcinoma in the whole-organ section (↗), distant from the main tumor site (wound cavity; ▲). H & E, × 1

Table 7. Residual carcinoma in secondary mastectomy specimens and size of the main tumor

Size of the main tumor	Total cases	Residual carcinoma	No residual carcinoma
0.5 cm or less	8 ⎫	5 ⎫	3 ⎫
1.0 cm or less	17 ⎬ 75	10 ⎬ 42	7 ⎬ 33
2.0 cm or less	50 ⎭	27 ⎭	23 ⎭
2.0–5.0 cm	21	15	6
More than 5.0 cm	2	1	1
Multiple sites	21	21	–
Unknown	45	33	12
Total	164	112	52

cases or 68% with residual carcinoma. In 52 cases or 32% no residual cancer was found in the conventional slides or in the large-area sections. Frequently macroscopic preparation and inspection with the naked eye revealed no tumor or suspicious tissue, but sometimes the radiographs of the whole-organ slides helped us to discover distinct tumorous foci. So we were able to identify − mostly incidentally − residual cancer on routine histological examination and in the large-area sections in 69 cases. However, in 43 cases, or 26% only complete scrutiny of the whole organ in large-area histological sections revealed residual tumor in the mammary gland. Most of these cancerous residues were microscopically very small, not being visible with the naked eye or palpable on macroscopic examination (Fig. 4). Surgical sutures, hemorrhages, or the development of resorptive granulation tissue at the margins of the previous tumor extirpation made their recognition possible. The size of the main tumor in cases of confirmed residual carcinoma ranged between 0.4 and 5.2 cm. There were five cases with a tumor size of 0.5 cm or less. In 10 cases the main tumor measured 1.0 cm or less, in 27 it was 2.0 cm or less, and in 15 cases, 5.0 cm or less. One case with a main tumor 5.2 cm across its longest diameter also showed residual carcinoma in the secondary mastectomy specimen. Finally there were 21 specimens with solely multiple tumor growth and in 33 cases the size of the previously excised main tumor was unknown.

Summing up, in 75 patients with mammary cancer of tumor stage I treated by tumorectomy and subsequent mastectomy we detected (mostly small) cancer residues within the secondary mastectomy specimen in 42 cases or 56%, while we were not able to find residual carcinoma tissue in 33 cases or 44%. A survey is given in Table 7.

Discussion

The prognostic assessment of breast cancer patients depends heavily among other diagnostic tools, on exhaustive histopathological examination of the tissue specimen. Not only excisional biopsies but also mastectomy specimens should be examined as a whole. The histotopographic study of large-area or whole-organ sections is the method of choice. These sections allow recognition of all histopathological features of the main tumor and diagnosis of multicentric occult noninvasive or invasive cancers or of residual carcinoma with no difficulty. Although the concept of multicentricity of breast cancer is generally accepted, such multiple sites of cancer in addition to the main tumor are usually underdiagnosed clinically and macroscopically. Restricted surgical treatment, i.e., tumorectomy or quadrantectomy, demands careful consideration of the short- or long-term infiltration potential or any residual cancerous tissue.

Multicentricity of breast cancer is reported frequently. Qualheim and Gall (1957) described multiple foci of breast cancer in 54% of cases, 17% limited to a single mammary quadrant and 37% in quadrants remote from the main tumor. Using serial whole-organ sections, Gallager and Martin (1969a, b) established multiple intraductal or invasive mammary carcinoma in a high percentage of their cases. They stated that concurrent invasion at multiple sites from pre-existing carcinoma in situ might be a common phenomenon. In 47% they were able to find multicentric carcinoma, sometimes separated by wide distances. Three of four mammary cancer cases of Hutter and Kim (1971) showed multiple lesions. Fisher et al. (1975) pointed out a correlation between the occurrence of multicentric cancers in different mammary quadrants and the demonstration of cancerous foci in the vicinity of the main tumor. Independently of the main tumor, de novo cancers appeared in 13% of their patient sample. Fisher also indicated an association between the maximum diameters of the main tumors and the appearance of multiple cancer sites. Multicentric cancers were found more often in grossly noncircumscribed main tumors with noninvasive cancers in their vicinity and in tumors with diameters greater than 4.1 cm. Zippel and Citoler (1976) also demonstrated an association between main tumor size and multicentricity. While they found no multiple lesions in breasts with tumors up to 0.5 cm, multicentricity was established in a different quadrant in 20% of patients whose main tumor measured 0.6−1 cm and in 26% with a tumor 1.1−2 cm in diameter. On the other hand, multicentricity occurred in 33% of patients with non-invasive intraductal breast cancer (Brown et al. 1976). Lagios (1977) found occult multicentric foci of carcinoma in 21% of his cases. Yet, he stated that on average the invasive cancers in breasts with multicentric tumors were significantly smaller in diameter than solitary invasive carcinomas. Rilke et al. (1978) observed multicentricity in 27% of their patients with invasive breast cancers. Multicentric carcinoma was associated with a main tumor size of more than 2 cm in a higher proportion of cases than with monocentric tumors. More than one quadrant was involved. Egan (1982) characterized the present system of histological staging of breast cancer as inadequate, since the usual histopathological features do not allow precise prediction of the course. Whereas tumor size, stage of disease, or tumor cell differentiation had only limited effects on the survival rate, the presence of multicentricity of the tumors and the heterogeneity of the histological types of carcinoma may influence and worsen the prognosis even if the stage of disease appears similar. In a combined clinical, radiographic, and histopathological study with whole-organ sections, Egan found multiple distant tumor sites in 60% and multiple tumor sites and multiple tumor types in 69% of his patients.

As is other studies described, the multicentric lesions usually are of microscopic size and some are noninvasive. In most cases it is impossible to decide whether these lesions are intramammary metastases, extensions of the tumor, or independently developing cancers. Although from the viewpoint of complete removal of cancerous tissue it is of minor importance for practical purposes, a distinction is made between multifocal and multicentric carcinoma. In our study we observed solitary cancer in 154 patients or 36%, as against multicentric cancer in 145, or 34%, and multifocal cancer in 110 or 26%. If surgical treatment consisted only in tumorectomy the complete removal of the cancerous tissue would be sufficient only in a third of all patients, and quadrantectomy would also leave cancers in the breasts of a third of patients. As other authors have stated, there is a correlation between the size of the main tumor and multicentricity. We observed multicentric cancers in 33 patients with a tumor measuring 2 cm or less in its maximum diameter against 75 patients with a tumor size above 2 cm. In 69% of the cases with multicentric carcinoma the main tumor was larger than 2 cm, while 31% had main tumors smaller than 2 cm. On the other hand, in patients with solitary carcinoma the longest diameter of the tumor was less than 2 cm in 65% and in 35% more than 2 cm in 35% of cases.

Another result of our study was gained from the examination of secondary amputated breast specimens. Though complete excision of the total cancer was intended in the first step of the operation, the diagnostic biopsy, extended histopathological examination of the secondary mastectomy specimens revealed residual carcinoma, of various sizes and in the same as well as in distant mammary quadrants, in 112 of the 164 patients. Our material shows a somewhat higher frequency than that of Rosen et al. (1975). We also saw a correlation between the size of the main tumor and the evidence of residual carcinoma: of 75 patients with a tumor size less than 2 cm, 42 had tumor residues in the secondary mastectomy specimen, i.e., 56% versus 70% of patients with a tumor size above 2 cm. More than half the patients harbored cancer residues in the breast tissue after diagnostic tumorectomy. They are generally neither clinically nor macroscopically detectable, only microscopical examination revealing them. Further, the detection of residual carcinoma is directly related to the quantity of histologically examined breast tissue. It is likely that it is not always detected in conventional slides in routine histopathological examination without extended investigation by means of whole-organ sections. In this study 38% of the residual carcinoma cases were demonstrated only by the aid of large-area sections. It is our opinion that large-area sections may improve the recognition of minute multiple cancers of the mammary gland in different kinds of mastectomy specimens. This method will be useful in the examination of breast carcinoma as a whole and will improve histopathological prediction with regard to the diagnosis and further treatment of the breast cancer patient.

The results of the study yielded a diagnosis of multicentric cancer in a high percentage, almost two-thirds of the cases. The results of the examination of secondary mastectomy specimens indicate the difficulties in precise identification and delimitation of breast cancer pre- and intraoperatively. If many breast cancers are multicentric in origin any modification of surgical treatment should be applied only with extreme caution and only if careful histopathological investigation of the tumor specimen is ensured (Kindermann and Ober 1978), and must also be confined to selected cases (Stegner 1982). More extensive studies are needed to judge the prognostic and therapeutic implications of multicentric breast cancers.

Summary

Whole-organ paraffin sections were prepared from 432 breasts removed surgically because of carcinoma.

Primary mastectomy was performed in 264 patients when the preoperative triple diagnosis supported by microhistology of fine − needle puncture material, was positive for cancer.

Beside the main tumor, multiple independent cancers, usually of microscopic size, were detected in 59% of the specimens (255 cases). Multicentric cancers were encountered in 34% (145 cases), and multifocal cancers in 25% (110 cases). In secondary mastectomy specimens (164 cases) residual carcinoma, in some cases in multiple independent foci, was evident in 68% (112 cases), and in 26% (43 cases) was present but only demonstrable by extensive histotopographic analysis.

The concept of breast cancer as a diffuse lesion is supported by these results. This diffuse breast involvement is rarely recognizable, on clinical examination.

Restriction of the surgical management of breast cancer should be decided on only with due consideration of its diffuse nature. Extensive histopathological examination by means of whole-organ or large-area sections may help in the selection of patients.

Acknowledgement. The authors thank Mrs. Stolz-Lou for technical assistance in preparing the whole-organ sections.

References

Brown PW, Silverman J, Owens E, Tabor DC, Terz JJ, Lawrence W (1976) Intraductal "noninfiltrating" carcinoma of the breast. Arch Surg 111: 1063−1067

Egan RL (1982) Multicentric breast carcinoma: clinical − radiographic − pathologic whole organ studies and 10-year survival. Cancer 49: 1123−1130

Fisher ER, Gregorio RM, Fisher B (1975) The pathology of invasive breast cancer. A syllabus derived from findings of the National Surgical Adjuvant Breast Project (Protocol no. 4). Cancer 36: 1−85

Gallager HS, Martin JE (1969a) The study of mammary carcinoma by mammography and whole organ sectioning. Early observations. Cancer 23: 855−873

Gallager HS, Martin JE (1969b) Early phases in the development of breast cancer. Cancer 24: 1170−1178

Hutter RVP, Kim DU (1971) The problem of multiple lesions of the breast. Cancer 28: 1591−1607

Kindermann G, Ober KG (1978) Radikalitätseinschränkungen bei der chirurgischen Behandlung des Mammakarzinoms? In: Schmähl D (ed) Behandlung und Nachbehandlung des Mammakarzinoms. Thieme, Stuttgart, pp 104−116

Köhler F, Kalbfleisch H, Schmidt U, Pries HH (1977) Über Erfahrungen mit histologisch verwertbaren Gewebsstückchen aus Schilddrüsenpunktaten. Verh Dtsch Ges Pathol 61: 480

Lagios MD (1977) Multicentricity of breast carcinoma demonstrated by routine correlated serial subgross and radiographic examination. Cancer 40: 1726–1734

Lüttges JE (1982) Morphometrische Untersuchungen über die Tumorgröße von Mammakarzinomen im histologischen Großflächenschnitt und Präparatradiogramm. Inaugural Dissertation, Marburg

Qualheim RE, Gall EA (1957) Breast carcinoma with multiple sites of origin. Cancer 10: 460–468

Rilke F, Andreola S, Carbone A, Clemente C, Pilotti S (1978) The importance of pathology in prognosis and management of breast cancer. Semin Oncol 5: 360–372

Rosen PP, Fracchia AA, Urban JA, Schottenfeld D, Robbins GF (1975) Residual mammary carcinoma following simulated partial mastectomy. Cancer 35: 739–747

Stegner HE (1982) Die Rolle des Pathologen in der stadiengerechten Therapie des Mammakarzinoms. Pathologe 3: 137–148

TNM Klassifikation der malignen Tumoren 3rd edn. (1979) Mammatumoren. Springer, Berlin Heidelberg New York, pp 45–52

World Health Organization (1981) Histologic typing of breast tumours. In: International histological classification of tumours, 2nd edn. World Health Organization, Geneva

Zippel HH, Citoler P (1976) Häufigkeit des lokal begrenzten Wachstums von Mammakarzinomen. Dtsch Med Wochenschr 101: 484–486

Bilateral Breast Cancer Revealed by Biopsy of the Opposite Breast

Jerome A. Urban

Memorial Sloan-Kettering Cancer Institute and Cornell Medical School,
215 E. 68th St., New York, New York 10021, USA

Introduction

The bilaterality of breast cancer is becoming increasingly evident and is generally recognized (Urban 1967, 1969). Not infrequently, one encounters simultaneous clinically apparent bilateral breast cancers. More often, these lesions appear to arise asynchronously. Foote and Stewart (1945) stated: "the most frequent antecedent of cancer in one breast is the history of having had cancer in the opposite breast." There is mounting evidence that bilateral breast cancer, simultaneous or otherwise, occurs most often in certain patients: in those with a strong family history of breast cancer, particularly patients whose mothers have had bilateral breast cancer before the age of 50; in those with multiple breast cancers in the dominant breast, in patients with in situ lobular carcinoma; and in younger women successfully treated for early localized cancer who have a good prognosis for long survival.

Leis et al. (1965) subjected a number of patients to prophylactic simple mastectomies. He applied this procedure to those patients who, in his opinion, had a high risk of developing a new cancer in the opposite breast. This group included those with early stage I cancers, with multiple primaries in the dominant breast, with in situ lobular carcinoma, and with a strong family history of breast cancer. In his series, 17% of the prophylactic simple mastectomy specimens contained carcinoma; two-thirds noninfiltrating and one-third infiltrating. Leis also pointed out that when a second primary cancer of the breast was detected through repeat clinical examinations and mammograms in a patient who had previously undergone mastectomy for breast cancer, the stage of disease found in the second breast was often no earlier or more localized than that of the first breast lesion, despite supposedly close clinical follow-up. We have had a similar experience. Newman (1963) demonstrated a particularly high incidence of bilaterality in patients with in situ lobular carcinoma of the breast. Others have substantiated this finding.

Robbins and Berg (1964) estimated that almost 1% of patients who had undergone mastectomy of one breast for breast cancer would develop a new cancer in the opposite breast during each year of follow-up. We were struck by the high incidence of new primary lesions in the second breast when we analyzed a follow-up study of our own patients treated by the extended radical mastectomy procedure (Urban and Castro 1971). Of the original 455 patients treated by this procedure, 9% developed a clinically apparent new primary breast cancer in the opposite breast during the 10-year follow-up. This corresponds to 15% of the patients who survived 10 years following the initial surgery.

Early Breast Cancer
Edited by J. Zander and J. Baltzer
© Springer-Verlag Berlin Heidelberg 1985

Since the stage of disease at the time of primary therapy is the most important prognostic factor, it is imperative to detect these lesions as early as possible, when they are most likely to be localized to the breast (Urban 1960). The need for early detection of second primary lesions in the contralateral breast cannot be overemphasized. Some patients already cured of breast cancer by their initial surgery have been lost through failure to recognize and treat new primary lesions of the second breast until late in their development. The usual follow-up program for patients treated by mastectomy for breast cancer has consisted of repeated careful physical examination, and early excisional biopsy of new findings. More recently, this has been supplemented by the use of repeated mammographies, which at times have detected new primary lesions before they developed the usual pathognomonic signs of breast cancer. Patients have also been instructed in the technique of breast self-examination, and have been urged to present themselves immediately on finding changes in the physical appearance of their breasts. Despite all these efforts, detection of early, localized breast cancer remains difficult and unreliable.

We have been increasingly impressed with the finding of occult breast cancers through generous excisional biopsy of persistent equivocal breast lesions. This has been particularly true when indefinite thickenings of the opposite breast were biopsied at the time of mastectomy for a known breast cancer in the dominant breast. During the last 18 years we have adopted a policy of routinely biopsying the contralateral breast at the time of mastectomy for a known cancer in the dominant breast. Between 1964 and 1975, we operated upon 1,204 patients with breast cancer. During this period 80% of the available contralateral breasts in these patients undergoing surgery for a known breast cancer were biopsied, and 12.5% of the contralateral breast biopsies were found to contain a new primary breast cancer. In addition, 10% of the benign biopsies contained markedly atypical hyperplasia of the ductal or lobular epithelium, which we consider to be a premalignant lesion (Urban et al. 1977).

Contralateral breast biopsy has been applied to three general categories of patients: (a) a small group of patients in whom bilateral carcinoma was suspected on the basis of preoperative physical and/or mammographic findings; (b) patients with breast cancer in a dominant breast who showed nonspecific thickenings or densifications in the opposite breast; and finally (c) a number of patients who showed no abnormal findings in the opposite breast, either on mammography or on physical examination. In the first group, in which carcinoma was suspected in the second breast, we found our highest incidence of

Table 1. Bilaterality of breast cancer in 1,204 cases (1964–1975, 80% biopsy of opposite breast)[a] by reason for biopsy procedure

No. of biopsies	Cancer		Benign
	Infiltrating	Noninfiltrating	
Random 301	5	18	278
Minimal signs 625	30	44	551
Positive signs 28	20	2	6
	55	64	835
Total 954		119	(88 atypia)

[a] 12.5% simultaneous bilateral carcinoma in breasts biopsied (119/954); 10% simultaneous bilateral carcinoma in total group (119/1204)

second primary breast cancers. Among 28 lesions, 20 proved to be infiltrating cancers, 2 were noninfiltrating, and 6 were benign. In the 625 patients with nonspecific areas of thickening or densification, 74 carcinomas were found, 30 infiltrating and 44 noninfiltrating. Finally, in the 301 patients who had no significant findings in the second breast, 23 cancers were detected by contralateral biopsy, 5 infiltrating and 18 noninfiltrating. This yields a total of 119 cancers revealed in the second breast by 954 biopsies performed in 1,204 patients, 12.5% simultaneous bilateral breast cancers found in the patients whose second breasts were biopsied at the time of mastectomy and 10% simultaneous bilateral breast cancer in the overall group (Table 1).

Technique

When positive physical and/or x-ray signs are present in the second breast, excisional biopsy of the suspected area is carried out, accompanied by specimen radiography when indicated. When an indeterminate thickening is noted in the second breast, or when x-ray mammograms show an area of densification of uncertain nature, these areas are excised widely and yield the highest take of occult lesions. Finally, when no significant lesion is present in the opposite breast, either by physical or mammographic examination, we remove anything from 20% to 25% of the breast parenchyma, removing a fusiform shaped area of glandular tissue through an incision that traverses and preserves all the overlying skin and subcutaneous fat. The latter tissues are then used to obtain a cosmetic closure and to minimize the operative defect. The wounds are closed in separate layers, approximating the superficial half of the breast parenchyma with interrupted heavy chromic catgut sutures, approximating the subcutaneous fat and dermis with interrupted fine chromic sutures, and finally the subcuticular tissue with fine chromic sutures and the skin with a subcuticular dexon closure. Although drainage with a Penrose drain was usually done routinely in the early years, this has been abandoned and we now very rarely drain these wounds. When the second breast appears to be normal, with no specific physical or x-ray signs, the tail of the breast and the mirror image of the primary lesion are usually excised. Carcinoma has been found in 8% of this group (32/301). These lesions are the earliest occult lesions found by us in this fashion, and are made up of 80% noninfiltrating and only 20% infiltrating lesions. In the combined group of occult lesions, 35 infiltrating cancers were found in the second breast, and only 3 (8.5%) had axillary node involvement.

Eighty-eight patients whose contralateral breast biopsies were considered benign, or approximately 10%, showed markedly atypical lobular or ductal hyperplasia. These are considered to be premalignant and are associated with a high risk of later development of breast cancer. These patients are monitored in a prospective clinic, with repeated physical examinations every 4 months and annual mammograms (Ashíkari R, personal communication). The latest review of activity in this clinic demonstrated that 8.8% of patients who had undergone mastectomy for cancer in one breast and who were found to have atypical hyperplasia of the epithelium by biopsy of the contralateral breast at that time subsequently developed cancer of the second breast within a 6-year follow-up period, 60% of these lesions being infiltrating and 40% noninfiltrating.

During this time interval (1964 to 1975), 70 asynchronous breast cancers were encountered (Table 2). In 50 patients who had previously undergone mastectomy and another 20 patients who had undergone mastectomy for a known breast cancer, and who had had a negative contralateral breast biopsy, a new cancer subsequently developed in the second breast. A good number of the patients in the latter group had had atypical epithelial

Table 2. Bilateral of breast cancer in 1,204 cases (1964−1975, 80% biopsy of opposite breast)[a] by dominant breast lesion

Dominant breast lesion	No. biopsied	No. benign	Simultaneous Ca.		Previous mastectomy	Subsequent mastectomy
			Infil- trating	Noninfil- trating		
Infiltrating Ca. 1049	838	741	51	46	33	15
Noninfiltrating Ca. 155	116	94	4	18	17	5
Total 1,204	954	835	55	64	50	20[b]
			Bilat. asynchronous		Bilat. asynchronous	

[a] 15.7% Bilateral Ca. (189/1204); 10% simultaneous (119/1204); 5.8% asynchronous (70/1204)
[b] Twenty patients with benign contralateral breast biopsies (four atypical) later developed cancer of second breast

Table 3. State of disease: Second primary breast cancers in 1,204 cases (1964−1975)

No.	Status	Infil- trating Ca.	Nodes +ve	Noninfil- trating Ca.
119	Simultaneous biopsy	55	10 (18%)	64 (54%)
97	Simultaneous biopsy random or minimal signs	35	3 (8.5%)	62 (60%)
22	Simultaneous biopsy with positive signs	20	7 (45%)	2 (10%)
50	Current mastectomy	46	14 (28%)	4 (8%)
50	Previous mastectomy	40	11 (28%)	10 (20%)
20	Subsequent mastectomy	18	9 (50%)	2 (10%)

hyperplasia in their original biopsy. In the entire group of asynchronous second bilateral breast cancers, 35% of infiltrating cancers had axillary node metastases and only 17% of the cancers were found at the noninfiltrating stage (Table 3).

When carcinoma is found in both breasts simultaneously the patients are treated by simultaneous bilateral mastectomy, the extent of mastectomy being based upon the extent of disease found in the breasts. Follow-up shows that 80% of these patients are living and well, being free of disease, 5 years after bilateral mastectomy.

We were not particularly impressed with the findings yielded by mammography in this group of patients. x-Ray mammography or xerox mammography was performed preoperatively in 75 patients in whom bilateral simultaneous breast cancers were subsequently found, and 34% had positive, or strongly suggestive, results bilaterally, 44% had positive results on the dominant side only, and 20% had negative results on both sides. Mammography is a valuable adjunct to physical examination, but it has its limitations and should not be relied upon to rule out the presence of a carcinoma. A negative mammogram should not preclude biopsy, particularly when a suggestive area is noted on physical examination (Table 4).

Table 4. Detection of contralateral breast cancer by x-ray mammograms in 1,204 cases (1964−1975)

No. of cases with x-ray mammograms	Dominant Ca. → opposite breast	++	+0	00
13	Noninfilt. → Noninfilt.	3	5	5
4	Noninfilt. → Infilt.	2	2	
22	Infilt. → Noninfilt.	5	12	5
36	Infilt. → Infilt.	14	14	8
Total 75		24	33	18

The relatively high incidence of breast cancer found in the opposite breast reflects the long silent history of this disease, its multicentricity, and the need for close cooperation between surgeon and pathologist. The multicentric nature of breast cancer was demonstrated unequivocally by the classic work of Gallager and Martin (1969). Mastectomy specimens performed for breast cancer were serially sectioned and whole-breast sections prepared for histopathological examination. The great majority of breast cancers were proved by these authors to be multicentric in origin. They also devised a rational scheme regarding the development of breast cancer and showed that many years intervene between the appearance of in situ non-infiltrating cancer and its subsequent development into infiltrating cancer. In order to succeed with contralateral breast biopsy, the surgeon must provide an adequate specimen for pathologic examination, at least 15%−20% of the breast parenchyma in our opinion, and committed pathologist must be willing to perform many sections of this tissue for adequate examination.

"Early detection of minimal lesions" confined to the breast, combined with adequate primary therapy, has achieved maximum survival of patients with breast cancer (Wanebo et al. 1974). *Contralateral breast biopsy at the time of mastectomy for a known breast cancer is another method of early detection of breast cancer.* A significant number of occult breast cancers have been detected in this manner, often in the absence of any positive physical or mammographic signs. A small number of patients in our group (2%) subsequently developed a second cancer in the remaining breast despite an initial benign contralateral biopsy. It is imperative that all patients treated for primary breast cancer be followed-up closely, with particular emphasis on examination and management of the remaining breast. The maximum detection of early lesions still in a favorable condition for successful treatment will be obtained by combining all current methods of detection.

References

Foote FW, Stewart FW (1945) Comparative studies of cancerous versus non cancerous breast, I and II. Ann Surg 121:6 (Part I), 197 (Part II)

Gallager HS, Martin J (1969) Early phases in the development of breast cancer. Cancer 1170−1178

Leis HP Jr, Mersheimer WL, Black NN et al. (1965) The second breast. NY J Med 62:2460−2468

Newman W (1963) In situ lobular carcinoma of the breast. Report of 26 women with 32 cancers. Ann Surg 157:591−599

Robbins GF, Berg SW (1964) Bilateral primary breast cancers. A prospective study − clinical
    pathological. Cancer 17: 1501−1527
Urban JA (1960) Treatment of early cancer of the breast. Postgrad Med 27: 389−393
Urban JA (1967) Bilaterality of cancer of the breast − biopsy of the opposite breast. Cancer
    20: 1867−1870
Urban JA (1969) Bilateral breast cancer. Cancer 1310−1313
Urban JA, Castro EB (1971) Selecting variations in extent of surgical procedures for breast cancer.
    Cancer 28: 1615−1623
Urban JA, Papachristou D, Taylor J (1977) Bilateral breast cancer − biopsy of the opposite breast.
    Cancer 40: 1968−1973
Wanebo HJ, Huvos AG, Urban JA (1974) Treatment of minimal breast cancer. Cancer
    33: 349−357

Histopathology and Frequency of Invasive Breast Cancer with Lipid Synthesis

R. Bässler and C. Eckardt

Institute of Pathology, Städtische Kliniken, Academic Hospital,
Pacelli-Allee 4, 6400 Fulda, Federal Republic of Germany

Introduction

The occurrence of lipids in the epithelial cells of the female breast is normally associated with pregnancy and lactation. In these periods their presence indicates secretory activity. Likewise the mammary epithelial cells are able to synthesize lipids in cases of hormonally induced hyperplasia, dysplasia, and mastitis caused by estrogens, gestagens, and prolactin. In carcinomas, the lipid production has usually been interpreted as a degenerative change, and therefore this phenomenon has received no attention for many years. Similarly, different types of breast cancer that develop in pregnancy or lactation reveal no secretory products in the cytoplasm, in particular no higher activity of lipid synthesis than in the surrounding parenchyma of the breast. Systemic histochemical studies of breast carcinoma have been concerned with mucosubstances, mucin, glycogen and enzymatic reactions, but there are few case reports and little information on lipid synthesis of cancer cells.

Aboumrad et al. (1963) described a case of a lipid-secreting mammary carcinoma associated with Paget's disease of the nipple. Both ducts and lobules were involved, and tumor cells contained vacuolated and foamy epithelial elements that stained with a fat-soluble dye. The authors assume that the vacuolization was caused by the presence of lipids and they estimate a frequency of lipid-secreting breast cancers of 1%. Further, they observed intracellular lipid in 8 of 12 other breast cancers.

Hood et al. (1973) investigated 13 metastases of breast cancer in the eyelids. In 8 cases they observed a histicytoid tumor pattern and suggest (without Oil Red staining) that lipid-rich cancers of the breast exhibit a more aggressive clinical behavior than other cancers.

Ramos and Taylor (1974) reported that 13 (1.4%) of 900 breast cancers had histopathological features of lipid synthesis. The median diameter of the tumors was 3.2 cm. Microscopically the authors classify as invasive cancer those cases with areas of intraductal cancer and lobular carcinoma in situ. Electron-microscopic examination revealed large intracytoplasmatic lipid droplets, glycogen, tonofilaments, and enlarged mitochondria with crystalloid inclusions. All the patients had nodal metastases at the time of mastectomy. Prognostically the tumors appear to be somewhat more aggressive than other types of breast cancer.

Van Bogaert and Maldague (1977) described ten new cases. The histopathological features suggested three different patterns of lipid-secreting carcinoma, which were all characterized by abundant intracytoplasmatic neutral fat deposits. Within lipid cell carcinoma the

Early Breast Cancer
Edited by J. Zander and J. Baltzer
© Springer-Verlag Berlin Heidelberg 1985

authors distinguished a histiocytoid type, a sebaceous type, and a carcinoma with apocrine extrusion of nuclei fulfilling the criteria of Hamperl (1977).

Lim-Co and Gisser (1978) published a case report of ulcerated breast cancer in a woman aged 43 years. It was a medullary type of breast cancer with lymphoid stroma. Electron-microscopic investigations reveal two cell types: dark cells, which contained lipid deposits and appeared more aggressive, and clear counterparts. The authors suggested that the former were myoepithelial cells, and were able to synthesize neutral fat.

In summary, there are about 20 well-documented cases of lipid-secreting breast carcinoma in the current literature. It is surprising that only one systemic investigation by Fisher et al. (1977) examined the lipid content of tumor cells of 65 breast cancers by fat-staining methods. The results of this study based on visual assessment revealed that approximately 70% of breast cancers contain some degree of intracytoplasmatic lipid; 25% of the carcinoma did not contain fat deposits; and in 6% there was a marked presence of lipid droplets consistent with grade 3 disease. Statistical analyses demonstrated a correlation between moderate and marked lipid synthesis in tumor cells and squamous metaplasia, low nuclear and high histological grade, and slight stroma. The cytoplasma of clear cell carcinomas of the eye contained only a few lipids; they were not generally lipid-secreting cancers.

The authors conclude that the features of breast cancer described may not constitute a distinct clinicopathological entity.

The above information suggests that a histometric investigation on the quantity and distribution of lipid deposits in cell of different breast cancers to distinguish between tumors of high and low lipid content referred to the various types of breast cancer might be valuable.

Materials and Methods

Specimens of 172 breast cancers treated by radical or modified mastectomy and specimens of biopsies were examined by a quantitative histometric method ($n = 112$ cases) and by a visual assessment of distribution and density of fat deposits in the cells of breast cancer ($n = 60$ cases) in studies similar to thoses of Fisher et al. (1977). Frozen sections of the tumors were stained with Sudan Black, Sudan Orange, or Oil Red for quantitative analyses and estimation of degree of lipid content. Counts were done using a Visopan (Reichert) projection microscope with a magnification of $\times 25$. To facilitate counting and to standardize the area a grid of 25 points was used. On each slide four areas of three specimens were counted, giving a total of 300 points ($3 \times 4 \times 25 = 300$) for each carcinoma. To adjust for differences between the areas of stroma and tumor cells more than 100 points of the specimen were counted, including tumor cells with and without fat deposits. For every case and group, the mean value, the standard variation, and the variance were calculated (Eckardt 1983). To give a better picture the results of the counts are expressed as histograms for each cancer group, with the quantities of lipid-containing cells as percentages (Figs. 1–4).

Results

Quantitative Analysis

Quantitative investigation by a histometric method reveals different degrees of lipid content in breast cancers. According to our own cytological grading of the quantity of intracytoplasmatic lipid droplets related to 100 tumor cells 25% of all cases did not contain

Table 1. Results of the quantitative analysis of the lipid content in breast cancer with grading

Quantitative	Examination	Results in %	Grading
0–3	Positive tumor cells	25	0
4–25	Positive tumor cells	45	1
26–70	Positive tumor cells	23	2
71–100	Positive tumor cells	6	3

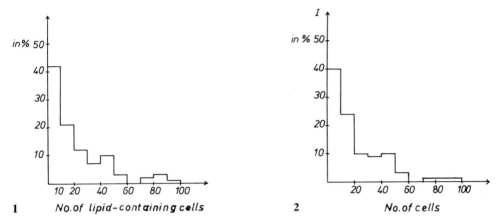

Fig. 1. Histogram of the lipid content of all cases of invasive breast cancer. *Abscissa*, percentage of lipid-containing tumor cells in relation to total cells. Thus, we found 0–10 lipid-positive cells in 42% and 90–100 lipid-positive cells in 1% of all carcinomas

Fig. 2. Histogram of the lipid content of the invasive ductal carcinoma

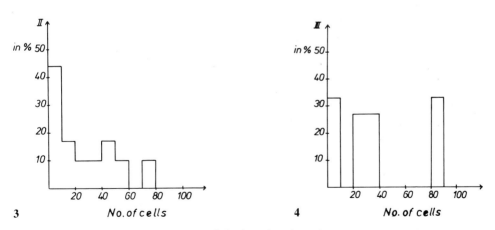

Fig. 3. Histogram of the lipid content of the intraductal carcinoma

Fig. 4. Histogram of the lipid content of the medullary carcinoma with lymphoid stroma (indicating a high histologic grading)

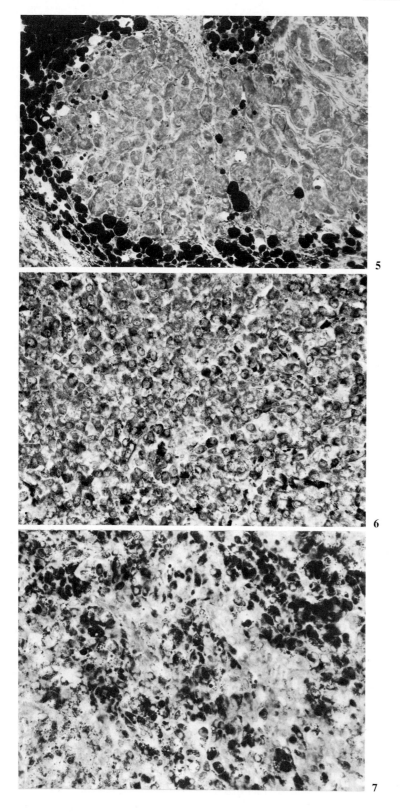

5

6

7

any lipid or only focal minimal droplets; in 45% of cases the lipid content was slight, in 24% moderate, and in 6% marked (Table 1).

The histometric results are presented in histograms for each group of breast cancer with respect to the lipid content (Figs. 1−4); the abscissa represents the percentage of positive tumor cells in the whole tumor, and the ordinate, the relative frequency. The histogram for all investigated breast cancers (Fig. 1) shows that 94% of all carcinomas contain 0−60% positive tumor cells and only 6% of the carcinomas contain 70%−100% positive tumor cells. Thus 0−10 lipid-positive cells are found in 42% of all tumors and 90−100 lipid-rich cells are found in 1% of all carcinomas (Fig. 1). This percentage corresponds to what is generally reported about the prevalence of lipid-rich breast carcinomas (Ramos and Taylor 1974; van Bogaert and Maldague 1977). Lipid-poor tumors are significantly more frequent. With increasing percentages of positive tumor cells the frequency of occurrence decreases. The histograms for the invasive ductal carcinomas (Fig. 2) and for the intraductal (invasive and noninvasive) carcinomas (Fig. 3) indicate a similar distribution with a quota of 6%−10% of cases containing 70%−100% of positive tumor cells.

The histological variants of invasive ductal carcinoma, i.e., types with a predominant fibrosis or adenoid pattern or mixed types, display a similar lipid content and distribution. This means that most carcinomas contain between 10% and 20% and between 40% and 50% positive tumor cells. Differing from this are medullary cancers with lymphoid stroma ($n = 6$) and the largely anaplastic invasive ductal cancer ($n = 11$), with high averages and a different distribution of positive tumor cells. The histograms for these carcinomas are very similar and indicate a wide distribution of positive cells between 20% and 40% and between 80% and 90% (Fig. 4).

Qualitative Analysis

At the same time as the quantitative tests were being run, 60 breast carcinomas of different types were being investigated qualitatively for lipid content. Frozen sections of various areas of the carcinomas were investigated by staining with Sudan Black and Oil Red. When the same histological methods were used in the different types of carcinomas wide differences in lipid production and fat distribution were found. Some of the carcinomas was totally fat free (Fig. 5) or had only minimal, small droplets of lipids in the tumor cells. Others contained focal or diffuse fat droplets (Fig. 6) or few or many large (globuled) lipid droplets (Fig. 7). As an aid to visual evaluation, the scheme shown in Table 2 was worked out. In this way it was possible to compare our values with those of Fisher et al. (1977). Our own visual evaluation revealed that 40% of the tumors were grade 0; 38% grade 1; 17%

◄

Fig. 5 (above.) Invasive ductal carcinoma free of intracellular lipid; in the surrounding black-stained fat tissue to grade 0. Formalin, frozen section, Sudan Black, × 320

Fig. 6 (middle). Invasive ductal carcinoma with a moderate, homogeneous lipid content in the tumor cells in a small-droplet pattern around the nuclei to grade 2. Formalin, frozen section, Sudan Black, × 300

Fig. 7 (below). Invasive ductal carcinoma with lipid secretion and deposits of large lipid droplets in the tumor cells. Marked and scattered lipid distribution corresponding to grade 3. Formalin, frozen section, Sudan Black, × 300

Table 2. Grading and distribution of lipids in breast cancer by visual evaluation

Degree of intensity	Distribution	Grading
Free or minimal lipid		0
Slight	Focal	1
Moderate	Scattered	2
Marked	Diffuse	3

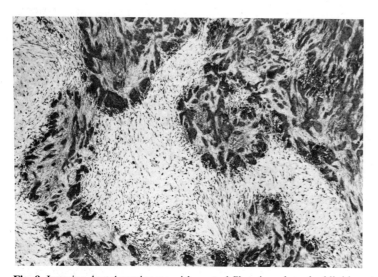

Fig. 8. Invasive ductal carcinoma with central fibrosis and marked lipid content at the tumor margin, caused by nutritional insufficiency and not by lipid secretion. Formalin, frozen section, Sudan Black, × 120

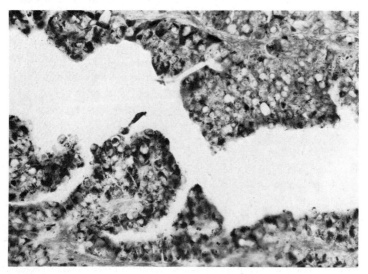

Fig. 9. Papillary carcinoma with a moderate lipid content in the tumor cells corresponding to grade 2. Formalin, frozen section, Sudan Black, × 260

grade 2; and 5% grade 3. The estimations for grade 0 are relatively high, since we included discrete minimal and territorially varying degrees of fat deposits in the tumor cells. The frequency of grade 1, on the other hand, was found to be low. In this case we consider there might be a more homogeneous pattern of the intracytoplasmatic fat droplets.

That meant that roughly two-thirds of the carcinomas had lipids in minimal and focal forms or were totally lipid free. Only 5%−6% exhibited pronounced lipid synthesis.

For the assessment of whether a lipid-secreting carcinoma is present it is important that signs of high lipid production by the tumor cells are recognizable *within the carcinoma homogeneously or in large areas.*

Focal lipid deposits in carcinomas are observed in the border areas or in the tumor centers, i.e., in zones of the tumor parenchyma in which insufficient metabolism, particularly hypoxia, is present. Pronounced fat deposits also occur in the cells of the tumor stroma (Fig. 8).

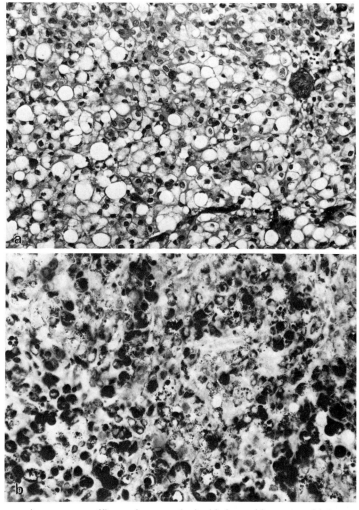

Fig. 10a, b. Lipid-secreting carcinoma: **a** paraffin section reveals the histiocytoid pattern with large, clear, vacuolated tumor cells; **b** staining with Sudan Black displays a marked lipid content with large lipid droplets and a homogeneous distribution. Formalin, frozen section, × 300

We were able to observe very wide variation in the grades of lipid production in *intraductal carcinomas,* particularly in comedocarcinoma. Higher grades of lipid production were found in *papillary carcinomas* (Fig. 9), while *mucinous carcinomas* were fully lipid-free, as were *lobular* and *secretory carcinomas* (Fig.10). In *apocrine carcinomas* we found lipids as fine droplets but no marked fat synthesis.

Discussion

Quantitative and qualitative studies should answer questions regarding the amount and form in which lipids occur in the cells of the more common breast carcinomas. Furthermore, the frequency with which lipids are produced in large quantities in breast cancer should be investigated to allow precise definition of the term "lipid-secreting carcinoma."

Quantitative investigations were conducted in 112 and qualitative investigations in 60 breast cancers of different types, and the lipid content was correlated with various histopathological parameters. The level of $P \leq 0.05$ was considered indicate to a statistically significant correlation. The results indicate that in 25% of cases no lipid was found; in 45% a low grade of lipid content (grade 1) was observed; in 24% a moderate amount (grade 2); and in 6% a marked grade (3) was demonstrated. Positive correlations between lipid content and carcinoma type existed with medullary carcinomas with lymphoid stroma and with highly anaplastic (undifferentiated) ductal carcinomas. This finding shows parallels with the results of Fisher et al. (1977), who also determined a high lipid content in carcinomas with a high nuclear grading (NG = 1) and a high histological grading. Comparison of the results of Fisher et al. (1977) and those of our own investigations reveals that the different methods have yielded consistent values.

Our own visual assessment of the lipid content differs in a shift of grade 0 to 1, since focal and minimal fat deposits in the tumor cells are subsumed under grade 0 (Table 3). In around 70% of cases the average values obtained in these investigations with various methods show either no lipid synthesis of only a low content of fat droplets in the cytoplasm. These proved to be non-type-specific with respect to cancer classification. The grade 3 carcinomas (Fig. 7) are invasive ductal carcinomas with a different histological grading.

It is obvious, however, that pronounced lipid synthesis in the tumor cells causes cytoplasmatic changes which, after embedding in paraffin, are seen as characteristic clear

Table 3. Results and comparison of the histometric analysis and the visual evaluation of the lipid content in breast cancer

Grading	Histometric analysis (own investigations)	Visual evaluation	Visual evaluation (Fisher)	Mean values
0	25%	40%	25%	30%
1	45%	38%	45%	42%
2	24%	17%	24%	21%
3	6%	5%	6%	6%
	$n = 112$	$n = 60$	$n = 87$	

cytoplasm or as vacuolization. On the basis of 15 cases, the carcinomas characterized by this feature were termed histiocytoid and sebaceous carcinomas by van Bogaert and Maldague (1977). It is an open question as to whether the so-called sweat cell carcinoma with nuclear extrusion described by Hamperl (1977) belongs to this group, since no lipid test was run and the secretory carcinomas are also lipid-free.

The frequency of lipid-producing carcinomas is reported to be 1%−5%. The marked lipid deposits we have determined in 6% of breast carcinomas indicate that around 4%−5% of carcinomas with high focal or diffuse lipid synthesis are not recognized as a result of the usual embedding in paraffin.

Summary

A quantitative and qualitative study of lipid production in 172 breast carcinomas is reported. Histometric investigation of 112 carcinomas of various types revealed no lipids in 25% of cases; small amounts in 45%; moderate amounts in 24%; and large lipid deposits in 6%. The values are consistent with the estimated values given in the literature. High lipid production in the cytoplasm of tumor cells is rare and could induce a clear or vacuolated cell pattern; in other words, a histiocytoid or a sebaceous type of breast cancer. Histopathological diagnosis requires staining of the tissues with specific dyes for neutral lipids.

References

Aboumrad MH, Horn RC, Fine G (1963) Lipid-secreting mammary carcinoma. Report of a case associated with Paget's disease of the nipple. Cancer 16: 521−525

Eckardt C (1983) Quantitative und qualitative histopathologische Untersuchungen intrazellulärer Lipide in Karzinomen der Brustdrüse. Inaug Diss, Marburg

Fisher ER, Gregorio R, Kim WS, Redmond C (1977) Lipid in invasive cancer of the breast. Am J Clin Pathol 68: 558−561

Hamperl H (1977) Das sogenannte Schweißdrüsenkarzinom der Mamma. Z Krebsforsch 88: 105−119

Hood CJ, Front RL, Zimmermann LE (1973) Metastatic mammary carcinoma in the eyelid with histiocytoid appearance. Cancer 31: 793−800

Lim-Co RY, Gisser SD (1978) Unusual variant of lipidrich mammary carcinoma. Arch Pathol Lab Med 102: 193−195

Ramos CV, Taylor HD (1974) Lipidrich carcinoma of the breast. A clinico-pathologic analysis of 13 examples. Cancer 33: 812−819

van Bogaert LJ, Maldague P (1977) Histologic variants of lipid-secreting carcinoma of the breast. Virchows Arch [Pathol Anat] 375: 345−353

Lobular Carcinoma In Situ and Its Relation to Invasive Breast Cancer

A. H. Tulusan, H. Egger, and K. G. Ober

Universitäts-Frauenklinik, Universitätsstrasse 23, 8520 Erlangen, Federal Republic of Germany

Introduction

The histological appearance of lobular carcinoma in situ (LCIS) in the breast is well defined. However, opinions differ on the interpretation of its biological nature and on how to treat the disease. Recommendations range from systematic follow-up to mastectomy (Haagensen et al. 1978; Rosen et al. 1981).

Is LCIS Truly a Carcinoma In Situ?

Our experience in the observation and treatment of *299* patients with LCIS between 1954 and 1982 in the Erlangen University Hospital for Women formed the basis of our attempt to find an answer to this question.

Analysing the types of invasive cancer found simultaneously with, previous to, and after LCIS, we observed that 46% of invasive cancers are of the *invasive lobular* or so-called small cell cancer type.

We previously reported on 43 LCIS patients monitored following surgery up to 1980 (Tulusan et al. 1982a). The indications for more extensive surgery in diagnosed LCIS have been guided by the extent of the disease, the age of the patients, and the assessability of the breasts. Perhaps the important difference between our study and those of others (Carter and Smith 1977; Rosen et al. 1979) is that we performed detailed histological examination of the tissue obtained from the surgical procedures, e.g., we divided the breast into four quadrants and a retromamillary area, and subjected the resected breast to total radial processing (Fig. 1) involving radiologic examination of each slice before embedding. We made only large-block sections, so that we were able to determine the topographic location of each lobular or ductal alteration found during the histological examination.

In the course of these procedures, 6 (16%) invasive cancers were detected in the breasts of 38 LCIS patients treated within 24 months after the diagnosis of LCIS, 10% being detected within the first 12 months. Four invasive cancers developed in the ipsilateral breast to the previous LCIS, and two in the contralateral breast.

The most important fact is that *five of the six* invasive cancers were clinically and mammographically *occult* (even in specimen radiography). These cancers had diameters of 3, 4, 7, 10, and 14 mm.

Early Breast Cancer
Edited by J. Zander and J. Baltzer
© Springer-Verlag Berlin Heidelberg 1985

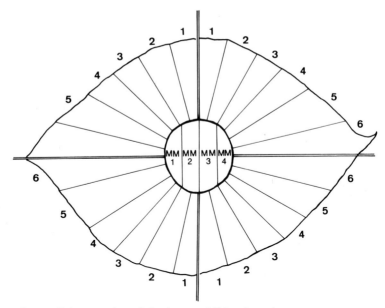

Fig. 1. Scheme for complete radial processing of the breast. *MM,* subareolar area

Table 1. Multicentricity of LCIS by primary site of biopsy and by extent in primary biopsy

LCIS diagnosed in the upper outer quadrant	38%
LCIS diagnosed outside the upper outer quadrant	64%
> 6 Separate lobules with LCIS	14/17 (= 82%)
Only 1 or 2 lobules with LCIS	2/18 (= 11%)

In the subsequent 2 years (1981, 1982) we treated 15 further LCIS patients within 24 months after the LCIS diagnosis. *Two* more occult invasive cancers (5 and 6 mm in diameter) were detected in the resected breast tissue.

In 7 LCIS patients with further surgery more than 24 months after diagnosis, 5 invasive cancers were detected (3 *occult:* diameters 2, 5, and multicentric 3−4 mm).

On the other hand, we have also observed 38 LCIS patients with no subsequent treatment after biopsy, and a follow-up of 2−24 years, who did not develop invasive cancer. Almost all of them had only LCIS lesions in one or two lobules.

An analysis of these observations revealed the following facts:

1) The multicentricity of LCIS varied with the location of the primary biopsy leading to the diagnosis of LCIS and with the extent of the disease in the primary biopsy (Table 1). Bilaterality (43%), in contrast, is not influenced by the extent of LCIS or by the presence of invasive cancer in the breast.

2) In the immediate vicinity of an LCIS lesion, but also in a completely different quadrant, we often found other atypical proliferations of the breast epithelium (12% ductal carcinoma in situ and 28% atypical proliferative mastopathy). In the other breast we found 6% ductal carcinoma in situ and 19% atypical proliferative mastopathy.

3) Even with our painstaking histological examination technique, carcinomas with a diameter of less than 2 mm might habe been overlooked, since we did not use a very

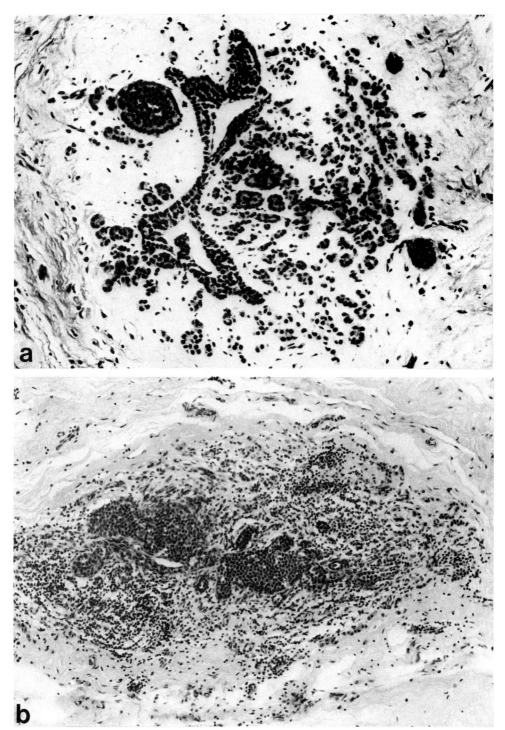

Fig. 2a, b. Early stromal invasion out of the LCIS in two cases, both about 1–2 mm in diameter. Note the radial single-cell infiltration and the incipient "Indian file" pattern unique for invasive lobular cancer

close serial sectioning procedure. But sometimes we were lucky enough to find "early stromal invasion" of the lobular cancer (Fig. 2). Stromal microinvasion in the terminal ductules or lobules is always accompanied by extensive changes in the basement membranes and a radial single-cell infiltration in this area (Tulusan et al. 1982b).

Summary

There is *no doubt* that *LCIS is a precursor of invasive lobular cancer* with its almost typical radial early invasion.

Because of the frequent coexistence of LCIS with atypical ductal proliferations, its multicentricity, and its bilaterality, the diagnosis of LCIS also means a *high risk* of subsequent invasive cancer in the breast. The degree of the risk depends on the extent of the LCIS lesion in the primary biopsy.

Our data and information on LCIS are still far from complete especially on those cases with small areas of infiltration. However, our findings supplement reports by other workers on further surgical treatment carried out shortly after establishment of the diagnosis of LCIS. If these observations are confirmed in larger numbers of patients we should probably revise our ideas about the time taken for a microscopically minute invasive lesion to become a clinically detectable tumor.

References

Carter D, Smith RL (1977) Carcinoma in situ of the breast. Cancer 40: 1189–1193

Haagensen CD, Nane N, Lattes R, Bodian C (1978) Lobular neoplasia (so-called lobular carcinoma in situ) of the breast. Cancer 42: 737–769

Rosen PP, Senie R, Schottenfeld D, Ashikari R (1979) Noninvasive breast carcinoma. Frequency of unsuspected invasion and implications for treatment. Ann Surg 189: 377–382

Rosen PP, Braun DW, Lyngholm B, Urban JE, Kinne DW (1981) Lobular carcinoma in situ of the breast: Preliminary results of treatment by ipsilateral mastectomy and contralateral breast biopsy. Cancer 47: 813–819

Tulusan AH, Egger H, Schneider ML, Willgeroth F (1982a) A contribution to the natural history of breast cancer. IV. Lobular carcinoma in situ and its relation to breast cancer. Arch Gynecol 231: 219–226

Tulusan AH, Grünsteidel W, Ramming I, Egger H (1982b) A contribution to the natural history of breast cancer. III. Changes in the basement membranes in breast cancers with stromal microinvasion. Arch Gynecol 231: 209–218

Essential Histological Findings in the Female Breast at Autopsy

The Frequency and Appearance of in Situ and Invasive Breast Carcinoma in 83 Unselected Cases

Johan A. Andersen[1], Maja Nielsen[2], and Jørn Jensen[3]

[1] Department of Pathology, University Hospital of Odense, Odense, Denmark
[2] Institute of Pathology, Frederiksberg Hospital, Copenhagen, Denmark
[3] Orthopaedic Hospital, Aarhus, Denmark

Introduction

The entity of breast cancer includes in situ and invasive carcinoma according to morphological criteria. Furthermore, proliferative lesions such as atypical ductal hyperplasia and atypical lobular hyperplasia, multiple papillomas, radial scar, juvenile papillomatosis, and cysts have all in some way been reported to be associated with breast cancer.

The lifelong cumulated incidence of invasive breast carcinoma in Danish women is 8.4%. In the county of Ribe, where the present study was performed, the figure is even higher, 9.4% (Jensen OM, 1983, personal communication).

Current figures on the frequency of in situ carcinoma in the female population are sparse and may be subject to some criticism. They are based on surgical material and a few autopsy investigations.

In nonscreening surgical materials the frequency of lobular carcinoma in situ is about 2%−3% but that of intraductal carcinoma is only 0.5%−1% (Andersen and Schiødt 1980). In autopsy studies, Frantz et al. (1951) found no cases of in situ carcinoma among 225 women, Kiær (1954) 4 cases of severe grade III fibroadenomatosis among 350 women, and Sandison (1962) registered only 1 intraductal carcinoma among 800 unselected autopsy cases. In the meticulous study of Kramer and Rush (1973) 3 cases with intraductal carcinoma and 3 cases with atypical ductal hyperplasia were found in a group of 70 women.

Therefore, a discrepancy between these supposed very low incidences of in situ carcinoma and the high, cumulated risk of invasive breast carcinoma seems obvious for the following reasons. In the last decade the prognosis of lobular carcinoma in situ has been well established (Andersen 1977; Haagensen et al. 1978; Rosen et al. 1978). Table 1 lists the three histologically comparable patient samples with exclusively biopsy-treated cases of lobular carcinoma in situ, all with a rather long follow-up, which in the sample treated by Andersen (1982) is now nearly lifelong. About 30% to possibly 35% of all patients with exclusively biopsy-treated lobular carcinoma in situ will later develop invasive carcinoma. Table 2 shows the same prognostic problems referred to intraductal carcinoma, not only illustrating a historical evolution but also indicating a wide difference in the biological significance of two totally different types of intraductal carcinoma. The old, selected, small samples of tumefacient cases of intraductal carcinoma (Dean and Geschickter 1938; Kiær 1954; Kraus and Neubecker 1962; Haagensen 1971) in the upper part of Table 2 seem to

Early Breast Cancer
Edited by J. Zander and J. Baltzer
© Springer-Verlag Berlin Heidelberg 1985

Table 1. Development of invasive carcinoma in 362 exclusively biopsy-treated cases of lobular carcinoma in situ

	No.	Invasive carcinoma %
Rosen et al. (1978)	99	32
Haagensen et al. (1978)	211	17
Andersen (1977, 1982)	52	33

Table 2. Development of invasive carcinoma in 114 exclusively biopsy-treated cases of intraductal carcinoma

	No.	Type	Invasive carcinoma %
Dean and Geschickter (1938)	8	Comedo-	75
Kiaer (1954)	8	Unspecified	75
Kraus and Neubecker (1962)	4	Papillary	50
Haagensen (1971)	11	Papillary	73
Farrow (1970)	25	Unspecified	20
Rosen et al. (1980)	30	Papillary	27
Page et al. (1982)	28	Papillary	25

have a very high frequency of later development of invasive carcinoma. This tumefacient type of intraductal carcinoma is probably very close to common invasive carcinoma of the type "invasive carcinoma with predominant intraductal component" (Sobin 1981). In contrast, in the unselected, consecutive samples with microfocal intraductal carcinoma (Farrow 1970; Rosen et al. 1980; Page et al. 1982) referred to in the lower part, the frequency of later development of invasive carcinoma seems to be similar to that reported for lobular carcinoma in situ. This microfocal type of intraductal carcinoma, therefore, seems to carry the same prognostic significance as lobular carcinoma in situ. All these investigations therefore indicate that 25%−35% of women with microfocal in situ carcinomas will develop invasive breast cancer at some time in their life. If we suppose that all invasive breast cancer cases develop from an in situ lesion, since we know that breast cancer mostly progresses rather slowly (Fournier et al. 1980; Spratt et al. 1981), we can use figures for the incidence of invasive breast carcinoma to estimate the incidence of in situ carcinoma in the general female population. Thus, with a known lifetime cumulated incidence of invasive carcinoma of 9.4% in the county of Ribe the calculated cumulated incidence of in situ carcinoma may be about three times higher, i.e., 25%−30%. Such a high incidence of in situ breast carcinoma may change our present view of breast cancer biology. Furthermore, it may be essential for an explanation and understanding of some of the results obtained in breast cancer marker and screening tests. It must be emphasized that the in situ carcinomas are at present the most reliable and important markers for breast cancer (Andersen and Mattheiem 1984).

These frequency figures are only hypothetical, however, and we therefore performed a systematic and comprehensive investigation of the occurrence of breast lesions in female autopsy cases.

Our Investigations in the County of Ribe

Materials and Methods

The sample is made up of 83 consecutive, unselected female autopsies performed at the Institute of Pathology, Esbjerg Central Hospital, Ribe county. The only criterion for exclusion was an age of less than 20 years. The hospital serves a stable population and autopsies were performed on 93% of inpatient deaths. This very high autopsy frequency corresponds to 52% of the total number of female deaths in the catchment area (Juul and Andersen 1977).

In addition to routine autopsy, bilateral total mastectomy with partial axillary dissection was performed. Afterwards, the breasts were divided into four quadrants including the areola and nipple zone. After fixation each quadrant was cut systematically from the nipple to the periphery into 3-mm-thick sections. All macroscopically visible glandular tissue was embedded in paraffin, resulting in a total of 15,692 blocks, varying from 57 to 166 per breast specimen. Sections from each block were stained with hematoxylin-eosin. Further information has appeared in a previous paper (Nielsen et al. 1984). The occurrence of the following pathologic entities was determined for each section: Infiltrating carcinoma (IBC), intraductal carcinoma (DCIS), lobular carcinoma in situ (LCIS), atypical ductal hyperplasia (ADH), and atypical lobular hyperplasia (ALH). Furthermore, the occurrence of age involution, diffuse fibrocystic disease, focal fibrocystic disease, and ductectasia was assessed (Table 5). Structural components of fibrocystic disease and papilloma and fibroadenoma were tabulated (Table 6). The conditions and lesions were classified according to *Histological Typing of Breast Tumours* (WHO 1981) and the criteria outlined by Azzopardi (1979). Only indisputably histologically confirmed cases were accepted as DCIS and/or LCIS. Only cases in whom there was a strong suspicion of in situ carcinoma were classified as ADH and ALH, respectively.

Besides the autopsy material all biopsies and mastectomy specimens removed surgically were available for re-evaluation except for two benign biopsies.

Results

Seven cases of IBC were found, 6 of which had appeared within the patient's lifetime and one was diagnosed at autopsy (Table 3). In another 14 women in situ carcinoma was detected, in every case at the postmortem examination. Thus, a total of 21 of the 83 female patients (25.4%) had or had had invasive and/or in situ breast carcinoma. Furthermore, one case of ADH and one of ALH were demonstrated at autopsy.

The histological types of carcinomas in the six women with clinical IBC are given in Table 4. In the breasts surgically removed because of IBC, in situ carcinoma was found in the tumor area in all cases, and in four as distant multicentric lesions in addition. In the contralateral breast one patient had LCIS in two of four earlier surgical breast biopsies. At

Table 3. Number of female patients with primary malignant breast lesions in 83 cases

Type	No.
Infiltrating carcinoma[a]	7
Intraductal carcinoma	8
Lobular carcinoma in situ	3
Intraductal carcinoma and lobular carcinoma in situ	3

[a] Six appearing within patients' lifetime

autopsy, two women harbored both invasive carcinoma and in situ carcinoma, and in another two LCIS was found. Thus, two-thirds of the women in this small series with clinical IBC had morphologically malignant breast lesions in the contralateral breasts. In the 77 women without clinical IBC, 2 patients had had multiple surgical benign breast biopsies. At autopsy, 1 case with IBC and 14 cases with in situ carcinoma were discovered. Furthermore, 2 women ad atypical lesions.

Table 5 shows a comparison of the general structural characteristics of the breast parenchyma between the 21 cases with primary malignant breast disease and the 62 cases without any primary malignant breast disease. When all breasts with fibrocystic disease, whether diffuse or focal, were compared, a significant difference between the two groups was found ($P < 0.001$; 15 of 21 women, as against 20 of 62 without primary malignancy). Thus, most cases of primary malignant breast disease were found in women with fibrocystic disease.

Table 6 shows a similar comparison for the morphological components of fibrocystic disease, papilloma, and fibroadenoma. Significantly increased frequencies of adenosis,

Table 4. Breast lesions in 6 women with clinical breast carcinoma

Type	Contralateral breast at autopsy
Ductal, DCIS	ADH
Ductal, DCIS, LCIS	Signet ring cell carcinoma, LCIS
Lobular, LCIS	LCIS, ADH
Mucinous, DCIS, LCIS	–
Ductal, DCIS	LCIS
Ductal, DCIS	Ductal carcinoma, DCIS

ADH, atypical ductal hyperplasia; LCIS, lobular carcinoma in situ; DCIS, intraductal carcinoma

Table 5. Comparison of the general structural characteristics of the breast between 21 women with and 62 women without primary malignant breast disease

Structural characterization of the breast	Primary breast malignancy		
	With ($n = 21$) %	Without ($n = 62$) %	Significance[a]
Age involution	10	21	NS
Age involution and duct ectasia	5	34	$P < 0.01$
Diffuse fibrocystic disease	5	–	–
Diffuse fibrocystic disease and duct ectasia	14	3	$0.05 < P < 0.10$
Focal fibrocystic disease and age involution	5	2	NS
Focal fibrocystic disease, age involution, and duct ectasia	48	27	$0.05 < P < 0.10$
Duct ectasia	10	10	NS
Pregnancy	–	2	NS
"Normal"	5	2	NS

[a] Chi-square test

epithelial hyperplasia, papillomatosis, and discrete papillomas were found in women with primary breast malignancy.

The in situ carcinomas were all microfocal with from 1 to 7 lesions per breast, with an average of 2 for LCIS and 1.6 for DICS. The multicentricity of LCIS and DCIS was 42.9% and 33.3%, respectively. The bilaterality was 16.7% and 9.1%. Figures 1 and 2 illustrate

Table 6. Comparison of the morphological components of fibrocystic disease, fibroadenoma, and papilloma between 21 women with and 62 women without primary malignant breast disease

| | Primary breast malignancy | | |
	With (n = 21) %	Without (n = 62) %	Significance[a]
Cyst	81	93	NS
Apocrine metaplasia	81	93	NS
Adenosis	85	50	$P < 0.005$
Intraductal and lobular hyperplasia			
Mild	86	48	$P < 0.005$
Severe	62	23	$P < 0.001$
Papillomatosis	86	47	$P < 0.005$
Discrete papilloma	62	21	$P < 0.0005$
Fibroadenoma	14	8	NS
Fibroadenomatoid hyperplasia	24	24	NS

[a] Chi-square test

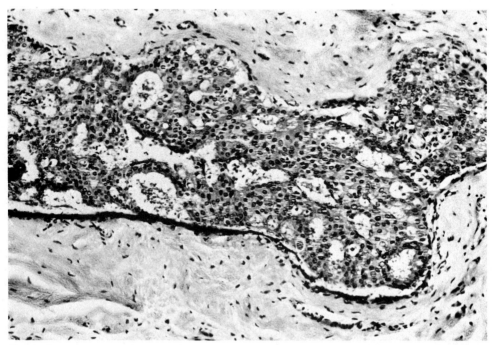

Fig. 1. Case no. 16/77, a 67-year-old woman. Atypical ductal hyperplasia with cribriform pattern of interlobular duct in the left breast. Otherwise atrophic parenchyma apart from some radial scars in both breasts. No other atypical or malignant lesions. H & E, *length scale* = 0.1 mm

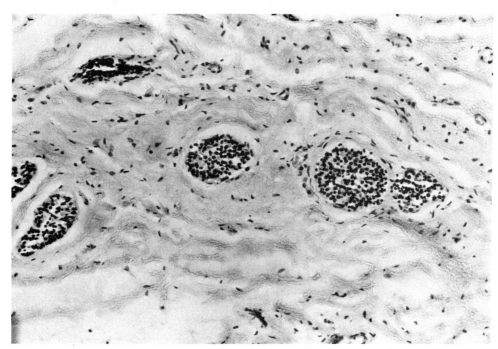

Fig. 2. Case no. 61/77, an 87-year-old woman. Left breast with area of atypical lobular hyperplasia. On both sides, atrophic breast parenchyma with no other atypical or malignant changes. H & E, *length scale* = 0.1 mm

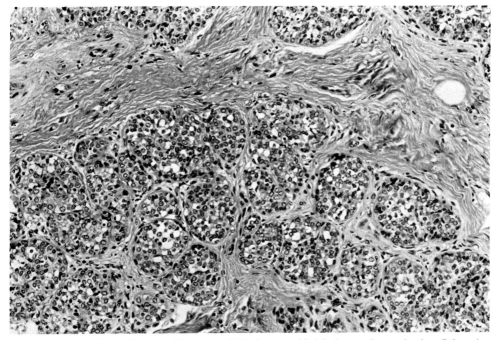

Fig. 3. Case no 21/76, a 48-year-old woman. Right breast with lobular carcinoma in situ. Otherwise both breasts showed chronic diffuse fibrocystic disease and multiple radial scars. H & E, *length scale* = 0.1 mm

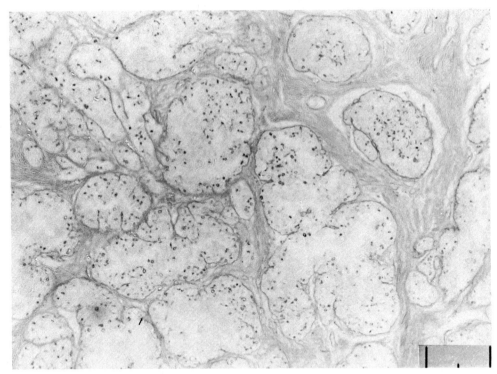

Fig. 4. Case no. 21/76. Same area as in Fig. 3. Lobular carcinoma in situ with many typical ring-like structures reflecting intracytoplasmic lumina. Picture is indicative of lobular carcinoma in situ. PAS/Alcian pH 2.7, *length scale* = 0.1 mm

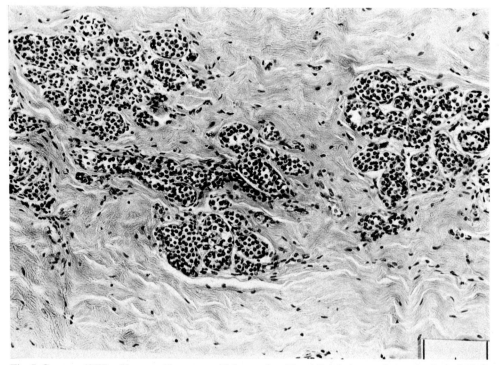

Fig. 5. Case no. 42/77, a 58-year-old woman with focus of multicentric lobular carcinoma in situ in the left breast. Areas of benign focal fibrocystic disease and some radial scars in the same breast. Right-sided mastectomy before autopsy due to invasive ductal carcinoma. H & E, *length scale* = 0.1 mm

our diagnostic level as regards atypical lesions. In the case shown in Fig. 1, PAS/Alcian staining revealed intracytoplasmic lumina strongly indicative of LCIS (Andersen and Vendelbo 1982). Due to our uncertainty about the case it was classified as atypical lobular hyperplasia. In Figs. 3–5 two clear-cut cases of LCIS are shown and in Figs. 6–10, five examples of DCIS representing different growth patterns of intraductal carcinoma, often in combination, i.e., cribriform, comedo-, papilliferous, and clinging types.

The median age of the 83 women was 67 years (range 22–89). No significant differences in age were found between the groups with and without primary malignant breast lesions.

Discussion

The results of this autopsy study confirm our hypothesis that 25%–30% of all women seem to harbor either in situ or invasive primary malignant breast lesions.

Our investigation probably reflects the frequency of primary malignant breast lesions in the general female population. The cases were unselected and collected consecutively, and our autopsy frequency corresponds to 52% of all female deaths within our catchment area. Furthermore, forensic materials from Denmark indicate no differences in the frequency of unexpected malignant disease between patients dying inside or outside hospital institutions (Asnæs and Paaske 1980).

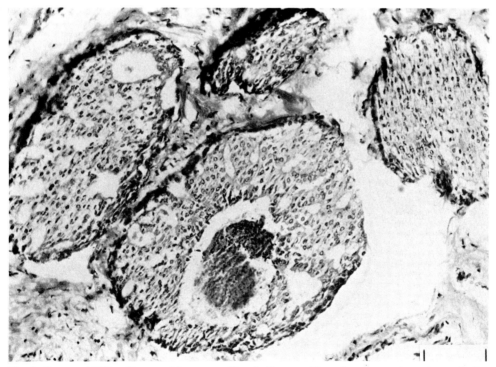

Fig. 6. Case no. 15/77, a 83-year-old woman with cribriform and intraductal comedocarcinoma in the left breast. Mild benign focal fibrocystic changes of both breasts. No other malignant lesions. H & E, *length scale* = 0.1 mm

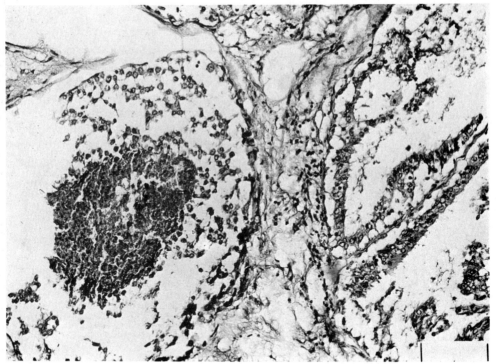

Fig. 7. Case no. 18/77, an 83-year-old woman with intraductal comedocarcinoma in the left breast. Clinging intraductal carcinoma and atypical ductal hyperplasia elsewhere in the same breast. Otherwise both breasts showed mild focal fibrocystic disease. H & E, *length scale* = 0.1 mm

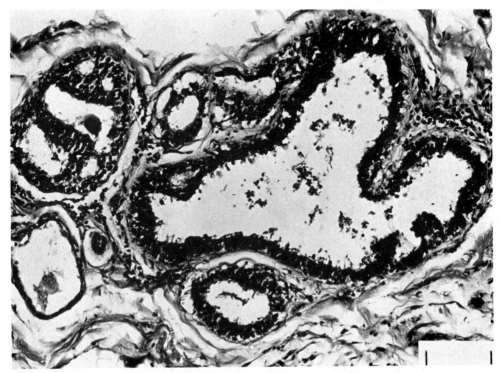

Fig. 8. Case no. 11/76, a 71-year-old woman. Area in the left breast with intraductal carcinoma with clinging and incipient cribriform pattern. Elsewhere in the same breast, area with lobular carcinoma in situ. On both sides atrophic parenchyma. H & E, *length scale* = 0.1 mm

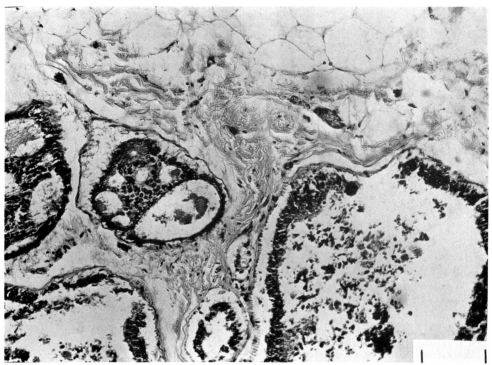

Fig. 9. Case no. 23/77, a 75-year-old woman with clinging and cribriform intraductal carcinoma in the right breast. Atypical ductal hyperplasia in another area of the same breast. Otherwise atrophic breasts with mild focal fibrocystic disease. H & E, *length scale = 0.1 mm*

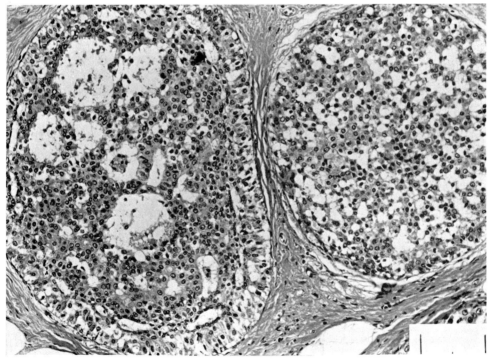

Fig. 10. Case no. 13/77, a 69-year-old woman with cribriform and solid intraductal carcinoma in the right breast. Micropapillary intraductal carcinoma and atypical ductal hyperplasia in the contralateral breast. Both breasts characterized by mild focal fibrocystic disease and some radial scars. H & E, *length scale = 0.1 mm*

The high frequency of in situ carcinoma in our study cannot be compared with previously published postmortem investigations, due to major differences in tissue sampling. Furthermore, differences in the morphological interpretation of these lesions, especially in the early studies may be the basis for some uncertainty (Azzopardi 1979).

The present investigation confirms earlier studies of the relationship between fibrocystic disease and cancer (Wellings et al. 1975). Fibrocystic disease is more frequently found in breast cancer cases than in other cases. These results do not indicate that fibrocystic disease is a precancerous condition, but probably only reflect some pathogenically common influences in the development of fibrocystic disease and breast cancer.

Our investigation confirms that only some of the patients harboring in situ carcinoma develop invasive breast cancer. This observation and the observed very high frequency of in situ carcinoma seem to be the most important results of our investigations.

References

Andersen JA (1977) Lobular carcinoma in situ of the breast: An approach to rational treatment. Cancer 39: 2597–2602

Andersen JA (1982) Pathologie und Prognose des Carcinoma lobulare in situ. In: Frischbier HJ (ed) Die Erkrankungen der weiblichen Brustdrüse: Epidemiologie, Endokrinologie, Histopathologie, Diagnostik, Therapie, Nachsorge, Psychologie. Thieme, Stuttgart, pp 54–58

Andersen JA, Mattheiem WH (1983) Markers and prognostic factors in breast cancer. Eur J Cancer 19: 1699–1705

Andersen JA, Schiødt T (1980) On the concept of carcinoma in situ of the breast. Pathol Res Pract 166: 407–414

Andersen JA, Vendelboe ML (1981) Cytoplasmic mucous globules in lobular carcinoma in situ: Diagnosis and prognosis. Am J Surg Pathol 5: 251–255

Asnaes S, Paaske F (1980) Uncertainty of determining mode of death in medicolegal material without autopsy: A systematic autopsy study. Forensic Sci 15: 3–17

Azzopardi JG (1979) Problems in breast pathology, vol 11. Saunders, London, pp 113–166, 192–257

Dean L, Geschickter CF (1938) Comedocarcinoma of the breast. Arch Surg 36: 225–234

Farrow JH (1970) Current concepts in the detection and treatment of the earliest of the early breast cancers. Cancer 25: 468–477

Fornier DV, Weber E, Hoeffken W, Bauer M, Kubli F, Barth V (1980) Growth rate of 147 mammary carcinomas. Cancer 45: 2198–2207

Frantz VK, Pickren JW, Melcher GW, Auchincloss H Jr (1951) Incidence of chronic cystic disease in so-called normal breasts: A study based on 225 postmortem examinations. Cancer 4: 762–783

Haagensen CD (1971) Diseases of the breast, 2nd edn. Saunders, New York, pp 528–544, 586–590

Haagensen CD, Lane N, Lattes R, Bodian C (1978) Lobular neoplasia (so-called lobular carcinoma in situ) of the breast. Cancer 42: 737–769

Juul A, Andersen J (1977) Rutineautopsier (Routine autopsy). Ugeskr Laeger 139: 323–325

Kiaer W (1954) Relation of fibroadenomatosis ("chronic mastitis") to cancer of the breast. Thesis. Munksgaard, Copenhagen

Kramer WM, Rush BF Jr (1973) Mammary duct proliferation in the elderly: A histopathologic study. Cancer 31: 130–137

Kraus FT, Neubecker RD (1962) The differential diagnosis of papillary tumors of the breast. Cancer 15: 444–455

Nielsen M, Jensen J, Andersen J (1984) Precancerous and cancerous breast lesions during lifetime and at autopsy: A study of 83 females. Cancer (in press)

Page DL, Dupont WD, Rogers LW, Landenberger M (1982) Intraductal carcinoma of the breast: Follow-up after biopsy only. Cancer 49: 751−758

Rosen PP, Kosloff C, Lieberman PH, Adair F, Braun DW Jr (1978) Lobular carcinoma in situ of the breast: Detailed analysis of 99 patients with average follow-up of 24 years. Am J Surg Pathol 2: 225−251

Rosen PP, Braun DW JR, Kinne DE (1980) The clinical significance of pre-invasive breast carcinoma. Cancer 46: 919−925

Sandison AT (1962) An Autopsy study of the adult human breast. Natl Cancer Inst Monog 8: 44−51

Sobin LH (1981) Histological typing of breast tumours, 2nd edn. WHO, Geneva

Spratt JS, Heuser L, Kuhns JG, Reiman HM, Buchanan JB, Polk HC Jr, Sandoz J (1981) Association between the actual doubling times of primary breast cancer with histopathologic characteristics and Wolfe's parenchymal mammographic patterns. Cancer 47: 2265−2268

Wellings SR, Jensen HM, Marcum RG (1975) An atlas of subgross pathology of the human breast with special reference to possible precancerous lesions. JNCI 55: 231−273

Stepwise Mammary Carcinogenesis: Immunological Considerations

Maurice M. Black[1] and Reinhard E. Zachrau[2]

Institute of Breast Diseases, Suite 1039, Macy Pavilion West, Westchester County Medical Center, Valhalla, NY 10595, USA

The literature provides ample evidence that mammary carcinogenesis is a nonrandom event influenced by such risk factors as ethnic group, family history, age, parity and, perhaps, nutritional factors (Lilienfeld 1963; Macklin 1959; Vakil and Morgan 1973). It is, therefore, not surprising that patients who develop a cancer in one breast are at a greatly increased risk of developing a second primary breast cancer (Harrington 1946; McCredie et al. 1975). In response to such observations some have gone so far as to recommend prophylactic removal of the "second" breast (Leis 1979). Certainly it is clinically and conceptually important to take note of the increased risk of second breast cancers. However, it may be of even greater importance to consider the paradox that among patients who have the necessary and sufficient requirements to develop breast cancer, only a small minority will develop a primary cancer in the second breast. This is all the more surprising in view of the similarity in microscopic structure, mammographic patterns, and physical proximity of the two breasts. Moreover, the relatively low incidence of second primaries persists regardless of the age at diagnosis of the first lesion, family history, parity, or any constellation of known risk factors.

The infrequent development of second primary cancers suggests the possibility that a significant proportion of postoperative breast cancer patients have a tumor-retarding mechanism which is not present in women without a prior breast cancer. It is noteworthy in this connection that more than two decades ago Black and Speer (1959) indicated that an immunologically mediated tumor-retarding mechanism was demonstrable in breast cancer patients. This conclusion was based on the preferential occurrence of distinctive types of lymphoreticuloendothelial (LRE) responses in the regional lymph nodes and in the primary tumors of those breast cancer patients who subsequently had prolonged disease-free survivals (Black 1965; Black et al. 1956). The cellular characteristics of the LRE responses in the lymph nodes, sinus histiocytosis (SH), and in the primary cancer, perivenous lymphoid cellular infiltrations (PVI), suggested that a cell-mediated type of immunity (CMI) was involved (Black 1975; Black et al. 1975b).

Previous publications from this laboratory have described distinctive in situ lessions which appeared to be part of a biological continuum eventuating in invasive breast cancer, i.e., precancerous mastopathy (PCM) → in situ carcinoma (ISC) → invasive carcinoma (Black and Chabon 1969). It is noteworthy that microscopically demonstrable LRE responses are

---

1 Professor of Pathology, New York Medical College
2 Associate Professor of Pathology, New York Medical College

Early Breast Cancer
Edited by J. Zander and J. Baltzer
© Springer-Verlag Berlin Heidelberg 1985

Table 1. Proportion of LRE-positive responses to precancerous mastopathy (PCM), in situ carcinoma (ISC), and invasive carcinoma of the breast

Lesions	Total	LRE-positive[a]
PCM, stage 0	83	24 (29)[b]
ISC, stage 0	62	49 (79)[c]
ISC with invasive Ca	217	141 (65)[c]
Invasive with (LRE+) ISC	141	93 (66)[d]
Invasive with (LRE−) ISC	76	10 (13)[b,d]

[a] Presence of diffuse lymphoid cellular infiltration and perivenous lymphoid cellular infiltrates; such responses are rarely ($< 3\%$) associated with normotypic lesions

[b] $p < 0.05$

[c] $p = 0.053$

[d] $p < 0.0005$

associated with approximately one-third of PCM cases, 70%–80% of ISC cases, and 40%–50% of unselected invasive breast cancer cases. Thus, LRE reactivity to breast lesions is not simply an epiphenomenon associated with advanced lesions. On the contrary, such LRE responses are most commonly localized in the region of ducts or lobules having preinvasive malignant changes. At the same time, adjacent areas of normotypic hyperplasia are devoid of LRE cell accumulations. These observations are consistent with the thesis that antigenic changes occur in association with the preinvasive phase of breast cancer. They further indicate that the host is responsive to such changes in antigenicity. If such LRE responses were not typically associated with malignant transformation, it would be unreasonable to postulate an association between mammary carcinogenesis and tumor antigenicity.

Further information on the biological significance of LRE responses to breast cancer is provided by examining breasts having both ISC and invasive cancer (Table 1). In breasts without LRE responses to ISC lesions, reactivity to invasive lesions is uncommon (13%). In contrast, in breasts with LRE reactivity to ISC foci, similar reactivity to the invasive foci is found in the majority of cases. Approximately 30% of breasts with LRE responses to ISC foci lack simultaneous reactivity to invasive areas. This suggests that the phenomenon of loss of antigen expression may occur. This interpretation is supported by direct measurements of CMI to foci of ISC and invasive cancer from the same breast (Black 1976).

The foregoing microscopic studies suggest that antigenic changes become manifest in the preinvasive phase of breast cancer. These changes stimulate a host response whose cellular features are consistent with CMI. In short, such changes are recognized as non-self and are clearly immunogenic.

The finding that a prognostically favorable type of immunity is commonly associated with the preinvasive phase of mammary carcinogenesis is inconsistent with the thesis that the development of breast cancer is dependent on a defect in immunosurveillance of a general or specific type. It seems reasonable to demand that our postulates be consistent with the realities which are readily observable in routine surgical pathology. In this regard it is also pertinent to note that the LRE responses to preinvasive breast cancer and the prognostically significant PVI responses to invasive breast cancer do not involve macrophage accumulations or direct evidence of cancer killing by cell-to-cell contact. In

Table 2. Characteristics of breast cancers arising after surgical removal of prior breast lesions, by type of prior breast pathology

Prior breast lesions	Subsequent breast cancer	
	Stage 0 ISC[a]	Invasive Pt surviving ≥ 5 years
None	16/291 (5)[b]	102/169 (60)[c]
Normotypic	8/ 62 (13)[d]	28/ 54 (52)[e]
PCM and stage 0 ISC	16/ 59 (27)[b, d]	29/ 33 (88)[c, e, f]
Invasive cancer	2/ 24 (8)	5/ 16 (31)[f]

[a] ISC, in situ carcinoma; [b] $p < 0.0005$; [c] $p < 0.005$; [d] $p = 0.087$; [e] $p < 0.005$; [f] p 0.0005

short, there is little in the actual appearance of prognostically significant in vivo LRE responses to in situ or invasive human breast cancer to support the thesis that nonspecific killer cells and phagocytic macrophages play a role in the biological behavior of human breast cancer.

If the ISC-associated immunogen(s) of different breast cancers are antigenically similar to one another, then patients having CMI to this antigen should behave as an immunized population with regard to the development and behavior of subsequent primary breast cancers. As judged by the aforementioned microscopic studies, such immunity is preferentially expressed in stage 0 patients as a group. Thus, asynchronous second breast cancers arising in stage 0 patients should be characterized by an increased tendency to be in situ and, when invasive, should exhibit unusually favorable survival characteristics. A test of this hypothesis is provided by comparing the characteristics of breast cancers developing after prior removal of different types of breast lesions. As reported by Black et al. (1972), breast cancers arising after removal of PCM or ISC lesions do have more favorable stage and survival characteristics than those arising after removal of normotypic breast lesions or invasive cancers or in patients without a prior breast lesion (Table 2). Analogous findings were also reported by Webber et al. (1981). Such findings are consistent with the thesis that there is antigenic similarity between the ISC-associated immunogens of different breast cancers which develop metachronously in the same patient.

Specific CMI to autologous breast cancer has also been assessed by means of direct in vivo and in vitro techniques, namely a skin window (SW) procedure and a leukocyte migration test (LMT), respectively (Black and Leis 1970, 1971, 1973; Black et al. 1974a). Both of these procedures indicate that reactivity to autologous breast cancer ist found in stage 0 > stage I > stage II patients and in LRE-positive > in LRE-negative cases (Black 1972; Black and Kwon 1978). More particulary, these techniques and blastogenesis procedures indicate that CMI to autologous invasive breast cancer is prognostically favorable (Akiyoski et al. 1978; Black and Zachrau 1979; Cannon et al. 1981). The prognostic significance of CMI to autologous breast cancer, as measured by the SW procedure, is documented in Table 3. It is evident that SW reactivity to autologous breast cancer, 4−14 months postoperatively, is significantly more frequent in patients with stage 0 breast cancer and in those invasive cancer patients who do not develop early recurrences, than in the patients who die of disseminated disease less than 4 years postoperatively.

Information regarding the relationships between biological behavior and SW reactivity at different postoperative intervals are also presented in Table 4. In SW tests performed 1−3, 4−12, and 13−24 months postoperatively, reactivity to autologous breast cancer was

Table 3. Skin-window reactivity of breast cancer patients to autologous cancer tissue; maximal response per patient during the 4- to 14-months postoperative interval

Skin window response	ISC stage 0	Invasive BCa	
		NED[a] 4−12 years	DOD[b] at < 4 years
Positive	10 (40)[c]	22 (33)[d]	1 (3)[d]
Intermediate	9 (36)	12 (18)	7 (24)
Negative	6 (24)	33 (49)	21 (72)
Total	25 (100)	67 (100)	29 (100)

[a] No clinical evidence of recurrent disease; [b] Dead of disseminated disease; [c] Numbers in parentheses are percentages; [d] $p < 0.005$

Table 4. Biological behavior and skin-window (SW) reactivity to autologous breast cancer at different postoperative intervals

SW (months postoperative)	ISC stage 0	Invasive BCa[a]	
		NED > 6 years	Metastases < 30 mo, p. SW[b]
1−3			
Positive	9 (35)	16 (31)	0
Intermediate	4	6	0
Negative	13 (50)	30 (58)	16 (100)
Total	26 (100)	52 (100)	16 (100)
4−12			
Positive	11 (42)	15 (37)	1 (4)
Intermediate	8	8	0
Negative	7 (27)	23 (56)	24 (96)
Total	26 (100)	41 (100)	25 (100)
13−24			
Positive	8 (47)	15 (34)	0
Intermediate	4	7	0
Negative	5 (29)	22 (50)	10 (100)
Total	17 (100)	44 (100)	10 (100)

[a] Nuclear grades I and II; [b] < 30 months after last SW test

commonly observed in stage 0 patients and in those nuclear grade I and II invasive breast cancer patients who subsequently remained disease-free for more than 6 years postoperatively. In contrast, among patients who developed metastatic disease less than 30 months after the reference SW, the SW in question was negative in almost all instances. In essence, Tables 3 and 4 demonstrate that among invasive breast cancer patients CMI to autologous breast cancer impedes progression of the disease. In addition, such reactivity is most regularly demonstrable among stage 0 patients at various postoperative intervals.

Table 5. Skin-window reactivity to gp 55 and autologous preinvasive and invasive breast lesions in clinically disease-free patients, 3–30 months postoperatively

CMI vs gp55	CMI vs autologous breast lesion			
	Positive	Negative	ND[a]	Total
Positive				
PCM	ND	ND	6	6
ISC	7	0	1	8
Invasive	15	4	12	31
Negative				
PCM	ND	ND	2	2
ISC	0	1	2	3
Invasive	0	13	5	18

[a] Not done

The particularly high frequency of postoperatively measured CMI to autologous stage 0 breast cancer is consistent with the microscopic studies cited above. Of particular interest is the ability of direct measurements to evaluate antigenic similarity between breast cancer tissue from different patients. Thus, in vitro measurements indicate that reactivity to autologous breast cancer is commonly associated with simultaneous reactivity to LRE-positive as compared with LRE-negative homologous invasive breast cancer tissue. It appears that a similar CMI determinant is expressed in LRE-positive breast cancers in general and in stage 0 ISC in particular (Black 1976, Black and Kwon 1980).

Further data bearing on the possibility of a common CMI determinant in immunogenic breast cancers is provided by studies of CMI to the gp55 component of the RIII-strain murine mammary tumor virus (MuMTV). In 1974, we reported that approximately one-third of breast cancer patients demonstrated in vitro CMI to RIII-MuMTV (Black et al. 1974b). Such reactivity was later shown to be selectively directed against its glycoprotein component, gp55 (Black et al. 1975a, 1978). Of particular interest is the finding that those postoperative breast cancer patients who lacked in vitro CMI to gp55, were rarely simultaneously responsive to autologous breast cancer tissue. On the other hand, breast cancer patients showing in vitro CMI to gp55 were simultaneously responsive to stage 0 autologous and homologous breast cancer > LRE-positive autologous invasive breast cancer > LRE-positive homologous invasive breast cancer ≫ LRE-negative homologous breast cancer (Black and Kwon 1980; Black and Zachrau 1979). Thus, it seems that the determinant responsible for prognostically favorable CMI in breast cancer tissues is similar to a CMI determinant of gp55. Accordingly, the CMI determinants of different stage 0 breast cancer tissues and of immunogenic breast cancers should be similar to one another. More recently we have examined CMI to gp55 by means of the SW procedure. As shown in Table 5, in vivo CMI to gp55 was found in 6/8 PCM, 8/11 ISC, and 31/49 recurrence-free invasive breast cancer patients. It seems that the developmental phase of breast cancer is associated with an immunogen which provokes CMI against gp55. It further appears that the lack of SW reactivity to gp55 ist usually associated with a lack of reactivity to autologous breast cancer. These observations, coupled with the aforementioned in vitro measurements and LRE responses, *all* support the view that the developmental phase of breast cancer is associated with the expression of a similar type of immunogen which

Table 6. Stage distribution of asynchronous second primary breast cancers, by stage at diagnosis of the first breast cancer (SEER data)

First breast cancer	Second primary breast cancer				
	Stage 0	Stage I	Stage II	Stage > II	Total
Stage 0	24 (46)[a, b]	24 (46)	3 (6)	1 (2)	52 (100)
Stage I	83 (14)[b]	380 (64)[c]	100 (17)	29 (5)	592 (100)
Stage II	54 (12)	209 (47)[c]	130 (29)	54 (12)	447 (100)
Total	161 (15)	613 (56)	233 (21)	84 (8)	1091 (100)

[a] Numbers in parentheses are percentages; [b] $p < 0.0005$; [c] $p < 0.0005$

provokes a prognostically favorable type of specific CMI that is directed against a determinant similar to that of gp55. Since such immunity is preferentially associated with preinvasive breast cancer, it follows that the development and progression of primary cancer should be impeded in women having CMI to ISC-associated immunogen(s) and/or gp55. As indicated above, this expectation was confirmed for second breast cancers by a comparison of the stage characteristics of asynchronous second primary breast cancers in relation to the stage characteristics of first breast cancers (Black et al. 1972). Similar observations were obtained more recently in a study of patients in the SEER program. It was again found that the stage distribution of second primary breast cancers is significantly better following stage 0 lesions than after invasive cancers (Table 6). Among stage 0 breast cancer patients who developed a second breast cancer, almost half the second, contra-lateral cancers were also in situ, and only 4% of the second cancers were ≥ stage II. The corresponding proportion of stage 0 lesions among second cancers developing in invasive breast cancer patients was 14% for stage I and 12% for stage II cases. However, second cancers among stage I cases were less commonly of an advanced stage, viz. 22% as compared with 41% in the stage II series.

The above data, coupled with those in Table 2, clearly demonstrate that the development and progression of second breast cancers is preferentially impeded in that group of patients which is characterized by a high level of CMI to the ISC-associated immunogen and/or gp55. Of eight second breast cancers developing among patients who were SW negative 4−12 months postoperatively, five developed second cancers less than 4 years postoperatively, while the remaining three cancers developed 53, 56, and 84 months postoperatively. All these second breast cancers were invasive. Of four second breast cancers which developed in SW-positive invasive breast cancer patients, one developed 24 months postoperatively and the others 59, 84, and 110 months postoperatively. It is noteworthy that the second cancer that developed 24 months postoperatively, was a stage 0 lesion.

Clinical observations, microscopic findings, and direct measurements of specific CMI, individually and collectively, support a working hypothesis that, *at any postoperative interval, CMI to the ISC-associated immunogen and/or gp55 should be associated with a reduced risk of developing a second primary invasive breast cancer.* If this prediction is indeed true, it should follow that a similar tumor-retarding potential would be engendered in control women with induced CMI against the ISC-associated immunogen and/or gp55 (Black 1973, 1977; Black and Zachrau 1978). In short, immunoprophylaxis of human breast cancer should be possible.

If spontaneous CMI against gp55, at any postoperative interval, impedes the development and progression of immunogenic autologous breast cancer, agents that are capable of inducing a negative-to-positive change in CMI to gp55 might be expected to have a similar prophylactic and prognostic significance. We have recently observed that high doses of vitamin A and high doses of vitamin E can induce negative-to-positive changes in SW reactivity to autologous breast cancer and/or gp55 in a majority of postoperative breast cancer patients (Black et al. 1983a, b). It remains to be determined, however, whether such induced reactivity has the same biological significance as spontaneous reactivity.

Considered in toto, data derived from diverse disciplines indicate that

1) mammary carcinogenesis is a stepwise phenomenon, involving recognizable preinvasive and invasive phases;
2) the in situ-to-invasive cancer progression is not obligatory;
3) the preinvasive phase is characteristically associated with the expression of some gp55-like CMI determinant(s), provoking measurable anti-gp55 CMI in the host;
4) such specific immunity impedes the development of de novo breast cancers and the progression of immunogenic invasive breast cancers;
5) it seems likely that induced anti-gp55 CMI will be prophylactically and therapeutically significant.

Attention has been drawn to observations supporting the existence and biological significance of CMI to autologous cancer in breast cancer patients. It is appropriate to note, however, that Hewitt has vigorously questioned the existence and significance of immunological responses to experimental tumors and, by inference, to human tumors (Hewitt 1982). Other investigators are equally vigorous in support of the use of animal models to clarify the nature and significance of tumor immunology (Herberman 1983). We submit that such polemics are not likely to add to our understanding of the nature and significance of CMI responses to the development of *human* breast cancer. We suggest that direct attention to correlations between biological behavior, structural variations, and analytical values in individual breast cancer patients are far more likely to add to our understanding and control of human breast cancers (Black and Kwon 1980). We are unaware of any index of CMI that fails to indicate that immunogenicity is associated with the developmental phase of human breast cancer. Nor do we know of any evidence that denies the prognostic significance of CMI to autologous human breast cancer. Finally, we reject the view that the occurrence of cancer is evidence that immunological responses are nonexistent or inconsequential in cancer patients. Such a non sequitur might equally be proposed for infectious diseases such as typhoid fever or smallpox.

Those who doubt the existence of immunological phenomena in human breast cancer would do well to examine the developmental phases of the disease and ponder the associated prognostically significant indices of CMI.

Acknowledgements. The work described in this paper was supported in part by USPHS grant no. 5R01 CA-25165, awarded by the National Cancer Institute, DHHS.

References

Akiyoski T, Nakamura Y, Kawaguchi M, Tsuji H (1978) Cellular hypersensitivity to autologous tumor extracts in patients with breast carcinoma. Jpn J Surg 8: 236–241

Black MM (1965) Reactivity of the lymphoreticuloendothelial system in human cancer. Prog Clin Cancer 1: 26–49

Black MM (1972) Cellular and biologic manifestations of immunogenicity in precancerous mastopathy. Natl Cancer Inst Monogr 35: 73–82

Black MM (1973) Human breast cancer. A model for cancer immunology. Isr J Med Sci 9: 284–299

Black MM (1975) Immunology of breast cancer: Clinical implications. Prog Clin Cancer 6: 115–138

Black MM (1976) Structural, antigenic and biologic characteristics of precancerous mastopathy. Cancer Res 36: 2596–2604

Black MM (1977) Immunopathology of breast cancer. Pathobiol Ann 7: 213–230

Black MM, Chabon AB (1969) In situ carcinoma of the breast. Pathol Annu 4: 185–210

Black MM, Kwon CS (1978) Prognostic factors. In: Gallager HS, Leis HP, Jr, Snyderman RK, Urban JA (eds) The breast. Mosby St. Louis, pp 297–319

Black MM, Kwon CS (1980) Precancerous mastopathie: Structural and biological considerations. Pathol Res Pract 116: 491–514

Black MM, Leis HP Jr (1970) Human breast carcinoma. III. Cellular responses to autologous breast cancer: Skin window procedure. NY State J Med 70: 2583–2589

Black MM, Leis HP Jr (1971) Cellular responses to autologous breast cancer tissue: Correlation with stage and lymphoreticuloendothelial reactivity. Cancer 28: 263–273

Black MM, Leis HP Jr (1973) Cellular responses to autologous breast cancer tissue: Sequential observations. Cancer 32: 384–389

Black MM, Speer FD (1959) Immunology of cancer. Surg Gynecol Obstet 109: 105–116

Black MM, Zachrau RE (1978) Immunotherapy of breast cancer? In: Gallager HS, Leis HP Jr, Snyderman RK, Urban JA (eds). The breast. Mosby St. Louis, pp 393–408

Black MM, Zachrau RE (1979) Antitumor immunity in breast cancer patients: Biologic and therapeutic implications. J Reprod Med 23: 21–32

Black MM, Speer FD, Opler SR (1956) Structural representations of the tumor-host relationships in mammary carcinoma, biologic and prognostic significance. Am J Clin Pathol 26: 250–265

Black MM, Cutler SJ, Barclay THC (1972) Post biopsy breast carcinoma: A natural experiment in cancer immunology. Cancer 29: 61–65

Black MM, Leis HP Jr, Shore B, Zachrau RE (1974a) Cellular hypersensitivity to breast cancer. Assessment by a leukocyte migration procedure. Cancer 33: 952–958

Black MM, Moore DH, Shore B, Zachrau RE, Leis HP Jr (1974b) Effect of murine milk samples and human breast tissues on human leukocyte migration indices. Cancer Res 34: 1054–1060

Black MM, Zachrau RE, Shore B, Moore DH, Leis HP Jr (1975a) Prognostically favorable immunogens of human breast cancer tissue: Antigenic similarity to murine mammary tumor virus. Cancer 35: 121–128

Black MM, Barclay THC, Hankey BF (1975b) Prognosis in breast cancer utilizing histologic characteristics, of the primary tumor. Cancer 36: 2048–2055

Black MM, Zachrau RE, Shore B, Dion AS, Leis HP Jr (1978) Cellular immunity to autologous breast cancer and RIII-murine mammary tumor virus preparations. Cancer Res 38: 2068–2076

Black MM, Zachrau RE, Dion AS, Katz M (1983a) Vitamin A stimulation of specific cell-mediated immunity in breast cancer patients. Fed Proc 42: 1197

Black MM, Zachrau RE, Dion AS, Katz M (1983b) Stimulation of prognostically favorable cell-mediates immunity of breast cancer patients by high dose vitamin A and vitamin E. In: Prasad KN (ed) Vitamins, Nutrition and Cancer. Karger Basel, 134–146

Cannon GB, Dean JH, Herberman RB, Keets M. Alford C (1981) Lymphoproliferative responses to autologous tumor extracts as prognostic indicators in patients with resected breast cancer. Int J Cancer 27: 131–138

Harrington SW (1946) Survival rates of radical mastectomy for unilateral and bilateral carcinoma of the breast. Surgery 19: 154−166

Herberman RB (1983) Counterpoint: Animal tumor models and their relevance to human tumor immunology. J Biol Resp Modif 2: 39−46, 217−226

Hewitt HB (1982) Animal tumor models and their relevance to human tumor immunology. J Biol Resp Modif 1: 107−119

Leis HP Jr (1979) Selective and reconstructive surgical procedures for carcinoma of the breast. Surg Gynecol Obstet 148: 27−32

Lilienfeld AM (1963) The epidemiology of breast cancer. Cancer Res 23: 1503−1513

Macklin MT (1959) Comparison of the number of breast-cancer deaths observed in relatives of breast-cancer patients, and the number expected on the basis of mortality rates. JNCI 22: 927−951

McCredie JA, Inch WR, Anderson M (1975) Consecutive primary carcinomas of the breast. Cancer 35: 1472−1477

Vakil DV, Morgan RW (1973) Etiology of breast cancer. II. Epidemiologic aspects. Can Med Assoc J 109: 201−206

Webber BL, Heise H, Neifeld JP, Costa J (1981) Risk of subsequent contralateral breast carcinoma in a population of patients with in situ breast carcinoma. Cancer 47: 2928−2932

Growth Rate of Primary Mammary Carcinoma and its Metastases

Consequences for Early Detection and Therapy

D. v. Fournier[1], W. Hoeffken[2], H. Junkermann[1], M. Bauer[1], and W. Kühn[1]

[1] Universitäts-Frauenklinik, Voßstrasse 9, 6900 Heidelberg, Federal Republik of Germany
[2] Strahleninstitut für Diagnostik und Therapie,
   Machabäerstrasse 19, 5000 Köln 1, Federal Republic of Germany

Estimations of the growth rate of breast cancer based on natural life expectancy of untreated patients were made by Bloom (1965). He calculated the mean duration of life in 1,091 untreated patients and found it to be 38.7 months, ranging from 3 months to over 30 years.

Richards (1948), using patients' reports on the duration of symptoms, estimated that a palpable tumor needs 3 months on average to increase in size by 1 cm.

In 1974 Haagensen commented that little was known about the growth rates of mammary carcinoma. From the scant data in the literature he estimated an average span of 5 years for the development of a palpable tumor from the first cancer cell.

Collins et al. (1956) suggested that the rate of doubling of a tumor mass reflects the rate of cell division and that volume-doubling time is constant, resulting in exponential growth.

They supported their hypothesis with measurements of pulmonary metastases of various tumors.

On the basis of this theoretical model, Gershon-Cohen et al. (1963) were the first to determine volume-doubling times of human mammary carcinoma from the increase in the tumor shadow in serial mammograms. Their volume-doubling times ranged from 23 to 209 days (18 cases).

Using the same method, Spratt et al. (1977) observed a mean doubling time of 325 days in 26 cases.

We (Fournier et al. 1976, 1980) observed a mean doubling time of 202 days in 100 cases of mammary carcinomas, relying on measurements in serial mammograms.

The gross doubling time of a tumor depends on:
1) The duration of the mitotic cycle.
2) The fraction of proliferating cells compared to dormant cells.
3) The rate of cell loss (hypoxia, necrosis, immunological defense).

Up to 50% of the cells in the tumor may die every day (Tubiana 1971). The effective tumor growth is the net result of cell proliferation and cell loss in a given tumor. In spite of the various influences effecting tumor growth in clinically measurable tumors exponential growth seems to be substantiated (Schwartz 1961).

In far advanced experimental tumors the growth rate slows down as the tumors reach a certain size (Laird 1965). In these cases tumor growth is best described by the Gompertz function: $V = k_0 \cdot \exp[k_1/k_2 \cdot (1 - \exp(-k_2 t))]$, where k_0 = initial value, k_1 = acceleration factor, and k_2 = deceleration factor (Fig. 1). In the early phase the Gompertz function is

Early Breast Cancer
Edited by J. Zander and J. Baltzer
© Springer-Verlag Berlin Heidelberg 1985

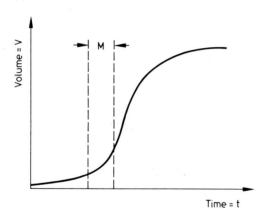

Fig. 1. The Gompertz function, a model describing growth. *M,* interval between mammographies

identical with an exponential function. There are indications that metastases of breast cancer correspond to the primary tumor in their speed of growth, but have a faster growth rate on average (Kusama et al. 1972; Spratt 1977).

Very little literature exists on the relation between growth rate of the primary tumor and histological parameters (Spratt et al. 1981), but there are several reports suggesting that histological findings correlate with survival rates (Bloom and Richardson 1967; Black 1975; Fisher 1977).

Estimation of Growth Rate from Tumor-Volume Doubling Time

We examined the doubling time of 200 primary carcinomas in the mammogram. Serial mammograms had been done in this population before definite treatment of the carcinoma, due to delay of the final diagnosis (neoplastic tumor could be identified only retrospectively), refusal of treatment, and other reasons.

Between 2 and 11 mammographies were performed in each case at different times. The time span of observation by mammogram lay between 0.2 and 16 years. In 128 further patients monitored with serial mammograms the tumor shadow was not measurable in previous screenings. These cases could not be used for measurements. Altogether 328 cases with previous mammographies had been collected from 28 clinics in Germany.

Measurement of the tumor diameter and the limitations of the method are discussed by Spratt (1977) and Fournier (1980). The method, in outline, is as follows. First, the tumor diameter is normalized by measuring the tumor nucleus shadow in 3 places. The volume doubling time is then calculated:

$$T_v = \frac{t}{9.97 \times I_g \dfrac{d_2}{d_1}}$$

where T_v = tumor volume doubling time, t = time in days between two observations, d_1 = normalized diameter of tumor at the beginning of observation, d_2 = normalized diameter of tumor at the end of observation. An example of the margin of error: tumor size 20–30 mm inaccuracy of measurement ± 0.75 mm error in doubling time 11.3%.

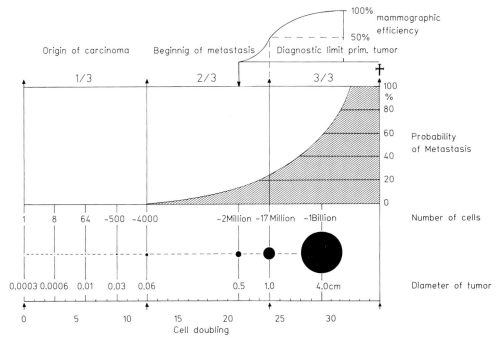

Fig. 2. Model of tumor growth behavior based on constant volume doubling times (Krokowski 1964; Oeser 1974)

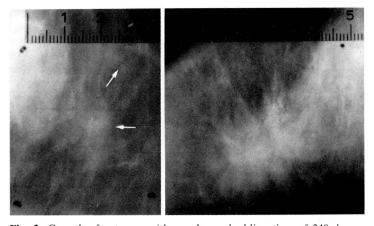

Fig. 3. Growth of a tumor with a volume doubling time of 240 days

Assuming that malignant growth begins with a single cell or a small cell cluster, and on the premise of a constant doubling time, the number of volume doublings necessary to reach a given tumor size can be calculated.

Using this method, growth rates and life-spans of tumors can be projected. Based on an exponential growth model beginning with a primary tumor cell 10 μm in diameter, 21 doubling times are needed to achieve a size of 0.06 cm (Fig. 2). At this point the tumor already has the potential ability to separate metastatic cells (Alvord 1975). It takes the tumor more than half its whole tumor life to reach 0.5 cm. To reach the clinically detectable

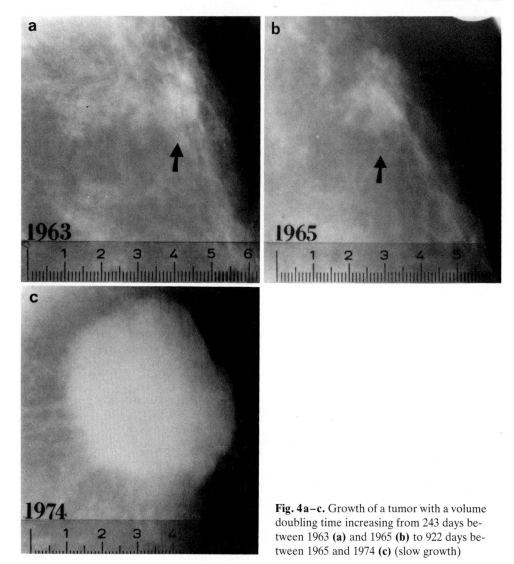

Fig. 4a–c. Growth of a tumor with a volume doubling time increasing from 243 days between 1963 **(a)** and 1965 **(b)** to 922 days between 1965 and 1974 **(c)** (slow growth)

size of 1 cm the tumor needs 30 doubling times. With this tumor size, detectable metastases are already found in 28% of patients with mammary carcinoma (Haagensen 1974).

Based on the exponential growth model we measured the tumor growth in the mammogram in a case of a moderately fast-growing tumor, as shown in Fig. 3 (doubling time = T_v = 240 days). Figure 4 shows the very slow-growing tumor of a patient who refused therapy from 1963 to 1974. Between 1963 and 1965 a doubling time of 243 days was calculated.

As one tumor grew larger between 1965 and 1974 the doubling time lengthened to 922 days (see Fig. 1), which would be in accordance with the Gompertz function.

Of the observed volume-doubling times (T_v), 95% were between 65 and 657 days. The shortest observed doubling time was 26 days, the longest approached a standstill of growth.

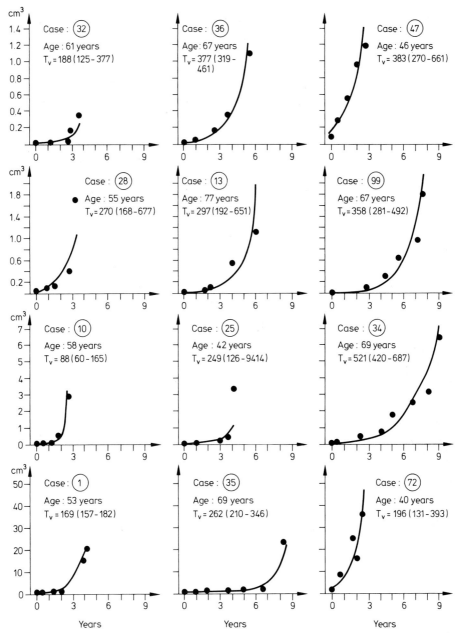

Fig. 5. Tumor growth as a function of time in 12 cases followed by mammography. *Points*, observed growth; *solid lines*, estimated exponential growth curves

Evaluation of 12 Cases with Five or More Mammographies per Case

Figure 5 shows the results of 12 cases with five or more single measurements from serial mammograms. The good fit of the observed growth to the estimated exponential growth curves indicates the applicability of the exponential growth model for the observed periods of tumor life in most cases.

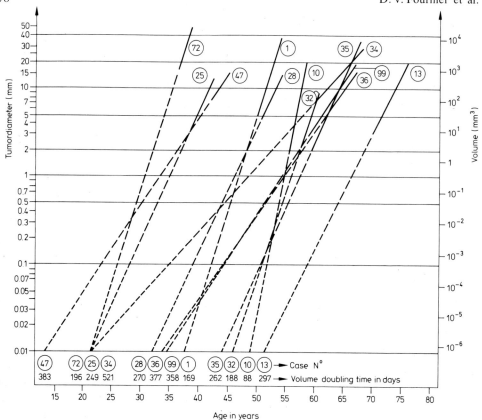

Fig. 6. Tumor function of same 12 cases as in Fig. 5 (5 and more measurements with consideration of age at the times of measurement). *Ordinates,* log tumor diameter (= volume); *abscissa,* time in years; ——— exponential growth curves; - - - -, calculated development of first tumor cell

Figure 6 shows the data from these 12 cases after logarithmic transformation so that the exponential growth curves result in straight lines. Assuming constant doubling times from the beginning of neoplastic growth it is possible to extrapolate to the time of the development of the first tumor cell. We estimated that it took on average more than 20 years for the tumor to reach a size of 20 mm from the initial cancer cell (average doubling time = 308 days in these 12 cases).

Different Tumour Diameters and Age of Patients

Based on the volume-doubling time it was estimated at what age women would have a tumor 0.01 mm in size (representing the first tumor cell), 0.1 mm, and so on up to 20 mm in size. It must be borne in mind that this hypothesis may not reflect the true situation in early cancer growth.

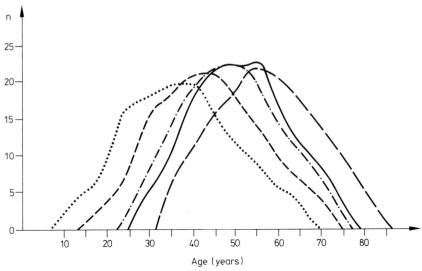

Fig. 7. Frequency distribution of estimated ages at extrapolation to tumor diameters of 0.01 mm
(· · · ·), 0.1 mm (- - - -), 1 mm (- · · · -), 2 mm (———), and 20 mm (– – –)

Figure 7 shows the frequency distribution of the age estimation with given tumor sizes.
Women with a 20-mm tumor had an average age of 58 years (maximum of the curve on the
right). The mean age of women with a 0.1-mm tumor was 44 years. The mean age for the
first tumor cell of 0.01 mm was 35 years (curve on the left). Extrapolation indicates that the
growth time for a palpable 20-mm tumor is close to 20 years on average and that in most of
our cases the growth of breast cancer will have started at the age of 30–40 years. This may
have important implications for the time interval between mammographies, the age at
which mammography should be started, and also the evaluation of therapeutic
results.

Fast, Moderate, and Slow Growth

Figure 8 shows the different groups of breast cancers according to their growth behavior.
Year by year we observe 3% extremely fast-growing tumors, of the inflammatory type for
instance. In these cases there is no measurable tumor shadow, and growth rates can be
estimated only on the basis of personal reports from the patients. From the visible tumor
enlargement as reported by the patient we estimated that it needed less than 3 years from
the first cancer cell to the clinical size in these cases (left curve in Fig. 8).
Very fast-growing tumors ($T_v \leq 100$ days) were observed in 15% of the measurable cases,
fast-growing tumors ($T_v = 101-149$ days) in 13%, moderately fast-growing tumors ($T_v = 150-299$ days) in 39%, and slow-growing cancers ($T_v \geq 300$ days) in 33%.
On the right-hand side in Fig. 8 an unknown number of breast cancers is indicated, which
have such a slow growth behavior that they never reach a clinically detectable size during
the patient's natural life-span.
These very slow-growing tumors can only be found by meticulous serial section methods, as
demonstrated by Andersen et al. (this volume), who report an incidence of about 25% for
invasive and noninvasive carcinomas of the breast in all women who died within 1 year in a

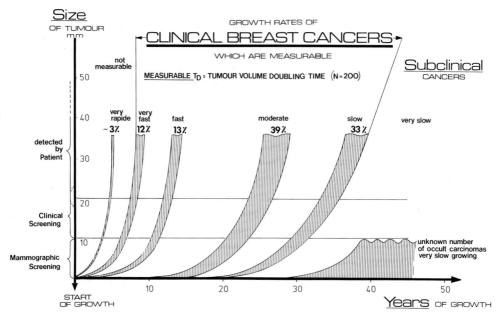

Fig. 8. Proportion of tumors with different growth rates and their clinical relevance (Fournier et al. 1980)

certain county of Denmark. According to Fisher (this volume) and Spratt et al. (1977) most of these tumors are cancers that will never reach clinical relevance.

In accordance with this, Müller (1982), in two comparable collectives of specimens from subcutaneous mastectomies, showed that the proportion of carcinomas detected (carcinoma in situ or invasive carcinoma) was 13.1% with a conventional method and 27.1% with a serial section method (Table 1).

Growth Rate of Primary Tumors and Histomorphological Character of the Tumor

We found (Kühn et al. 1983) a correlation between the calculated tumor growth rate and the histological tumor grading (Bloom and Richardson 1957; Table 2).

Growth Rate of Primary Tumors and Hormone Receptor Status

In a group of our cases with slow growth on average, we found that tumors positive for estrogen receptors showed significantly slower growth rates than those that were estrogen-receptor-negative (Table 3).

Growth Rate of Primary Tumors and Growth Rates of Metastases

In seven cases the doubling time of the primary tumor and the doubling time of one to three lung metastases could be observed. If the measurement of the primary tumor and

Table 1. Diagnosis of premalignant and malignant lesions in subcutaneous mastectomy

	Conventional work up (percentage) $n = 130$	Work up in serial 2.5-mm thick sections (percentage) $n = 70$
Mastopathy with atypias	7.7	24.3
Lobular or ductal in situ carcinoma	10.8	17.1
Invasive carcinoma	2.3	10.0

Table 2. Histological grading[a] and growth rates of 61 mammary carcinomas

Type of tumor	n	Very fast	Fast	Medium	Slow	Mean tumor doubling time (days)
Grade-1-Ca	8	0	2	4	2	470
Grade-2-Ca	32	3	2	19	8	270
Grade-3-Ca	13	2	5	5	1	193
Lobular Ca	3	0	0	3	0	200
Mucinous Ca	1	1	0	0	0	90
Papillary Ca	3	0	0	2	1	372
Ductal Ca in situ	1	0	0	1	0	261

[a] Grading according to Bloom and Richardson (1957)

Table 3. Growth rates and estrogen-receptor status in 59 cases with slow average growth rates

Estrogen receptor	n (= 59)	Average doubling time
Positive	39	580 days
Negative	20	403 days

metastases are extrapolated to their origin (Fig. 9) the results indicate that most lung metastases start their growth many years before diagnosis of the primary tumor.

In 16 cases we found a correlation between the growth rate of the metastases and that of the primary tumor (Fig. 10). Fast-growing tumors seem to produce fast-growing metastases and slow-growing tumors, slow-growing metastases.

After mean observation times of 2½ years after operation we found that fast-growing tumors had a higher rate of distant metastases (22%) than moderately fast-growing (14%) or slow-growing tumors (6%) (Fig. 11).

These data should not be interpreted as an indication of a higher metastatic potential of fast-growing tumors, because the already established metastases of the slow-growing tumors need a longer time to reach a clinically detectable size. To answer the question as to whether there is a correlation between growth rate and metastatic potential it is necessary to have a much longer observation time. Assuming that the tumor is able to spread out metastatic cells after as few as 21 doubling times, as mentioned above (Fig. 2), the so-called

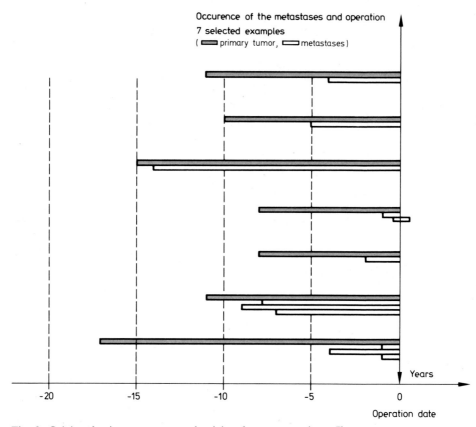

Fig. 9. Origin of primary tumors and origin of metastases ($n = 7$)

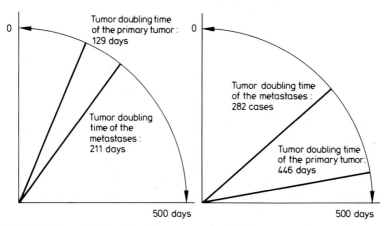

Fig. 10. Growth rates of primary tumors and of metastases ($n = 16$)

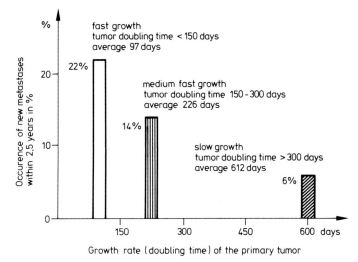

Fig. 11. Growth rates of primary tumors and probability of distant metastases. Mean observation period: $2^1/_2$ years after operation

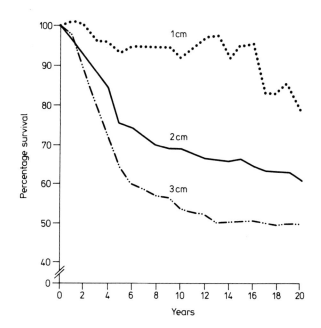

Fig. 12. Age-corrected survival rates for women treated for breast cancer up to 3.0 cm in diameter. (Duncan and Kerr 1976)

early detection in breast cancer with the help of sophisticated methods (mammography) may be biologically late (MacDonald 1951).

In an individual case we are merely able to reveal the terrifying diagnosis to our patients a few years earlier, while the remaining life-span may already be predetermined by the progressing occult metastases. This is exemplified by the studies of Duncan and Kerr (1976), who showed that women with small tumors up to 2 cm in size die of metastatic disease even after 20 years of follow-up (Fig. 12). In contrast to women with tumors 3 cm or more in size, women with small tumors cannot be called cured even if they have survived

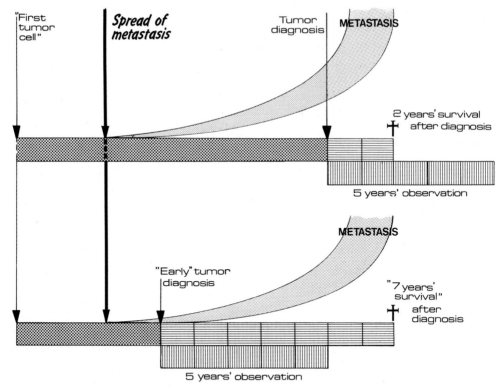

Fig. 13. Effect of so-called early diagnosis in some cases

for 20 years. It is obvious that in the majority of cases, metastases start to spread when the tumor reaches 0.5 mm in size (see Fig. 9). For instance, if a clinically palpable tumor had been diagnosed 5 years earlier by mammography, there would have been no benefit if metastasis had already occurred. Though survival time from detection would have been 5 years greater (Fig. 13), actual life-span would not have been increased.

Discussion

The evaluation of tumor growth behavior by the concept of constant doubling times, i.e., exponential growth up to the clinical phase of the tumor, allows us to give a sound explanation for some strange phenomena in the behavior of breast carcinoma (Fig. 14).

Theoretical considerations show that it takes the tumor about three-quarters of its life-span to achieve a size at which it can be detected clinically; this means that what we call "early diagnosis" is actually diagnosis in a late phase of tumor growth. Metastases may have spread at a much earlier preclinical stage of the tumor. The establishment of metastases before the diagnosis of the primary tumor predetermines the life-span of the host. Local therapy does not cure the patient in this case.

The appearance of metastases many years after diagnosis of the primary breast cancer has been attributed to the possible existence of dormant cells. The evaluation of the growth

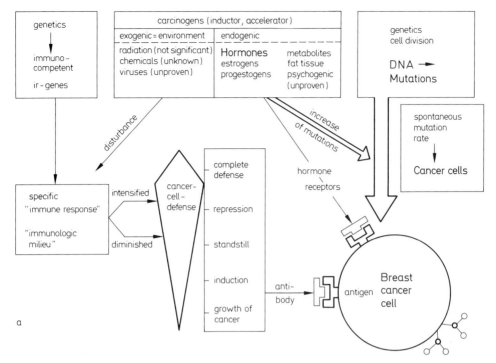

Fig. 14. Factors which can influence the growth behavior of breast cancer cells

rate with rather long doubling times explains the sometimes long latency period between primary tumor and the appearance of metastases. Thus the hypothesis of dormant cells can be dismissed. Our knowledge of tumor growth behavior has implications for the clinical management of patients:

The majority of mammary carcinoma grow at a moderately fast or a slow rate.

Theoretically they need on average 15–20 years to grow from the first malignant cell to a clinically detectable tumor 2 cm in size.

Women are 35 years old on average when the growth of their breast carcinoma begins.

Methods for early detection of breast carcinoma should not be first applied at the age of the highest incidence of carcinoma, 40–50 years, onward, but at the time when carcinoma most frequently begins, i.e., in women 30–40 years old.

The interval between two mammographies should be between 1 and 2 years. Control mammographies at shorter intervals than 6 months are usually not useful because of the growth behavior of the tumors.

Therapeutic effects, especially definite cure rates, can be evaluated after 20 years or later.

The predetermination of the life-span by occult metastases in most cases gives us a rationale for use of nonmutilating treatments.

Whether systemic chemotherapy or hormonal therapies have an effect on the definite cure rate of the disease can be decided only after an observation period of 10–20 years. Improved 5- or 10-year survival may only mean that the course of the disease is slowed down somewhat while definite cure rates remain unaffected.

References

Alvord EC Jr (1975) When do carcinomas of the breast begin to metastasize? Cited in: Spratt JS (1977) Growth kinetics in mammary cancer. In: Stoll BA (ed) Secondary spread in breast cancer. Heinemann Medical, London

Black MM (1975) Cell mediated response in human mammary cancer. In: Stoll BA (ed) Host defence in breast cancer. Heinemann Medical, London, p 48

Bloom HJG (1965) The influence of delay on the natural history and prognosis of breast cancer. Br J Cancer 19:228

Bloom HJG, Richardson WW (1957) Histological grading and prognosis in breast cancer. A study of 1,409 cases of which 359 have been followed for 15 years. Br J Cancer 11:359

Collins VP, Loeffler RK, Tivey H (1956) Observations on growth rates of human tumours. AJR 76:988

Duncan W, Kerr GR (1976) The curability of breast cancer. Br Med J IV:781

Fisher ER, Redmond C, Fisher B (1977) A perspective concerning the relation of duration of symptoms to treatment failure in patients with breast cancer. Cancer 40:3160

Fournier D v, Kuttig H, Kubli F, Prager P, Stolpe H, Maier A, Hüter J (1976) Wachstumsgeschwindigkeit des Mammakarzinoms und röntgenologische "Frühdiagnosen". Strahlentherapie 151:318

Fournier D v, Weber E, Hoeffken W, Bauer M, Kubli F, Barth V (1980) Growth rate of 147 mammary carcinomas. Cancer 45:2198−2207

Gershon-Cohen J, Berger SM, Klickstein HS (1963) Roentgenography of breast cancer moderating concept of "biologic predeterminism". Cancer 16:961

Haagensen CD (1974) Diseases of the breast, 2nd ed. Saunders, Philadelphia, p 501

Krokowski E (1964) Betrachtung zur Dynamik des Geschwulstwachstums. Krebsforsch Krebsbekämpfung 5:189−192

Kühn W, Fournier D v, Leppien G, Rummel HH, Müller A, Dick G (1983) Korrelation morphologischer Kriterien mit der Wachstumsgeschwindigkeit beim Mammakarzinom. Geburtshilfe Frauenheilkd 43:24−29

Kusama S, Spratt JS, Donegan WL et al. (1972) The gross rates of growth of human mammary carcinoma. Cancer 30:594

Laird AK (1965) Dynamics of tumour growth and comparison of growth rates. Br J Cancer 19:278

MacDonald I (1951) Biological predeterminism in human cancer. Surg Gynecol Obstet 92:443

Müller A, Tschahargane C, Kubli F (to be published) Zum Problem der subkutanen Mastektomie. Die Bedeutung der histopathologischen Aufarbeitung des Mastektomiepräparates. Dtsch Med Wochenschr

Oeser H (1974) Krebsbekämpfung: Hoffnung und Realität. Thieme, Stuttgart, pp 12−30

Richards GE (1948) Mammary cancer. Part 1. Br J Radiol 21:109

Spratt JS Jr, Kaltenbach ML, Spratt JA (1977) Cytokinetic definition of acute and chronic breast cancer. Cancer Res 37:226

Spratt JS, Hauser LS, Kuhns JG, Greenberg R, Polk HC (1981) Association between the actual doubling times of primary breast cancer with histo-pathologic characteristics and Wolf's parenchymal mammographic patterns. Cancer 47:2265−2268

Tubiana M (1971) The kinetics of tumour cell proliferation. Br J Radiol 44:325

Diagnosis

Identification of a High-Risk Population

H. Maass

Universitäts-Frauenklinik
2000 Hamburg 20, Federal Republik of Germany

To identify groups of women with an increased risk of developing breast cancer within a given population it is necessary to characterize so-called risk factors. The first hints are given by epidemiological examinations of the geographic distribution of breast cancer. These examinations are followed by observations of etiological and pathological factors, which lead to a series of hypotheses. So far none of these hypotheses has been confirmed by analytical, especially hormone analytical, investigations. Moreover — apart from small subgroups — no specific and clear discrimination between a high-risk and low-risk population is possible.

First of all we can point out a higher breast cancer incidence in western nations. This increase is independent of age, although it is slightly higher in women over 45 (Vorherr 1980). This result is based on standardized incidence rates, which are adjusted for different age distributions. Moreover, with the increased median life expectancy the incidence rate is correspondingly higher.

The geographic variation in incidence is an accepted fact. Breast cancer is more frequent, by a factor of 7, in western countries than in Japan (Maass and Sachs 1972). Although published studies deal only with small numbers, it can be expected that breast cancer is even more rare in Third World countries. Examination of the distribution by age in different countries shows that the differences in incidence are related mainly to the postmenopausal group (Fig. 1). In Japan the incidence decreases with age. In countries within median incidence rates the curve slopes downward, and in countries with a high incidence a linear increase with age can be seen (MacMahon et al. 1973).

The different age curves suggest the existence of factors exerting their main influence in the peri- and postmenopausal periods. Obviously the adaption to forms of western civilization is of importance. This is illustrated by two examples:

Second-generation Japanese women immigrants in the United States of America have a significantly higher incidence of breast cancer than the first generation (Table 1).

The life style in Iceland has risen from a low standard up to 1930 to a high western standard now. Correspondingly, the incidence rate for breast cancer has changed from a low- to a high-risk profile that is typical for western nations (Fig. 2).

The geographic distribution is influenced by genetic factors. The genetic disposition of breast cancer is an accepted fact. In particular, if a woman develops breast cancer during the premenopause, there is a high risk of breast cancer for her daughters. In general, women with breast cancer in their families have a higher risk of developing cancer of the breast themselves (Table 2).

Early Breast Cancer
Edited by J. Zander and J. Baltzer
© Springer-Verlag Berlin Heidelberg 1985

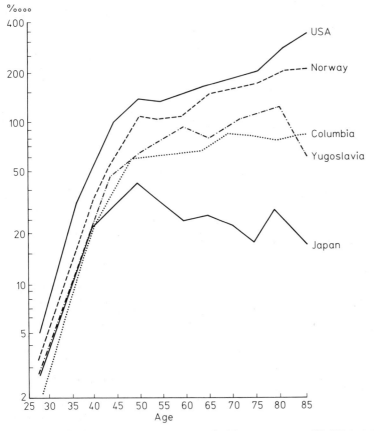

Fig. 1. Standardized annual breast cancer incidence rates per 100,000 females in several countries. (MacMahon et al. 1973)

Table 1. Average annual breast cancer death rates (per 100,000 women) for Japanese and white women in California during two time periods

	Japanese				Whites	
	Issei (immigrants)		Nisei (2nd generation)			
	1956–1962	1968–1972	1956–1962	1968–1972	1959–1961	1969–1971
Number of deaths	14	7	11	33	6,024	7,990
Age-adjusted death rate[a]	7.4	11.5	14.6	22.8	45.7	48.4

[a] For women from 35 to 64 years of age

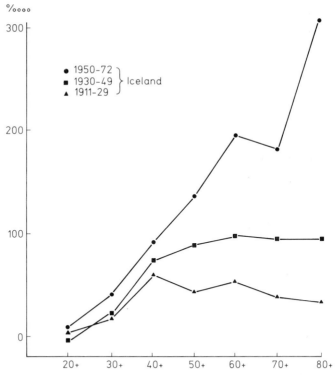

Fig. 2. Annual incidence rates in the female population of Iceland (per 100,000 females) 1911–1929; 1930–1949; and 1950–1952. (Nagel-Studer et al. 1978)

Table 2. Risk factors in daughters of breast cancer patients (Anderson 1971; Petrakis 1977)

Breast cancer of the mother	Risk factor	Increment of risk during life[a]
Premenopause	3.1	18.6%
Postmenopause	1.5	9.0%
Bilateral	5.4	32.4%
Bilateral premenopause	8.8	52.8%
Bilateral postmenopause	4.0	24.0%

[a] Average risk 6%

Different geographic and age distributions are explained primarily by specific habits, especially different nutritional habits. In 1968 Carroll reported a significant correlation between breast cancer incidence and high-calorie and high-fat nutrition. Thus dietetic factors seem to be of great importance in the development of breast cancer. Any discussion of this question must include consideration of the positive correlation between breast cancer and colon cancer.

In the cities of The Hague and Rotterdam De Waard (1975) observed an increased incidence rate within a group of women consuming very high-calorie diets. Moreover, in animal experiments a coincidence of breast cancer with fatty nutrition can be seen.

Wynder (1978) expected a direct connection with carcinogenic cholesterol metabolites. Furthermore, adipose tissue is able to metabolize steroid hormones in the periphery. From endometrial cancer we know that an increased proportion of adipose tissue may lead to a higher risk.

These epidemiological factors point to an endocrine mechanism in the genesis of breast cancer. Breast cancer is known to be a hormone-dependent tumor. This is documented by the demonstration of steroid hormone receptors in breast cancer cells. In view of these facts there is strong evidence that a hormone imbalance is associated with elevated breast cancer risk in humans. Great importance seems to attach to ovarian function. There is no doubt that a decreased risk of developing breast cancer follows early ovariectomy.

By analogy with endometrial cancer it has been postulated by Kaiser and Zippel (1980) and by Korenman (1980) that the risk of developing breast cancer is elevated in women with anovulatory cycles and with luteal phase deficiency. These results produced support for their gestagen deficiency hypothesis.

Among other factors associated with breast cancer, late age at first delivery is one of the most constant, and can be observed in all subgroups. First published by McMahon and Cole (McMahon et al. 1973) this phenomenon has now been reported by many other groups (e.g., Pauli and Trotnow 1973). This factor is involved in both high-risk and low-risk populations. Since in western countries late age at first pregnancy is a common situation this must be considered an important risk factor.

As mentioned above, epidemiological data have led to numerous hypotheses. Doubtless endocrine imbalance is of major importance. Nonetheless, so far no group has been able to characterize this imbalance. The so called Guernsey study published by Bulbrook et al. (1971) is well known. It is a prospective study of the relationship between androgen and corticosteroid metabolite excretion and risk of breast cancer in a large normal population in Guernsey. In the second prospective study, started in Guernsey in 1969, blood was obtained from 4,600 normal women aged 30−40 years. So far the only conclusion that can be derived from this study is that there was a shift in the balance between androgens and estrogens in favor of estrogens in the group of women developing breast cancer. Furthermore, a slightly decreased plasma progesterone level during the luteal phase was observed and moderately higher prolactin levels. On the premise that breast cancer needs a long time for manifestation, even slight differences in the endocrine balance may affect the risk of breast cancer. It is difficult to detect these slight differences.

It should be possible to use epidemiological data to identify risk groups. The definition of risk groups would permit a better selection of women for a screening program for early detection of breast cancer. Overall the risk factors are two- or three-fold. Only a small subgroup of women who have a known family history of breast cancer (mother with breast cancer in the premenopause) and women who have themselves already had breast cancer is known to be linked with a significantly increased risk. The same is true for women with proliferating mastopathy. Another important point which is mentioned too seldom is the increased risk with age (Table 3).

Besides these parameters we are still not able to characterize a specific group of women who would benefit from a screening program. The Health Insurance Plan (HIP) study (Shapiro et al. 1973) showed that one and/or two risk factors are present in 79% of the screened normal population, and only 67% of patients developing breast cancer belong to a subpopulation with less than three risk factors. Three and more risk factors were found in 21% of the control population, and only one-third of this high-risk group developed cancer, while two-thirds did not. So the difference from the healthy group is rather small (Table 4). Farewell (1977) established a mathematical model for definition of a subpopulation for

Table 3. Risk factors for breast cancer

Risk groups	Risk factors
1. Nulliparous	1.5–2.3
2. Advanced age at first birth	~ 3
3. Early menarche and late menopause	~ 2
4. Obesity, esp ecially in postmenopause	2–3
5. History of breast cancer	> 10
6. Family history of breast cancer	2–9
7. Increasing risk with age	–
8. Fibrocystic disease	~ 2
Without atypia	1
With atypia	2–4
8. Estrogen replacement in postmenopause	1.5–(2)

Table 4. Analysis of risk factor[a] data in the Health Insurance Plan study, New York (Shapiro et al. 1968)

	Percentage of normals	Percentage of those developing cancer
Less than three risk factors	79	67
Three or more risk factors	21	33
Total	100	100

[a] Risk factors: (1) Menarche at age 15; (2) Three pregnancies; (3) First pregnancy at age 30 or more; (4) Sister with breast cancer; (5) Prior breast disease

selected screening purposes. Even the introduction of endocrinological parameters derived from the Guernsey study led to disappointing results.

Thus, in conclusion we have to say that the situation has not changed since 1969, when Dunn stated:

> "None of these variables or their combination, with the exeption of age, concentrates a large enough proportion of all mammary cancers into a high-risk segment of the population to warrant dichotomizing the population of women between those who will be and those who will not be examined periodically for asymptomatic cancer of the breast."

References

Anderson DE (1971) Some characteristics of familial breast cancer. Cancer 28: 1500–1504

Bulbrook RD, Hayward JL, Spicer CC (1971) Relation between urinary androgen and corticoid excretion and subsequent breast cancer. Lancet II: 395–398

Carroll KK, Gammal EB, Plunkett ER (1968) Dietary fat and mammary cancer. Can Med Assoc J 98: 590–594

Farewell VT (1977) The combined effect of breast cancer risk factors. Cancer 40: 931–936

Kaiser R, Zippel HH (1980) Die Wirkung oraler Kontrazeptiva auf die weibliche Brust. Intern Prax 20: 449–458

Korenman SG (1980) Oestrogen window hypothesis of the aetiology of breast cancer. Lancet I: 700—701

Maass H, Sachs H (1972) Epidemiologie des Mammacarcinoms. Internist 13: 326—331

Maass H, Sachs H, Pauka B (1969) Epidemiologische Untersuchung bösartiger Neubildungen in Hamburg 1960—1962. Z Krebsforsch 73: 1—45

MacMahon B, Cole P, Brown J (1973) Etiology of human breast cancer: a review. JNCI 50: 21—42

Nagel-Studer E, Staub JJ, Nagel GA (1978) Zur Biologie des Mammakarzinoms. Ansatzpunkte für die aktuelle Therapieforschung. Schweiz Med Wochenschr 108: 2050—2059

Pauli HK, Trotnow S (1973) Zur Epidemiologie des Mammacarcinoms. Arch Gynecol 213: 271—282

Petrakis NL (1977) Genetic factors in the etiology of breast cancer. Cancer 39: 2709—2715

Shapiro S, Strax P, Venet L, Fink R (1968) The search for risk factors in breast cancer. Am J Public Health 58: 820—835

Vorherr H (1980) Breast cancer. Urban und Schwarzenberg, Baltimore

de Waard F (1975) Breast cancer incidence and nutritional status with particular reference to body weight and height. Cancer Res 35: 3351—3356

Wynder EL, Chan P, Cohen L, MacCornack F, Hill P (1978) Etiology and prevention of breast cancer. In: Grundmann L, Beck L (eds) Early diagnosis of breast cancer. Cancer campaign, vol 1. Fischer, Stuttgart, pp 1—28

Developments in Methods for Early Detection of Breast Cancer

J. Lissner, M. Kessler, G. Anhalt, D. Hahn, T. Wendt, and M. Seiderer

Radiologische Klinik und Poliklinik der Universität, Klinikum Großhadern, Marchioninistr. 15, 8000 Munich 70, Federal Republic of Germany

Up to 90% of all women with breast cancer discover their condition, now as always, themselves (Haagensen 1971; Strax 1976). Palpation findings are the prerequisite for all further diagnostic procedures, because 16% of minimal cancers would not have been detected otherwise (Moskowitz 1982). But for diagnosis of early breast cancer in the remaining 84% of cases methods have still to be developed.

Of all these methods mammography is the only one by which a carcinoma can be reliably diagnosed regardless of size (Feig et al. 1977a).

An unbelievable wealth of literature on the diagnostic accuracy of mammography has appeared. Since the examination has been performed with a variety of techniques, the possibility of proper detailed comparison is questionable. Despite this fact, however, we would still like to attempt it.

We have tried to take into account the varying conditions between the United States of America and Europe (Tables 1 and 2). The overall diagnostic accuracy differs; being 62%−89% in America and 81%−96% in Europe. The varying accuracy rates may be due to several factors:

In America, most of the examinations performed were of a general screening nature, in contrast to Europe, where specific diagnostic procedures were carried out.

America has always been the Mecca of medicine for us. Developments usually came along first there, but not only positive ones. Bailar, for instance, raised the question of radiation risk in mammography back in 1977 (Bailar 1977). In America this has been discussed even more exhaustively than in Europe. The emphasis of risk versus benefit, especially among the general public, is recognizable in the relation between dosage and image quality − or at least it seems so to us.

In America, approximately 63% of the examinations are carried out with xeroradiography; the rest, almost without exception, are done with low-dose x-ray (Jans et al. 1972, 1982). We did not care for the low-dose system.

Approximately 50% of x-rays are still performed with industrial film, in spite of the high radiation doses involved. Since grids were introduced they have been combined with high intensifying film/screen systems in 20% of cases, and in a further 20% with high-resolution film/screen systems. In the Encyclopedia of Medical Radiology we learn at the very start that the most frequent false diagnoses in mammography are due to poor image quality and not to misinterpretation (Barth et al. 1982).

If we keep in mind what we are looking for in the x-ray image this can be reduced essentially to microcalcifications or a dense patch in the parenchyma. In a fatty breast this is

Early Breast Cancer
Edited by J. Zander and J. Baltzer
© Springer-Verlag Berlin Heidelberg 1985

Table 1. Diagnostic accuracy of mammography in detection of breast cancer (USA)

Author	Year	Carcinomas (n)	T1 < 1 cm		Accuracy (%)
			(n)	(%)	
Hicks	1979	113	37	33	62
McLelland	1978	–	–	–	65
Moskowitz	1977	119	29	24	–
Letton	1977	32	–	–	71.8
Egeli	1978	778	–	–	72.5
Cole-Beuglet	1981	79	–	–	74
Feig	1977	139	36	26	78
Pagani	1980	53	–	–	84
Sayler	1977	97	–	–	85
Dodd	1977	3,661	–	–	87
Egan	1977	53	–	–	87
BCDDP	1982	3,557	–	–	88.9

Table 2. Diagnostic accuracy of mammography in detection of breast cancer (Europe)

Author	Year	Carcinomas (n)	T1 < 1 cm		Accuracy (%)
			(n)	(%)	
Fournier	1974	259	–	–	81
Kriedemann	1981	312	–	–	82.4
Kratochwill	1975	62	–	–	89.7
Bjurstam	1973	185	–	–	92
Frischbier	1977	788	–	–	92
Schmidt	1981	53	20	41	92
Andersson	1980	451	230	51	93
Barth	1982	197	–	–	93.4
Thiel	1982	90	–	–	94.2
Tabar	1980	235	97	41	94.5
Grosse-Vorholt	1979	67	–	–	95.5
Otto	1980	264	–	–	95.8
Hüppe	1977	277	–	–	96

not too difficult, but it can be almost impossible in a dense fibrocystic breast (Fig. 1). Thus the diagnostic accuracy of mammography is independent of tumor size, but declines with increasing density or advancing fibrocystic disease (Feig 1977b).

As the number of calcifications increases, the probability rises that it is a carcinoma (Menges et al. 1973). But recognition of the five calcifications that should be the definitive indication for a biopsy is ultimately dependent on image quality (Hoeffken et al. 1981).

If we take industrial film as a standard, different methods have been applied to reduce the radiation dose in mammography (Friedrich 1975, 1977, 1978).

1) The use of so-called high-resolution film/screen systems, or low-dose systems. The reduction in dosage leads to a loss of informative detail (Fig. 2).

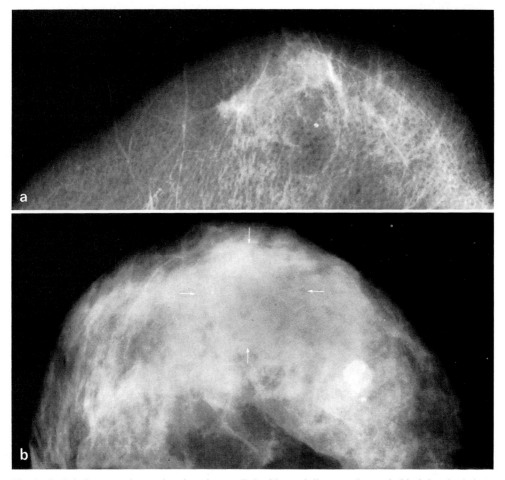

Fig. 1a, b. Scirrhous carcinoma in a fatty breast. Palpable medullary carcinoma behind the nipple in a dense breast

2) The scatter radiation grid. The grid reduces the scattered radiation to approximately one-third, which is involved about 50% in imaging. The grid technique is combined with the so-called high-resolution single-coated or with the actual high-resolution double-coated film/screen-systems. The second gives the better image contrast, especially in dense breasts. Dense structures become more transparent, and microcalcifications are easier to recognize.

It should be pointed out that this is a sophisticated system. In other words, the film/screen combination exposure and development data must be finely tuned if a dose reduction is to be achieved.

3) Selective filter techniques (Fewell 1978). Combined with a grid, these might become the method of the future. The optimal radiation energy is a function of the object's thickness. In thick and dense breasts a large portion of low-voltage energy offering a good contrast is absorbed. The overall contrast is only a little weaker, but the dose can be reduced considerably, if the molybdenum spectrum is not filtered with aluminium or molybdenum, as at present, but instead the tungsten spectrum is filtered with rhodium

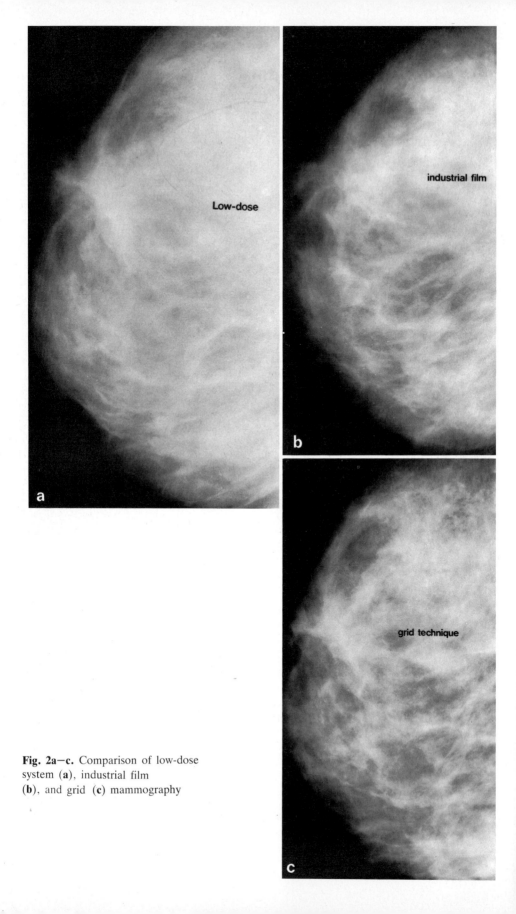

Fig. 2a–c. Comparison of low-dose
system (**a**), industrial film
(**b**), and grid (**c**) mammography

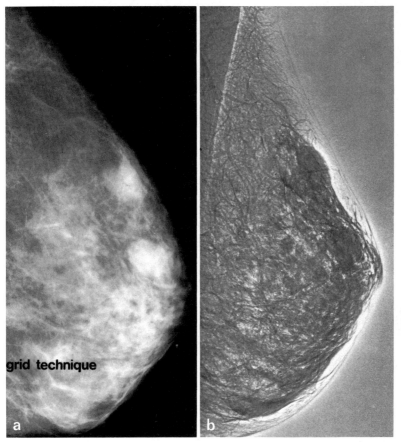

grid technique

a b

Fig. 3a, b. Benign cysts. Comparison of grid mammography (**a**) with xeroradiography (**b**)

    or palladium. Thus the characteristic density and thickness of the parenchyma is taken into account.
4) and 5) XERG and magnification mammography. Since it is obviously problematic to introduce these methods into routine work they are not covered here, but in unclear cases magnification mammography can be of value (Muntz 1979; Muntz et al. 1977).

According to the Bent study, 63% of the examinations in America are carried out using xeroradiography. This is said to be mainly due to the reduced radiation exposure and the better contrast representation of microcalcifications, particularly in dense parenchyma (Gros et al. 1975a; Wolfe et al. 1972). However, before grids were introduced, Egan et al. (1977) showed that x-ray mammography is superior to xeroradiography with regard to the visualization of microcalcifications, regardless of tumor size and breast density.
We abandoned xeroradiography in favor of the grid system 2 years ago. Since we cannot carry out control examinations on microcalcifications, we can show the contour contrast enhancement of xeroradiography compared with grid mammography only in benign cysts (Fig. 3).
The literature contains no data on the diagnostic accuracy of low-dose mammography directly compared with grid mammography, but consideration of the two parts of Fig. 4 should provide convincing evidence.

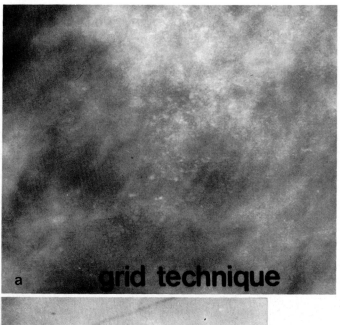

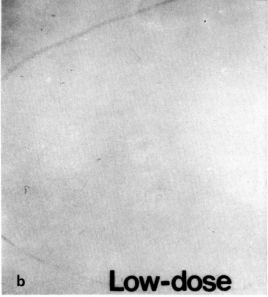

Fig. 4a, b. Clustered microcalcifications in fibrocystic disease of the breast visualized by grid mammography (**a**) and low-dose system (**b**)

Once more, let us consider the dose: The mean mid-breast dose in grid mammography is less than 2 cGy/examination, thus lying between the dose needed with industrial film and that given in xeroradiography (F. E. Stieve, Present View of the Benefit-Risk Rate in Mammography, this volume). We compromise by accepting this dose and the radiation risk it entails for the sake of the benefit we consider to accrue from the use of radiologic methods.

However highly developed the technique of mammography, it can never achieve an accuracy of 100%. This is partly due to human error, but this factor cannot be completely avoided (Cahill et al. 1981; Kalisher 1979; Martin et al. 1979). Furthermore, even with

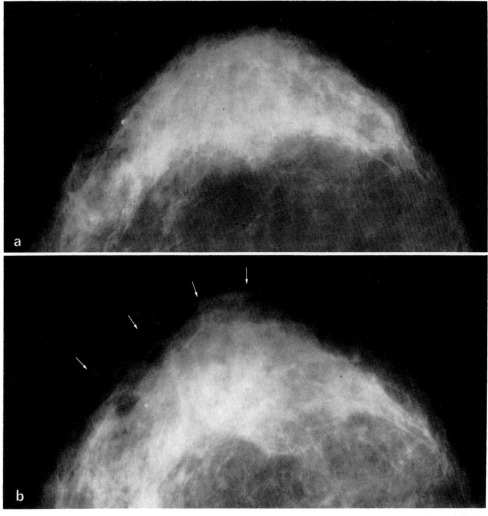

Fig. 5a, b. Inflammatory carcinoma of the breast. Six weeks before the diagnosis, except for mastopathy there were no pathologic findings

optimal techniques, error also results from the pattern and density of the breast (Feig et al. 1977b).

Only about 60% of all carcinomas show pathognomic calcifications (Fournier et al. 1975). If they are absent early breast cancer cannot be differentiated in dense parenchyma or in the pattern of benign fibrocystic disease.

In the case illustrated in Fig. 5 the mammogram, even when viewed retrospectively, does not reveal a malignant growth although 6 weeks later an inflammatory carcinoma was found.

In addition, mammography is blamed for a great many false-positive findings. As shown previously, it is true that the positive predictive value increases with the number of calcifications (Menges et al. 1973). But 60%−80% of all biopsied microcalcifications turn out to be noncarcinomatous (Hoeffken et al. 1981; Lanyi et al. 1981) (Fig. 6). Also, the differential diagnosis of smooth round lesions is only possible to a limited extent. But we

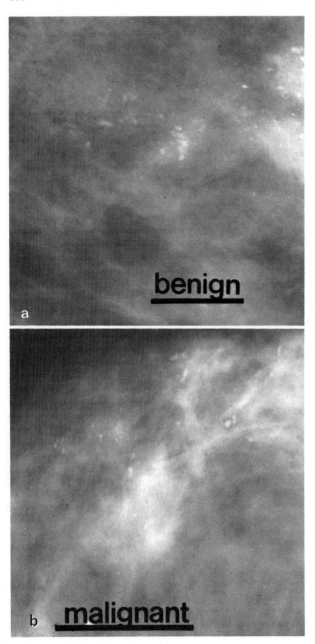

benign

malignant

Fig. 6a, b. Differentiation of benign (**a**) and malignant (**b**) microcalcifications is not always possible

cannot dismiss mammography without considering the alternatives available and the risks they involve.

Ultrasound

Since the physical parameters used in ultrasound diagnostic techniques have shown that tissue damage is unexpected, there has recently been a great deal of discussion about its use AJUM 1976.

Table 3. Diagnostic accuracy of automated breast scanning

Author	Year	Carcinomas (n)	Accuracy %	
			X-Ray	Ultrasound
Cole-Beuglet	1981	79	83	79
Jellins	1980	112	–	84
Kobyayshi	1979	112	83	87
Wagai	1974	281	–	88
Pluygers	1980	285	82	90
Kossoff	1978	82	–	91
Schmidt	1981	53	92	87
Gros	1978	443	–	95
Harper	1982	43	95	95

Table 4. Diagnostic accuracy of manual breast scanning

Author	Year	Carcinomas (n)	Accuracy %	
			X-Ray	Ultrasound
Damascelli	1970	21	–	57
Fields	1980	44	–	75
Teixidor	1977	33	94	79
Van Kaick	1980	36	–	80
Jellins	1975	21	–	81

Table 5. Diagnostic accuracy of ultrasound in relation to tumor size

Author	Year	Carcinomas		Accuracy		
		n	n T1	%	% T1	T1 < 1 cm
Furuki	1970	165	–	90	89	56
Kossoff	1978	82	34	91	88	–
Pluygers	1980	285	12	90	83	58
Kobayashi	1979	112	–	87	80	–
Wagai	1974	281	72	88	78	–
Gros	1978	443	13	95	77	38
Schmidt	1981	53	24	87	75	–
Fujii	1970	103	–	82	70	–
Cole-Beuglet	1981	79	24	79	46	–

The acoustic velocity of sound, specific impedance, and attenuation by absorption, reflexion, and scattering are the acoustic properties of the parenchyma of the breast. For instance, expressed as a percentage difference compared with water, the relative acoustic velocity of fatty, normal, or pathologically altered tissue may be different (Glover 1977).

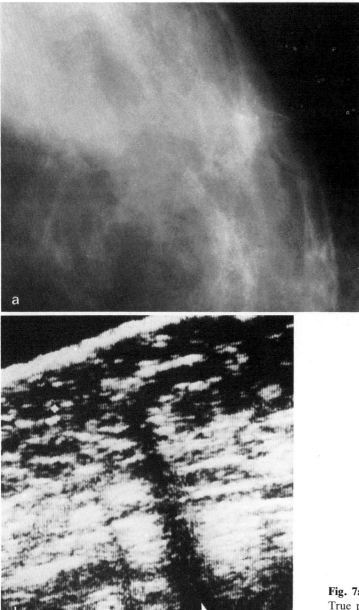

Fig. 7a, b. Carcinoma in situ. True positive sonogram with central shadowing

Acoustic properties provide the basis for the analysis of masses (Cole-Beuglet et al. 1975, 1980; Kobayashi et al. 1979; Kobayashi 1980). In addition, there are indirect criteria. The study of these criteria has brought about a series of publications that have resulted in the unfortunate public opinion that many x-ray examinations of the breast can now safely be replaced by ultrasound. We should, therefore, examine the actual relevance of ultrasound in breast diagnostics.

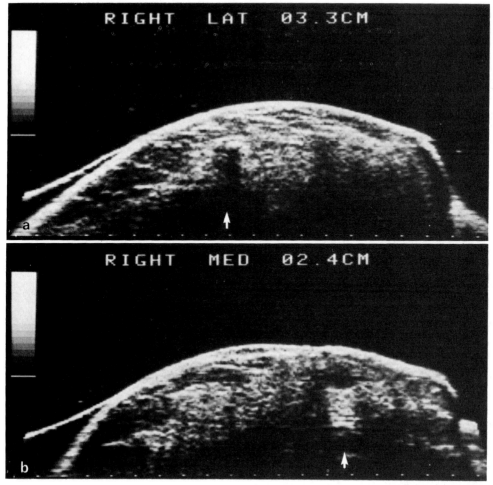

Fig. 8. a Fibroadenoma with central shadowing due to calcifications; **b** distal enhancement of a medullary carcinoma in the same patient

Improvements in technical equipment have made two methods available:
1) Automated water-path scanners offering reproducible and complete morphological representation of the breast with 79%−95% accuracy (Tables 3−5).
2) Commercial compound and real-time apparatus with and without water coupling, allowing specific visualization of palpable masses or mammographically suggestive findings. This technique is 57%−81% accurate.

The diagnostic accuracy is reduced by 6%−30% when palpation findings are not included in the evaluation. When the tumors are staged accuracy in stage T1 is 1%−33% lower and ranges between 46% and 89%. The sparse data available on T1 tumors smaller than 1 cm indicate a diagnostic accuracy of only 38%−58%.

Aside from differences in construction modes, the limited diagnostic value of automated apparatus in detecting early breast cancer is mainly due to the poor resolution. In manual methods, axial and lateral resolution are sufficient in principle and allow the representation of the smallest lesions analogous to mammography. In our opinion, this is also true for microcalcifications, which theoretically lie below the limits of ultrasound resolution (Kessler et al. 1983). In fact, they do not appear themselves alone but always in conjunction with histopathological alterations in tissue (Fig. 7).

In addition, the diagnostic value of the criteria mentioned varies. Although the central shadowing is very specific, it appears in less than 50% of carcinomas. On the other hand, weak internal echoes in a lesion are very sensitive, but the specificity for benign or malignant lesions is very low. Astonishingly enough, the distal enhancement so typical for cysts is very specific in carcinomas, especially medullary ones (Fields 1980). This can lead to misinterpretation, as seen in Fig. 8 for example, which illustrates a case of medullary carcinoma with distal enhancement and fibroadenoma with attenuation that presented simultaneously in the same patient.

The initial euphoria about breast ultrasound is waning. Improved resolution in the automated apparatus is expected, and problems of documentation and reproducibility need to be solved.

Considering the results obtained, mammography cannot be replaced by ultrasound in our opinion at present.

Thermography

Two procedures are currently available:
1) Infrared thermography.
2) Plate thermography.
Both methods allow visualization of a breast carcinoma if it contains abundant cells with a high metabolic activity, in contrast to collagen-rich tumors, which have less infrared emission.

The criteria of malignancy in thermography are measurable quantities, on the one hand, and are morphologically tangiable on the other (Amalric et al. 1976). In true positive carcinomas a combination of delta T2 equal to or higher than $1.5°$ with an image of anarchic vessels is typical (Frischbier et al. 1977).

The diagnostic accuracy of the methods ranges between 29% and 97% and between 61% and 100%, respectively. In the literature the maximum accuracy of the method in stages T0 to T1 is quoted as 72% (Tables 6−8).

It should be noted that approximately 10% of confirmed carcinomas are not detected until thermography is applied (Amalric et al. 1976).

Thermography can indeed be valuable in dense fibrocystic breasts when estimating risk factors (Stark 1976). Another important application is evaluation of the prognosis of carcinomas already diagnosed; the degree of malignancy increases with rising temperature (Amalric et al. 1976; Dodd 1976; Jones et al. 1975). Moreover, thermography is useful in postoperative care following unilateral ablation if a baseline thermogram exists (Gros et al. 1975a).

However, in conclusion it must be stressed that neither of the criteria mentioned above specifically confirms or excludes malignancy.

Computed Tomography

Shortly after the adoption of body computer tomography as a routine diagnostic technique the first results obtained in the breast were published.

Table 6. Accuracy of infrared thermography in the diagnosis of breast carcinoma

Author	Year	Carcinomas (n)	Accuracy (%)
Egan	1977	53	29
Dodd	1977	46	29
Bothmann	1979	132	33
Feig	1977	139	39
Lohbeck	1982	62	48
Jones	1975	363	68
Isard	1972	306	72
Gros	1971	468	73
Stark	1982	−	79
Wallace	1969	195	85
Raskin	1976	49	88
Amalric	1974	1,103	91
Gershon-Cohen	1967	200	92
Melander	1968	232	92
Pistolesi	1973	108	93
Aarts	1972	93	97

Table 7. Accuracy of plate thermography in the diagnosis of breast carcinoma

Author	Year	Carcinomas (n)	Accuracy (%)
Barth	1977	182	61
Goldberg	1981	17	65
Bothmann	1975	132	74
Grosse-Vorholt	1979	67	77
Hüppe	1976	146	77
Müller	1974	59	78
Frischbier	1975	83	84
Geissler	1974	46	87
Lauth	1975	109	92
Tricoire	1974	78	100

Table 8. Accuracy of infrared (I) and plate thermography (P) according to tumor size

Author	Year	Method	T0−T1 (%)
Bothmann	1974	I	21
Raskin	1976	I	29
Lohbeck	1978	P	33
Bourjat	1972	I	40
Barth	1977	I/P	37/49
Lohbeck	1978	I	52
Moskowitz	1982	P	55 (Stage I)
Frischbier	1977	P	58
Hüppe	1976	P	37/65
Amalric	1976	I	72

Table 9. Comparison of diagnostic accuracy of mammography and CT/M

Author	Year	Carcinomas (n)	Detected by			
			Mammography		CT/M	
			(n)	%	(n)	%
Gisvold	1977	41	38	93	39	95
Chang	1981	93	75	77	87	94
Chang	1982	17	12	71	16	94

Studies were carried out using a special breast scanner with and without contrast medium. In 93 cases of breast carcinoma in a total of 1,846 examinations, 94% of the carcinomas were verified by CT/M, as against only 71%–77% with low-dose mammography (Chang et al. 1980) (Table 9).

Remarkably enough, in dense fibrocystic structures, Chang was able to detect only 3 of 14 carcinomas when using low-dose mammography, while with CT/M he detected all 14. Furthermore, it is noteworthy that atypical epithelial proliferation and similar benign, purely proliferative alterations could be correctly differentiated when contrast medium inducing an increase in iodine concentration was used (Chang et al. 1982). The technical data concerning computed tomography mammography are as follows: without contrast medium − 6 slices, slice thickness of 10 mm; with contrast medium − 300 ml contrast medium. The average mid-breast radiation dose for six slices was 0.175 cGy.

Meanwhile, CT examinations of the breast have been carried out with body scanners. The results are comparable to those of CT/M (Fig. 9).

Irrespective of the examiner there is digital representation of the density data.

A critical evaluation of the results obtained so far suggests that the merit of CT in breast diagnostics is doubtful. The average radiation dose in mid-breast with six slices is 0.175 cGy and is therefore acceptable. But we consider that IV administration of 300 ml contrast medium, i.e., a dose greater than is used on average for a complete abdominal angiography, is a significant factor, at least in light of the other methods available.

Nuclear Medicine

In contrast to the morphologically oriented mammography, breast scintigraphy makes use of the pathophysiological differences between normal glandular and fatty tissue compared with malignant tumors.

Various radionuclides have been used. The high organ dose held up the development of the method when 197-mercury was used. The arrival of 99-m-technetium resulted in a lower radiation exposure and renewed interest in this little used method. The average organ dose for both breasts is 0.2 cGy with 300 MBq 99-m-technetium-DTPA (Table 10). The technical data concerning scintigraphy of the breast with 99-m-Tc-DTPA were as follows: single-photon-emission computed tomography (SPECT) − (A) 30′ PI, (B) 120′ PI; transversal reconstruction; quantitative evaluation by ROI technique.

Up to now, breast scintigraphy has mostly been carried out with a planar gamma camera, but this method is inadequate for investigation of small tumors or those close to the chest

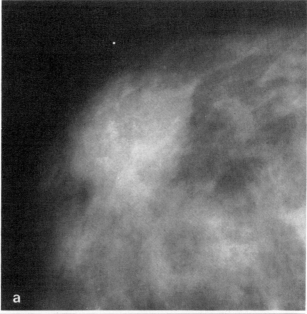

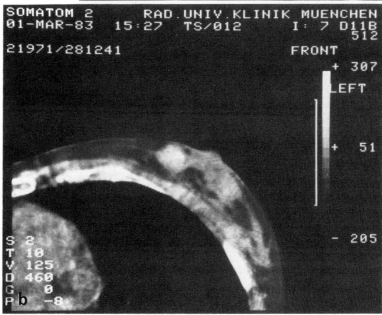

Fig. 9. a x-Ray mammography and **b** CT of a T1 carcinoma of the breast

wall. However, this is not the case in the transversal single-photon-emission method of computed tomography now in use (Wolfe et al. 1971).

This method provides transversal reconstructions of both breasts 30 min after injection. A carcinoma induces a hot spot (Fig. 10). This nuclide accumulation can be evaluated quantitatively in regions of interest. Besides accumulation, the temporal increase in radioactivity is a further criterion.

Table 10. Accuracy of scintigraphy in the diagnosis of breast cancer

Author	Year	Nuclid	Examination (*n*)	Carcinoma (*n*)	Accuracy (%)
Buchwald	1969	$^{197}HGCL_2$	36	18	50
Richmann	1979	67-GA	10	5	50
Wendt	1983	99M-TC-DTPA	13	10	77
Richmann	1979	99M-TC-O$_4$	16	14	88
Sanazzari	1972	$^{197}HGCL_2$	10	9	90
Cuschieri	1981	99M-TC-DTPA	32	10	94
Rossi	1975	99M-TC-DTPA	13	13	100

It must be pointed out that a diagnosis is not made, as in mammography, on the bases of many years of experience, but rather from reproducible measured data. The prerequisite, however, is a healthy contralateral breast.

Nuclear Magnetic Resonance

Nuclear magnetic resonance (NMR) is based on the interaction of magnetic and electrical fields with the magnetic nuclear momentum of hydrogen present in the body (Loeffler et al. 1981). Unlike other imaging procedures, this method allows not only imaging, but also spectrum analysis. This indeed will open up new diagnostic horizons.

In 1973, in vitro examinations in biopsies of the breast were performed by NMR for the first time. The first in vivo examinations of breast carcinoma date back to 1979 (Mansfield et al. 1979). The results obtained up to now show that the differentiation of a malignancy from normal or fibrocystic tissue is possible in 85%−95% of in vitro examinations (Table 11). In vivo examinations, however, do not allow accurate identification.

With the expected technological developments, this will be the method of the future, primarily because of the new dimension of spectral analysis, mentioned above. Recent studies indicate no risk for the patient whatsoever (Budinger 1981). But like all new procedures, nuclear magnetic resonance will only confirm its merit through large-scale clinical studies.

So much for the alternatives. Let us return to the actual everyday routine.

Conclusions

This review of the literature demonstrates that, as mentioned initially, mammography is so far the only method by which a carcinoma can be reliably diagnosed regardless of size.

Mammography does not screen out further carcinomas. But this method does help to detect incident carcinomas as prevalent ones (Dodd 1976; Andersson et al. 1979; Frischbier 1982; Moskowitz 1981, 1982; Moskowitz et al. 1977), thus improving not only the 5-year but also the long-term survival. For this reason we endorse "aggressive diagnostics", which means: *clinical examination plus mammography for women over 30 years*. Since currently 20% of all women operated on for breast cancer in our hospital are under 40 years of age.

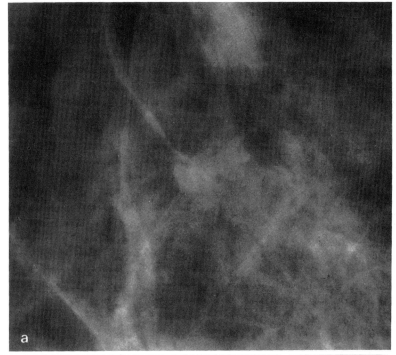

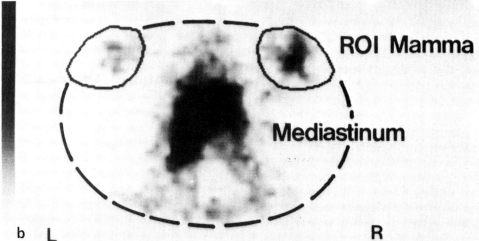

Fig. 10. a Transversal single-photon-emission computed tomography; **b** hot spot induced by a ductal carcinoma

Table 11. Accuracy of NMR for in vitro diagnosis of breast cancer

Author	Year	Examinations (n)	Accuracy (%)
Goldsmith	1978	119	95
Medina	1975	55	85

When we weigh radiation risk in relation to image quality, the high-resolution film-screen system in combination with a grid seems to us to be the method of choice at present. With this combination we have a diagnostic accuracy of 92%−96% according to tumor size.

All other methods mentioned are supplementary procedures, which can be of the greatest value in individual cases or in differential diagnosis, especially, again according to tumor size, in the missed 4%−8%.

References

Amalric R et al. (1976) Value and interest of dynamic telethermography in detection of breast cancer. Acta Thermographica 1: 89

American Institute of Ultrasound in Medicine (AJUM) (1976) Biological effects of ultrasonic energy in living mammals. Ultrasound Med Biol 2: 351

Andersson I et al. (1979) Breast cancer screening with mammography − A population-based, randomized trial with mammography as the only screening mode. Radiology 132: 273

Andersson I et al. (1980) Breast cancer screening in Sweden − The single modality approach. Radiologe 20: 608

Bailar JC (1977) Screening for early breast cancer: Pros and cons. Cancer 39: 2783

Barth V et al. (1982) Mammatumoren. In: Diethelm L (ed) Spezielle Strahlentherapie maligner Tumoren. Springer, Berlin Heidelberg New York (Handbuch der medizinischen Radiologie, vol 19, part 2, pp 1−65)

Budinger ThF (1981) Nuclear magnetic resonance (NMR) in vivo studies: Known tresholds for health effects. J Comput Assist Tomogr 5: 800

Cahill CJ et al. (1981) Features of mammographically negative breast tumours. Br J Surg 68: 882

Chang JCH et al. (1980) Computed tomography in detection and diagnosis of breast cancer. Cancer 46: 939

Chang CHJ et al. (1982) Die Computertomographie der Brust. In: Frischbier HJ (ed) Die Erkrankungen der weiblichen Brust. Thieme, Stuttgart, p 119

Cole-Beuglet et al. (1975) Continuous ultrasound B-scanning of palpable breast masses. Radiology 117: 123

Cole-Beuglet et al. (1980) Atlas of breast ultrasound. Telles, Philadelphia

Dodd G (1976) Pathophysiology of heat production in breast cancer. NCI, Breast Cancer Task Force 5: 5

Egan RL et al. (1977) Conventional mammography, physical examination, thermography and xeroradiography in the detection of breast cancer. Cancer 39: 1984

Feig StA et al. (1977a) Thermography, mammography, and clinical examination in breast cancer screening. Radiology 122: 123

Feig StA et al. (1977b) Analysis of clinically occult and mammographically occult breast tumors. AJR 128: 403

Fewell TR (1978) A comparison of mammographic X-ray-Spectra. Radiology 128: 211

Fields SJ (1980) Ultrasound mammographic histopathologic correlation. Ultrasound imaging 2: 150

Fournier VD et al. (1975) Häufigkeitsverteilung der Malignitätszeichen bei der Mammographie. Med Welt 26: 2211

Frischbier HJ et al. (1977) Frühdiagnostik des Mammakarzinoms. Thieme, Stuttgart, p 216

Frischbier HJ (1982) Die Erkrankungen der weiblichen Brustdrüse. Thieme, Stuttgart, p 78

Friedrich M (1975) Der Einfluß der Streustrahlung auf die Abbildungsqualität bei der Mammographie. Fortschr Röntgenstr 123: 556

Friedrich M (1977) Bildqualität in der Mammographie – Einfluß der Streustrahlung und der Bildaufzeichnungssysteme. Fortschr Röntgenstr 36: 4

Friedrich M (1978) Neuere Entwicklungstendenzen der Mammographietechnik: Die Raster-Mammographie. Fortschr Röntgenstr 128: 207

Glover GH (1977) Computerized time-of-flight – ultrasonic tomography for breast examination. Ultrasound Med Biol 3: 117

Gros CM et al. (1975a) Xéroradiographie mammaire. J Radiol Electrol 56: 471

Gros C et al. (1975b) Prognosis and posttherapeutic follow up of breast cancer by thermography. Thermography, Basel, Biol Radiol 6

Haagensen CD (1971) Diseases of the breast. 2nd edn, Saunders, Philadelphia

Hoeffken W et al. (1981) Erkrankungen der Brustdrüse. In: Schinz (ed) Lehrbuch der Röntgendiagnostik, vol II, 2, Thieme, Stuttgart, p 969

Jans RG et al. (1979) The status of film/screen mammography. Radiology 132: 197

Jans RE et al. (1982) Bent-Study, 30. 9. 82: Breast exposure: Nationwide trends. U.S.-Department of Health and Human Services TDA, Bureau of Radiological Health, 5600 Fishers Lane, Rockville, Maryland 20857

Jones CH et al. (1975) Thermography of the female breast: a five-year study in relation to the detection and prognosis of cancer. Br J Radiol 48: 532

Kalisher L (1979) Factors influencing false negative rates in xeromammography. Radiology 133: 297

Kessler M et al. (1983) Ergebnisse von Mammographie und Mammasonographie mit manuellem und automatisiertem Scanvorgang. In: Otto RC, Jame IX (eds) Ultraschall-Diagnostik 82. 6. gemeinsame Tagung d. deutschsprachigen Gesellschaft für Ultraschall. Thieme, Stuttgart, p 362

Kobayashi T (1980) Current status of breast ultrasonography and ultrasound tissue – characterization of breast cancer. In: Lindberg DAB, Kaihara S (eds) Medifino 80. IFIP, North Holland, Amsterdam, p 205

Kobayashi T et al. (1979) Differential diagnosis of breast tumours. The sensitivity graded method of ultrasonotomography and clinical evaluation of its diagnostic accuracy. Cancer 33: 940

Lanyi M et al. (1981) Differentialdiagnose der Mikroverkalkungen bei kleincystischer (blunt duct) Adenose. Fortschr Röntgenstr 134: 225

Loeffler W et al. (1981) Physical principles of NMR tomography. Eur J Radiol 1: 338

Mansfield P et al. (1979) Carcinoma of the breast imaged by nuclear magnetic resonance (NMR). Br J Radiol 52: 242

Martin JE et al. (1979) Breast cancer missed by mammography. AJR 132: 737

Menges V et al. (1973) Korrelation zahlenmäßig erfaßter Mikroverkalkungen auf dem Mammogramm und dadurch diagnostizierter Carcinome und Mastopathietypen. Radiologe 13: 468

Moskowitz M (1979) Screening is not diagnosis. Radiology 133: 265

Moskowitz M (1981) Mammographic screening: Significance of minimal breast cancers. AJR 136: 735

Moskowitz M (1982) Reihenuntersuchung zur Diagnostik des Mammakarzinoms. Wie wirksam sind unsere Untersuchungsmethoden? In: Frischbier HJ (ed) Die Erkrankungen der weiblichen Brustdrüse. Thieme, Stuttgart, p 69

Moskowitz M et al. (1977) The breast cancer screening controversy: a perspective. AJR 537

Muntz PE (1979) Focal spot size and scatter suppression in magnification mammography. AJR 133: 453

Muntz PE et al. (1977) Preliminary studies using electron radiography for mammography. Radiology 125: 517

Stark AM (1976) The significance of an abnormal breast thermogram. Acta Thermographica 19: 87

Stieve FE (this volume) Present view of the benefit-risk rate in mammography.

Strax P (1976) Result of mass screening for breast cancer in 50,000 examinations. Cancer 37: 30

Strax P (1982) Die Zielsetzung bei der Durchführung von Reihenuntersuchungen zur Früherkennung des Mammakarzinoms. In: Frischbier HJ (ed) Die Erkrankungen der weiblichen Brustdrüse. Thieme, Stuttgart

Strax P et al. (1973) Value of mammography in reduction of mortality from breast cancer in mass screening. AJR 117: 686

Wendt TG et al. (1983) Emission computed tomography in benign and malignant tumors of the breast. Nuclear Med Commun 4: 5

Wolfe JN et al. (1971) Xeroradiography of the breast: A comparative study with conventional film mammography. Cancer 28: 1569

Wolfe JN et al. (1972) Xeroradiography of the breast. Thomas, Springfield I 11

Morphologic Analysis of Microcalcifications

A Valuable Differential Diagnostic System for Early Detection of Breast Carcinomas and Reduction of Superfluous Exploratory Excisions

M. Lanyi

Gummersbach Radiological Institute,
Kaiserstrasse 19, 5270 Gummersbach 1, Federal Republic of Germany

Introduction

Almost 30 years ago, Gershon-Cohen et al. (1955) were the first to report on the mammographic detection of clinically occult carcinomas of the breast. Since then, mammography has come into use all over the world, so that preclinical carcinomas are discovered daily everywhere. In my institute alone, these cases made up 18% of the total of 519 carcinomas diagnosed from 1 October 1974 to 30 June 1983. More than half of these occult carcinomas ($n = 50$) were diagnosed solely on the basis of microcalcifications; microcalcifications are thus the most important leading symptom in mammographic detection of preclinical carcinomas. All physicians using mammography are naturally concerned to draw therapeutic conclusions from this diagnosis. Only a nonmutilating treatment appropriate to the stage of early cancer can justify the major expenditure entailed by mammography. However, what is the meaning of "early cancer"? No generally valid definition is found in the literature. Even the fact that a carcinoma is clinically occult does not by any means imply that an early cancer is involved, since even relatively large carcinomas can remain clinically occult in large breasts.

In the American literature, the terms "early cancer" and "minimal cancer" were coined for the very tiny incipient carcinomas with an exceedingly good prognosis. Bässler (1978) regards the term early cancer as inappropriate, because it can also be taken to include early stages in the sense of precancers.

Gallager and Martin (1971) refer to minimal cancer when the tumor is not larger than 0.5 cm. Urban (1976) raises the uppermost limit and refers to minimal cancer when the tumor is not larger than 1 cm, provided that lymph node metastases cannot be palpated. According to Kindermann (1977) and Zippel et al. (1981), early cases are all noninfiltrating carcinomas irrespective of their extent and infiltrating carcinomas up to 0.5 cm in diameter. The true rating of the microcalcifications in the detection of early carcinomas depends on which of the above definitions is regarded as correct. Of the 519 mammary carcinomas, 12 cases were a maximum of 0.5 cm in size (2.3% of all carcinomas) and were thus minimal cancers according to the definition of Gallager and Martin (1971); of these, 5 cases (0.96% of all carcinomas) were diagnosed on the basis of microcalcification. According to the criteria drawn up by Urban, I found 56 minimal cancers (10.7% of all carcinomas) 12 of these (2.3%) on the basis of microcalcifications alone. However, when I used the definition of Kindermann (1977) or of Zippel et al. (1981) I found 31 early cases (5.9%), 23 of these (4.4%) on the basis of microcalcifications. Irrespective of the definition one accepts, the

Early Breast Cancer
Edited by J. Zander and J. Baltzer
© Springer-Verlag Berlin Heidelberg 1985

number of early cancers/minimal cancers/early cases is very small. The proportion of cases discovered on the basis of microcalcifications is even smaller. However, what price must be paid for these cancers with good prognosis with respect to microcalcifications? If the number of exploratory excisions because of suggestive or dubious microcalcifications is compared with the number of early cancers/minimal cancers/early cases discovered in this way, then the question arises as to whether the effort has a reasonable relationship to the result. In my material, 756 exploratory excisions were carried out because of palpable nodes with any radiologic symptoms at all or because of clinically occult radiologic alterations extending to microcalcifications, and 426 cancers were found; 44% of the exploratory excisions were thus superfluous. On the other hand, without palpatory findings, 294 exploratory excisions were carried out solely because of microcalcifications, and 50 carcinomas were found; 83% of the exploratory excisions were thus superfluous here. The proportion of early cancers/minimal cancers/early cases discovered on the basis of microcalcifications in relation to the exploratory excisions carried out because of microcalcifications is 1.7%, 4.0%, or 7.8%, depending on the definition. Even with the "most generous" definition, more than 92% of the exploratory excisions carried out because of microcalcifications are superfluous with regard to diagnosis of early breast cancer. Citoler (1978) arrived at a similar result. He evaluated the histological diagnoses of the cases operated on at the University Department of Gynecology and Obstetrics in Cologne because of microcalcifications. He found noninfiltrating ductal carcinomas in only 4.4%–5.3% of all exploratory excisions.

The question thus arises as to whether such a "result" must be accepted or whether one should attempt to improve it. However, in my opinion a better differential diagnosis of microcalcifications can only become possible if we achieve a better definition of what microcalcifications of malignant or benign genesis look like.

Since the discovery of microcalcifications in breast cancer by Leborgne in 1951, these have been characterized in many ways (or "grouped") in the literature. A critical analysis of these descriptions reveals that mere impressions are given in 14 of 17 descriptions. Besides repeated references to punctiform microcalcifications, the following formulations are used: "Salt grain" (Leborgne 1951; Willemin 1972); "sand grain" (Egan 1965); "crystalline" (Gershon-Cohen 1970; Hoeffken and Lanyi 1973); "stone smashed with a hammer" or simply "crumbly" (Hoeffken and Lanyi 1973, 1981; Lanyi 1977b); "needle-shaped" or "like broken-off needle tips" (Gros 1963; Ingleby and Gershon-Cohen 1960; Barth 1977); "bizarre" or "irregular" (Egan 1965; Hoeffken and Lanyi 1973; Barth 1977; Frischbier and Lobeck 1977; Bjurstam 1978); "drop-like" (Lanyi 1977b); and "tip-like" (Egan 1965).

Only three papers have been found whose authors have attempted to describe the various configurations of "cancer-specific" microcalcifications: according to Moskowitz (1979) the diagnosis of a carcinoma is almost certain when the calcifications are in the form of lines or branches, and less certain when the calcifications are small, punctiform, angular, dispersed between larger irregular calcifications, or localized in one or several groups. The diagnosis is also less certain when small numerous irregular calcifications are found in an area of less than 1 cm². The chance of diagnosing a carcinoma is very slight when an isolated group of small irregular or smooth dense or hollow microcalcifications is present.

Le Gal et al. (1976) have compared the microcalcifications in 27 carcinomas with those in 33 benign alterations and classified these into five groups depending on their form: (a) annular (exclusively in benign cases); (b) punctiform (mainly in carcinomas, but also in benign cases); (c) very fine, hardly visible (also in both carcinomas and benign alterations); (d) punctiform, irregular; and (e) worm-like (exclusively in carcinomas). Egan et al. (1980)

have arrived at the conclusion that the relatively fine calcifications with major variations in form indicate a carcinoma. However, the symptoms are so unspecific that all punctiform microcalcifications detected radiologically have to be investigated histologically.

My objective was to search for principles allowing better differentiation of "benign" and "malignant" microcalcifications by means of an objective, precise, and reproducible analysis of their form. This was achieved with a set of technically perfect mammograms taken from a sample which was specified as precisely as possible histological by I means.

On the basis of the analysis of 153 microcalcifications groups or 5,641 individual microcalcifications in malignant lesions and 136 microcalcification groups in benign lesions, an attempt was made to create a system of differential diagnosis which permits a better yield.

In all cases submitted to analysis the sole radiologic symptom was grouped microcalcification and radiography of the excised material had preceded its histological examination. A further requirement was likewise that the calcifications were situated within the histological sections and that their relationship to the pathologic process concerned was described.

Two characteristics of grouped microcalcifications were analyzed:

1. The configuration of the group as a whole ("configuration"), describing its shape and contours.
2. The form of the single microcalcification ("form").

Analysis of Configuration and Contour of Microcalcification Groups in Intraductal Carcinomas

The form and the shape of 153 microcalcification groups were analyzed and systematized in 114 patients. In 16 cases, 2–8 groups were found (Lanyi 1977a, 1982). The microcalcifications delimiting the groups and situated on their outside borders were linked together by crayon lines under four-fold lens magnification. A proportion of the cases was analyzed using photographic magnification. Seven types of configurations can be differentiated (Fig. 1). The triangular or trapezoid configuration (Figs. 2–5) was found in 65% of groups. A square/rectangular configuration (possibly with a sharp end) is detected in 9.5% (Fig. 6), bottle and club shape in 4% each (Fig. 7a and b), propeller or stellate form (Fig. 8) in 5.5%, rhomboid configuration in 5.5% (Fig. 9), and finally line or branch form in 4% (Fig. 10a and b). In 3%, the microcalcification groups cannot be classified into any of these configurations. No roundish or ovoid calcification groups were found. In the vast majority of the cases the groups show the same configuration in both planes. However, in a number of cases the configuration was different in the two planes (Fig. 11A and B).

When the group form is related to the group size, it can be shown that larger groups are more likely to be triangular or trapezoid in form, whereas in groups with under 100 mm² surface a triangular or trapezoid configuration was found only in half the cases.

(65%)   (9.5%)   (4.0%)   (5.0%)   (4.0%)   (5.5%)   (4.0%)   (3.0%)

Fig. 1. Different configurations of microcalcification groups in intraductal carcinomas

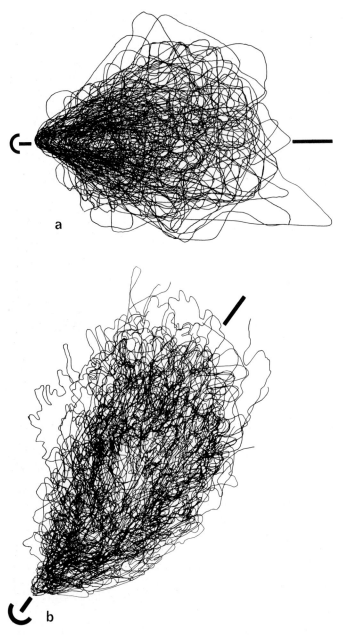

Fig. 2. a Superposition of the contours of 153 microcalcification (mc) groups in patients with intraductal carcinoma as seen in mediolateral mammograms. Each group was magnified to a standard size by means of a projection system, and all groups were superimposed on a drawing board. As can be seen from the drawings, mc groups in intraductal carcinomas most commonly have a triangular configuration. **b** Superposition of the contours of 60 lactiferous ducts contrasted during galactography. Technique as described in Note similarity of **a** and **b**

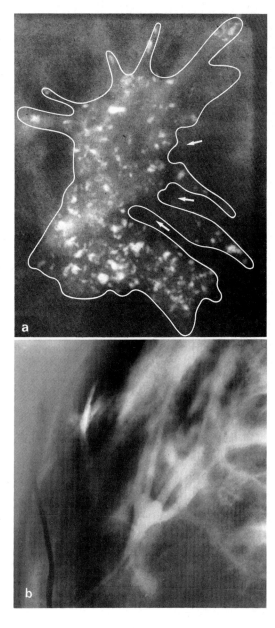

Fig. 3. a Triangular group of polymorphic mcs with firtree-like processes and indentation directing posteriorly towards the chest wall (swallow tail) (*arrows*). Noninfiltrating comedocarcinoma (2 cm diameter). Such indentations and processes are very rarely seen in such small carcinomas. **b** The histoanatomical basis of the processes and indentations can be explained by the galactogram showing the anatomical course and distribution of the lactiferous ducts

There are almost always firtree-like processes in the larger groups of malignant genesis and indentations resembling swallow tails pointing towards the chest wall (Fig. 5). In the smaller groups these phenomena are found less frequently (Fig. 3a). Whereas the microcalcifications in the small groups are densely packed and distributed homogeneously, they are scattered less homogeneously with islet-like gaps free of microcalcifications in the large groups (Fig. 4a and 7b). All these variable signs mentioned above can be explained by the three-plane anatomical arborization of the lactiferous duct system and its mammographic representation in two planes.

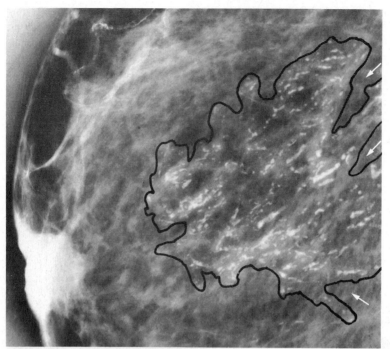

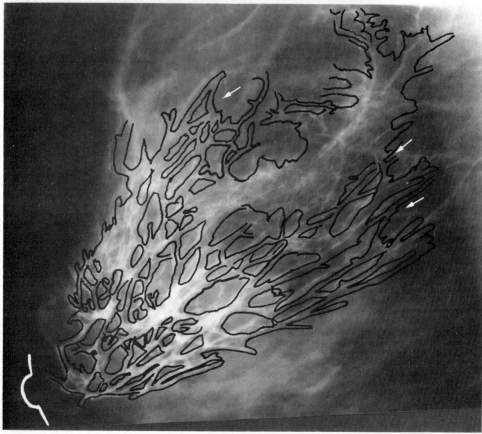

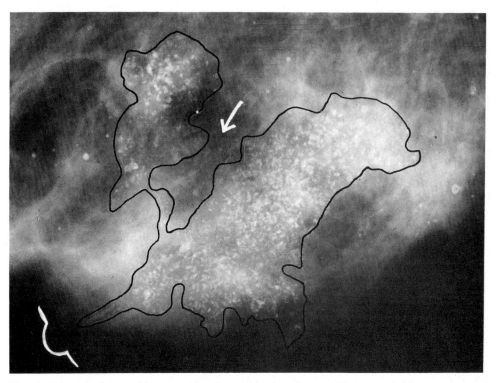

Fig. 5. Triangular/trapezoid group of polymorphic, largely punctiform mcs with processes and swallow-like indentation (*arrow*), the tip of the triangle pointing towards the nipple. Complete involvement of the lobus; calcium deposits in sebaceous glands. Histology mixed cribriform and comedocarcinoma

Since the microcalcifications in intraductal carcinomas are cast stones of the lactiferous ducts, they depict their course. Hence, the larger the group is, the more marked the lactiferous system character with its triangular/trapezoid configuration will be, and vice versa. The smaller the microcalcification group, the more often configurations other than these forms will occur. However, the configurations of small groups can also be determined by the anatomy: the line/branch form arises when only a small region of the lactiferous duct is infiltrated by the carcinoma and consequently calcified. The club-bottle configuration corresponds to an anatomical variant (Fig. 7). The propeller configuration and the dragon form may be due to the projection (Fig. 8). The contour processes which give the larger groups a firtree-like appearance as well as the swallow-tail phenomenon and the islet-like gaps which correspond to interductal fat tissue islets are all symptoms which can be explained on the basis of many galactographies (Fig. 4b).

◀

Fig. 4. a Comedocarcinoma. Mammogram: triangular trapezoid group of polymorphic mcs, predominantly lines and branches. Note the islet-like gaps within the group, its indentations (*arrows*) and processes; **b** galactogram (a different case): the islet-like gaps correspond to interductal fat tissue, the lactiferous ducts diverging from the swallow-like processes and indentations in between pointing dorsally to the chest wall (*arrows*)

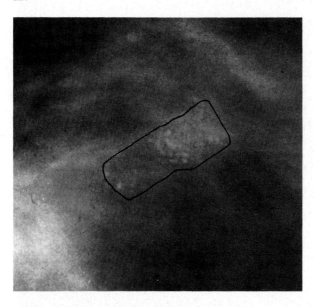

Fig. 6. Square/rectangular group of mcs with moderate polymorphism and branched mcs on the center of the group. Histology: mixed papillary and comedocarcinoma

Analysis of Configuration and Contour of Microcalcification Groups of Benign Genesis

To check the specificity of the above group configurations found in intraductal carcinomas, the configurations of 136 microcalcification groups of histologically benign genesis (in 107 patients) were also analyzed (Lanyi 1982). Since the microcalcification groups of benign origin (like those of malignant genesis) have no uniform etiology, their shapes also had to be arranged and analyzed in terms of histopathological diagnoses. Three different entities can be differentiated:

Microcalcification Groups of the Lactogenic System (n = 92)

These include the microcalcification groups localized within the cystically dilated acini of the lobules or in the mastopathic calcium-milk cysts. These microcalcifications are calcium-containing secretions that have coagulated to varying degrees; in the mammogram

▶

Fig. 7. a Group of polymorphic mcs with a bottle-like configuration. Discrepancy between large extension of the mixed papillary and comedocarcinoma histologically and only small number of mcs in the mammogram. Localization of the mcs within lactiferous ducts is proven by the linear and branched form of the individual mcs and by the orientation towards the nipple of the tip of the group. This corresponds with the malignant infiltration of the main duct found histologically. **b** Mcs in all parts of a comedo carcinoma spreading across a complete lobus. The configuration of the mc group is similar to that in **a**. According to the histological type, there is marked polymorphism with linear and branched mcs, gaps within the group, processes and indentations, the tip of the group pointing to the nipple. The latter phenomenon corresponds to malignant infiltration of a main duct histologically. **c** In the galactogram of an other case, the bottle-like or club-like formation of mc groups can be explained anatomically by secondary lactiferous ducts arising like fingers from the main duct

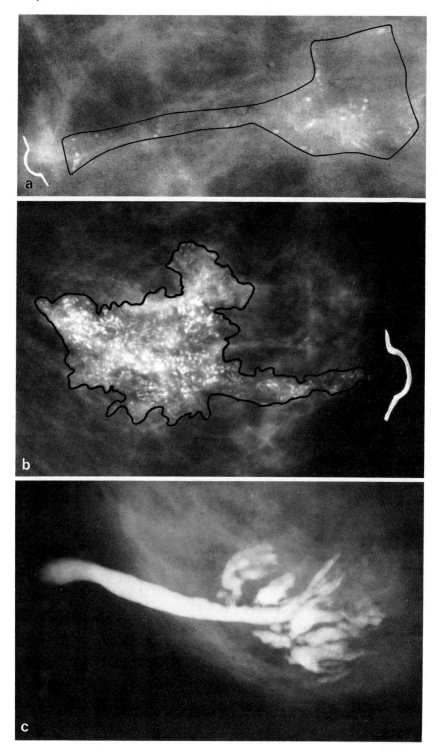

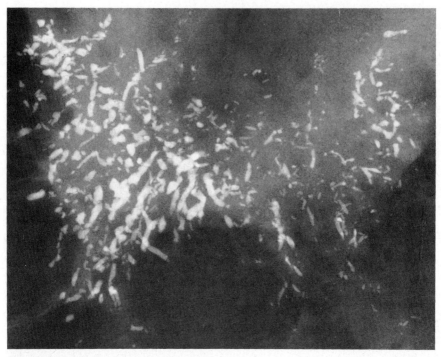

Fig. 8. Propeller- or butterfly-shaped group of polymorphic, predominantly branched mcs in a comedocarcinoma

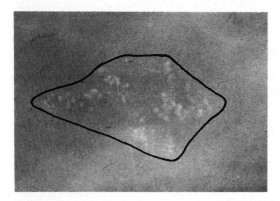

Fig. 9. Rhomboid group of mcs with moderate polymorphism in a mixed lobulaer and comedocarcinoma

they mark the shape and size of the cystic cavities they fill. These cysts arise in the lobules (Fig. 12). The stages of cyst development from the normal acini in order are lobular hypertrophy; blunt duct adenosis (Foote and Stewart 1945); microcystic adenosis; finally, when the lobule boundaries are exceeded, microcyst; cyst. (The multilobulated cysts still retain the original acinar structure.) The specific histological form of sclerosing adenosis (fibrosing adenosis) (Foote and Stewart 1945; Hamperl 1939; Urban and Adair 1969) arises by proliferation of the myothelia in the surrounding periacinar intralobular tissue and leads to compression of the acini.

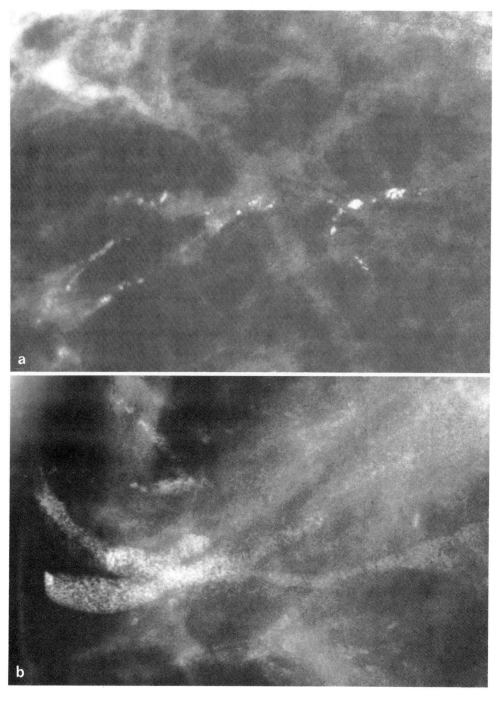

Fig. 10. a Branched group of predominantly punctiform, occasionally linear mcs in an occult in situ comedocarcinoma. Many of the densely packed punctiform mcs are still single-standing, but later they will clot and coalesce to form lines and branches; **b** lactiferous ducts completely filled with multiple, mostly punctiform mcs: cribriform carcinoma

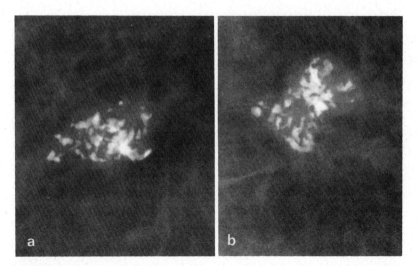

Fig. 11a, b. The form of the mc group varies with the projection: craniocaudal view, triangle (**a**), mediolateral view, propeller (**b**)

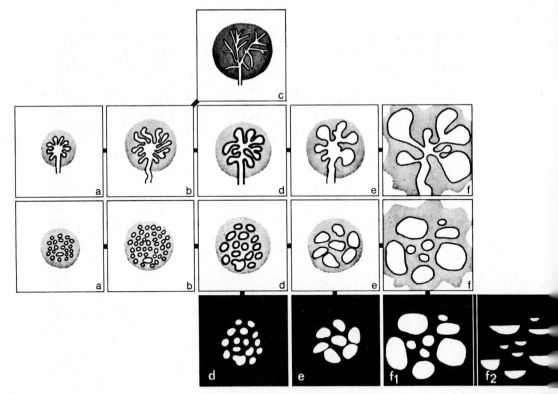

Fig. 12. Schematic of development of mammary dysplasia: *Top,* longitudinal sections. *a* normal lobules; *b* lobular epithelial hyperplasia; *c* sclerosing adenosis; *d* blunt-duct adenosis; *e* microcystic adenosis; *f* microcystic mammary dysplasia; *middle,* same stages as above; cross section without sclerosing adenosis; *bottom,* mcs in blunt-duct adenosis (*d*), microcystic adenosis (*e*), microcystic mammary dysplasia (calcium-milk cysts) in the craniocaudal (f_1) and mediolateral (f_2) view) (tea-cup phenomenon)

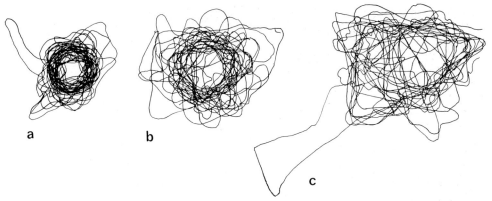

Fig. 13. a Superposition of the contours of 58 mc groups in blunt-duct and sclerosing adenosis, lateral views (technique as in Fig. 2a). Configuration of the mc group is predominantly roundish or oval (43/58 cases). **b** Superposition of the contours of 34 mc groups in patients with calcium-milk cysts; craniocaudal views. In most cases, the configuration of the mc groups is roundish or amorphous. In cases of triangular groups, there are never lateral processes which are typical for larger intraductal carcinomas. **c** Superposition of the contours of 29 mc groups in benign intraductal lesions (epithelial hyperplasia, stasis of secretion, plasma cell mastitis). There was a triangular group in 26/29 cases

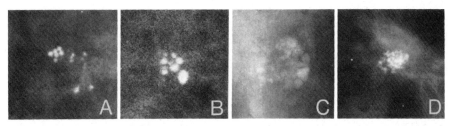

Fig. 14A−D. A set of microcystic foci of blunt-duct adenosis (original size, 3−5 mm). **A** Only a fraction of the dilated blunt acini contain calcium deposits. The configuration of the mc group tends to be oval. The septa between the acini can be seen very clearly at the top; **B** oval group of mcs with good visibility of the intercystic septa trough the contrasting calcium secretions; **C** roundish group of mcs in microcystic adenosis. The dilated acini look more cystic than blunt, the borders of the lobule are still respected. "Facetted" mcs (morula); **D** predominantly blunt-duct adenosis, partly sclerosing adenosis, at the bottom a few linear mcs. Despite minimal polymorphism of the individual mcs, roundish form of the group avoids incorrect diagnosis of a malignant process

The configurations of 92 histologically confirmed intracystic grouped microcalcifications (58 microcystic (blunt duct) or sclerosing adenosis and 34 grouped calcium-milk cysts) were analyzed. In small or microcystic (blunt duct) adenoses and sclerosing adenoses the configuration was roundish/oval in 43 cases, and amorphous in four cases; a triangular form was detected in only 11 cases (Figs. 13 and 14). The groups consisting of calcium-milk cysts had roundish and amorphous configurations in two-thirds of the cases (Fig. 15a, b) and triangular configurations in one-third. The firtree-like processes and the indentations of the group, as described in the intraductal carcinomas, however, are not seen even in the larger triangular groups of benign origin. Instead, the contours are smooth or only slightly undulant. This is because the intracystic microcalcifications are not related to the lactiferous duct system and thus do not follow its lumina, but have the size and form of a lobe or lobule (Fig. 15c).

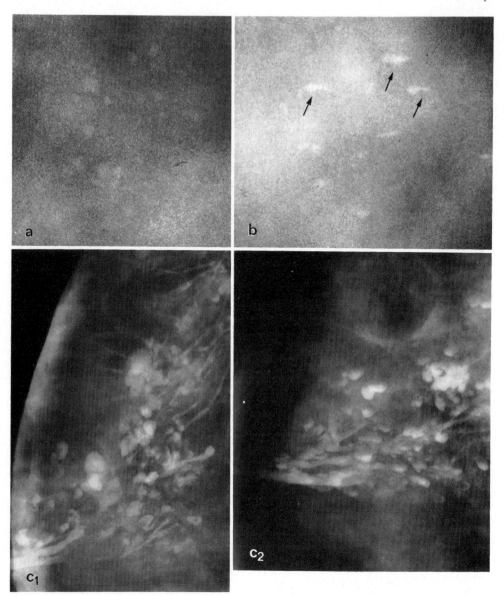

Fig. 15a–c. Grouped calcium milk cysts (original diameter of the group 18 mm). **a** Craniocaudal view: pale roundish mc forming a rounding group; **b** mediolateral view: change of shape of the individual mcs: some linear, some tea cup shape; **c** galactographic demonstration of numerous small terminal cysts: c_1 craniocaudal view (roundish), c_2 mediolateral view (several tea cups. Similarly, the appearance of the small cysts changes if they are filled with calcium milk instead of radiologic contrast agent

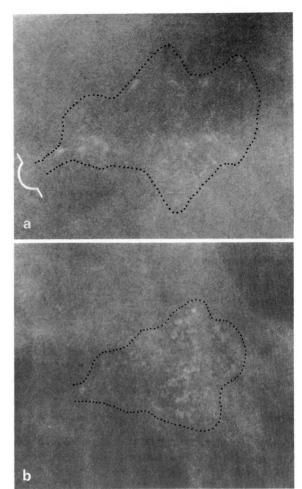

Fig. 16. a Triangular group of pale, somewhat polymorphic microcalcifications in severe papillomatosis with focal atypias, the tip of the triangle pointing towards the nipple; **b** triangular/rhomboid group of markedly pale predominantly monomorphic mcs in a plasma cell mastitis, histologically localized within the walls of the obliterated ducts, thus outlining their course

Microcalcification Groups of the Milk-Draining System (n = 29)

Benign microcalcifications of the lactiferous system arise due to calcium impregnation of the congested secretions with or without epithelial proliferation of various degrees, or in comedomastitis. Of the 29 cases of this type investigated, 26 groups had the mostly triangular shape described in the intraductal carcinomas (Fig. 16), i.e., the "triangular principle" is not characteristic for carcinoma, but for the intraductal localization.

Microcalcification Groups Outside the Milk-Draining System (n = 15)

Of the eight groups of microcalcifications with histologically proven fibroadenoma, five were roundish/oval (Fig. 17) and one was amorphous. Of the seven adipose tissue necroses, two were circular and two amorphous. The remaining cases had shown similar configurations to that of the intraductal processes.

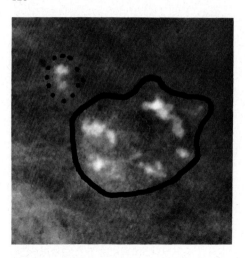

Fig. 17. Two neighboring roundish groups of slightly polymorphic mcs, punctiform, clumpy, and also some branched mc. Histology: peri- and intracanalicular fibroadenoma

Of the 107 microcalcification groups investigated that were not localized intraductally, 79 had a roundish/oval or amorphous configuration. If any configuration of the calcification group except roundish, oval or amorphous were to be taken as an indication for exploratory excision, many such operations (79/107 in this mater could be avoided.

Analysis of the Form of Individual Microcalcifications in Intraductal Carcinomas

For more precise characterization of the microcalcifications in malignant lesions, the individual microcalcifications were investigated for characteristics of their form. In all 5,641 individual microcalcifications from 100 histologically verified intraductal carcinomas were analyzed (Lanyi 1983). The microcalcifications were projected onto a drawing board (magnification 20 times) and their outlines drawn on paper. Four readily definable and frequently recurring forms were detected (Fig. 18):
1) Punctiform, of varying size.
2) Bean form.
3) Undulaling line of various lengths (already described earlier by Le Gal et al. 1976 and by Willemin 1972).
4) Branching form (also described by Moskowitz 1979) or V, W, X, Y, or Z form.
In addition, microcalcifications were found in 55% of the groups whose form could not be classified under one of the above configurations. It was characteristic that monomorphism of the punctiform microcalcifications was found only in 5% of the microcalcification groups of malignant genesis: these carcinomas were mainly of the papillary/cribriform type histologically, and the groups were very small (5–15 microcalcifications). Beyond 15 microcalcifications not a single group had exclusively punctiform microcalcifications. In 95% of all groups polymorphism of the microcalcifications was detected, which varied in degree (Fig. 19a–c).
An attempt was made to analyze the percentages of the individual microcalcification forms in relation to group size (i.e., the number of microcalcifications) but independently of the histological categories (Fig. 19). It was shown that the smaller the group, the larger the number of punctiform microcalcifications. On the other hand, the percentage of bean-,

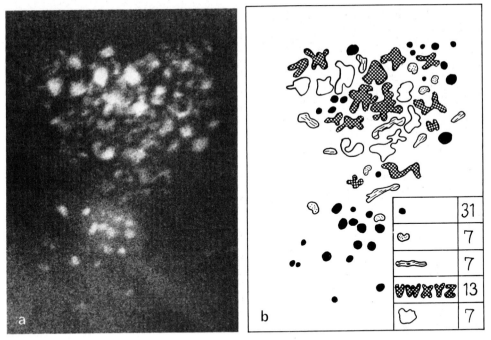

Fig. 18. a Triangular group of polymorphic microcalcifications in an intraductal carcinoma; **b** schematic showing technique for analysis of form of individuals mcs

line-, and branch-shaped and amorphous microcalcifications also shows a certain tendency to increase with increasing group size. In the carcinomas with predominantly comedo parts (Fig. 20B) the number of punctiform microcalcifications is somewhat lower, whereas in the carcinomas with predominantly papillary/cribriform parts (Fig. 20C) the picture is dominated by punctiform microcalcifications. The ratio between the punctiform and remaining configurations appears to be subject to the specific histological characteristics of the lactiferous duct carcinomas. This phenomenon can be explained by the different localization of the microcalcifications in the different histological types. In comedocarcinomas, the punctiform, bean-shaped, line-shaped, branching, and amorphous microcalcifications are in the center of the lactiferous gland lumina, because they are calcifications of the centrally necrotized tumor tissue. The line-shaped microcalcifications arise from the fusion of punctiform and bean-shaped microcalcifications and the various branching microcalcifications, when the process takes place in the region of the branches (Figs. 21 and 22A).
On the other hand, in cribriform carcinomas, the punctiform microcalcifications are situated within the lacunae of the sponge-like carcinoma tissue, the vesicular form of these cavities determining the size (around 0.1 mm) and shape of these microcalcifications (Fig. 22B). Since pure forms of the basic histological types probably practically never occur, at least one line-shaped calcification (Fig. 19a) is also seen in the smaller papillary cribriform carcinomas. The fact that from 17 microcalcifications upwards no single case (of whatever ultrastructure) showed monomorphism is likely to be especially important for the differential diagnostic considerations in benign cases with numerous monomorphic punctiform microcalcifications.

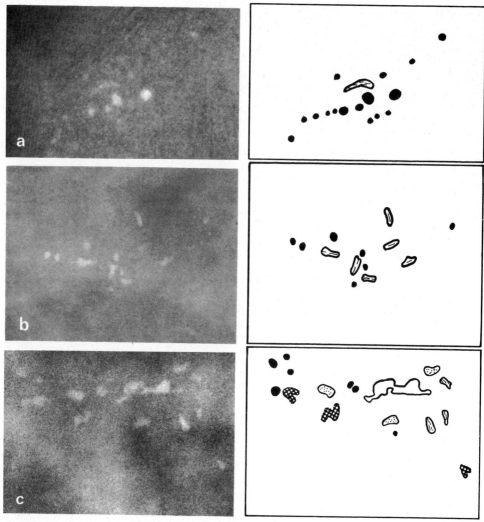

Fig. 19. a Flat triangular group of punctiform mcs. There is also one single linear mc which gives rise to the suspicion of intraductal localization as does the configuration of the whole group. Occult comedocarcinoma; **b** rhomboid group of mcs with an equal number of punctiform and linear mcs. Occult comedocarcinoma; **c** flat propeller-like mc with considerable polymorphism (points, lines, branches, V, Z, amorphous). Occult comedocarcinoma

The Form of Microcalcifications of Benign Genesis

The form of microcalcifications in benign processes also depends on the localization and pathomorphological conditions.

1) When the calcified secretion is localized within the cystically dilated acini of microcystic/blunt duct adenosis the calcifications are roundish or "faceted" on the contact surfaces. The intercystic septa become visible through the contrast of the calcium secretion (Fig. 14) (Lanyi and Citoler 1981).

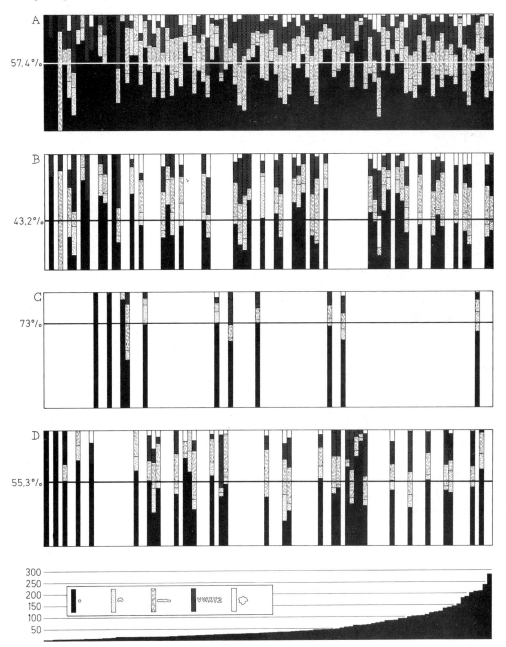

Fig. 20A–D. Each column represents one of 100 mcs: **A** all groups, irrespective of histological subtypes: punctiform mcs 57.4%, all other mcs 42.6%; **B** only comedocarcinomas: inversion of the ratio of mcs; **C** papillary and cribriform carcinomas: nearly 75% of all mcs are punctiform; **D** mixed types (some comedocarcinoma, some papillary and cribriform): nearly equal numbers of mcs punctiform and other mcs

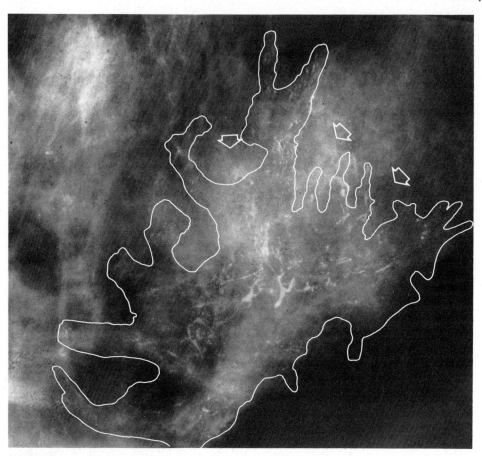

Fig. 21. Noninfiltrating comedocarcinoma. The large group of polymorphic mcs has a triangular configuration with several processes, indentations directed towards chest wall (*arrow*) and islet-like gaps corresponding to interductal fat tissue. There are punctiform, linear and branched mcs

2) When the acinar cysts develop and extend beyond the lobule boundaries, the calcium milk can either give rise to roundish, chiefly pale, microcalcifications in one or both planes or it can show the form change characteristic for calcium-milk cysts, depending on the direction of the x-ray. In the latter case, roundish, pale calcifications with somewhat blurred contours are seen in the craniocaudal projection, whereas in the lateral projection calcifications rounded off towards the bottom, forming a flattened niveau at the top, are to be seen. This picture, resembling a tea cup, is due to sedimentation of the calcium particles in the calcium milk in the upright position, only marking the floor of the cyst in the lateral projection, and leaving the upper contour of the cyst unmarked. On the other hand, on the craniocaudal projection the outer contour is marked all around by calcium milk (Lanyi 1977; Sickles and Abele 1981) (Fig. 15).

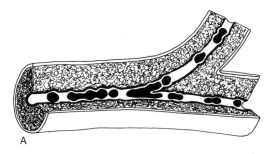

Fig. 22A, B. Schematics showing the pathogenesis of different mcs in the two subtypes of intraductal carcinomas: **A** Comedocarcinoma. Solid tumor with the calcifications localized centrally within the necrotic tissue. There is a tendency for punctiform mcs to coalesce to smaller or longer, sometimes undulated linear branches; **B** cribriform/papillary carcinoma. The mcs are situated within the lacunae of the sponge-like carcinoma tissue

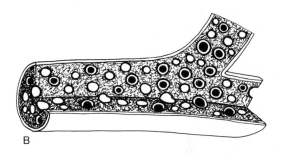

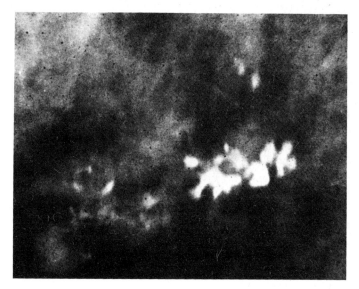

Fig. 23. Polymorphism of the mcs with intracanicular fibroadenoma

3) In the mainly intracanalicular fibroadenoma, the calcifications are due to necrobiosis. They are clumpy with rounded edges (Fig. 17). On the other hand, secretion calcifications in mainly intracanalicular fibroadenomas can show the same polymorphism as is usually seen in intraductal comedocarcinomas (Fig. 23). This is because in intracanalicular fibroadenomas the calcifications are also situated in the branching lactiferous ducts and are cast stones of the ducts, as they are in comedocarcinomas.

Table 1. Results of a study of 297 patients in whom surgery was performed (University of Cologne) solely on the basis of grouped microcalcifications with no knowledge of the histology

42 Malignant	correct positiv	41
	false negativ	1
255 Benign	correct negativ	187
	false positiv	68

Sensitivity: 97.6%

Specificity: 73.3%

4) A picture which can be confused with incipient small intraductal carcinoma will arise in a benign process, fibrosing adenosis. This phenomenon requires further detailed analysis. However, it can be assumed that the elongated, deformed acini are marked here by calcified secretions, and thereby simulate the polymorphism of the small intraductal carcinoma.
5) Whereas many fibroadenomas and fibrosing adenoses cause appreciable difficulties in the differential diagnosis of microcalcifications, the secretion calcifications of plasma cell mastitis are mostly recognized without difficulty as such on the basis of their elongated, linear appearance and their arrangement resembling tracer munition.

The Touchstone

To test the efficiency of the system of differential diagnosis sketched above, 297 cases from the University of Cologne operated on solely on the basis of grouped microcalcifications were investigated without knowledge of the histology (Lanyi and Neufang 1984).

According to the results (Table 1) the sensitivity is 97.6%, the specificity 73.3% and 63% of the exploratory excisions could have been dispensed with. The false-positive cases are mostly fibrosing adenoses, small, mainly intracanalicular fibroadenomas, and liponecroses. The grouped calcium-milk cysts and the calcium deposits in the foci of blunt duct adenosis are readily screened out as not requiring exploratory excision. A further analysis of the microcalcifications in fibrosing adenosis, fibroadenoma, and liponecrosis would probably make even better results possible. In this way, the false-positive diagnoses mentioned above could be reduced, without neopardizing the detection of early cancers.

References

Barth V (1977) Atlas der Brustdrüsenerkrankungen. Enke, Stuttgart
Bässler R (1978) Pathologie der Brustdrüse. In: Doerr V, Seifert G, Uehlinger E (eds) Spezielle pathologische Anatomie, vol II/11. Springer, Berlin Heidelberg New York
Bjurstam NG (1978) Radiography of the female breast and axilla. Acta Radiol [Suppl] 357

Citoler P (1978) Microcalcification of the breast. In: Early diagnosis of breast cancer. 8th International Symposium of the BGK Düsseldorf, June 1976. Fischer, Stuttgart

Egan RL (1964) Mammography. Thomas, Springfield Illinois

Egan RL, Sweeney MB, Sewell CW (1980) Intramammary calcifications without an associated mass in benign and malignant diseases. Radiology 137 : 1

Foote FW, Stewart FW (1945) Comparative studies of cancerous versus non cancerous breasts. Ann Surg 121 : 6

Frischbier HJ, Lohbeck HV (1977) Frühdiagnostik des Mammakarzinoms. Thieme, Stuttgart

Le Gal M, Durand JC, Lauvent M, Pellier D (1976) Conduite à tenir devant une mammographie rérélatrice de microcalcifications groupées, sand tumeur palpable. Nouv Presse Med 5: 1623

Galleger HS, Martin J (1971) An orientation of the concept of minimal breast cancer. 28: 1505

Gershon-Cohen J (1970) Atlas of mammography. Springer, Berlin Heidelberg New York

Gershon-Cohen J, Ingleby H, Hermel MB (1955) Occult carcinoma of breast. Arch Surg 70: 385

Gros C (1963) Les maladies du sein. Masson, Paris

Hamperl H (1939) Über die Myothelien (Myo-epithelialen Elemente) der Brustdrüse. Virchows Arch Pathol Anat 305: 171

Hoeffken W, Lanyi M (1973) Röntgenuntersuchung der Brust. Thieme, Stuttgart

Hoeffken W, Lanyi M (1981) Erkrankungen der Brustdrüse. In: Schinz R, Bansch WE, Frommhold W, Glauner R, Uehlinger F, Wellaver J (eds) Lehrbuch der Röntgendiagnostik, vol II2. Thieme, Stuttgart

Ingleby H, Gershon-Cohen J (1960) Comparative anatomy, pathology and roentgenology of the breast. University of Pennsylvania Press, Philadelphia

Kindermann G (1977) Über Definition, Diagnostik und Behandlung der sogenannten "Frühfälle" des Mammakarzinoms. Geburtshilfe Frauenheilkd 37: 829

Lanyi M (1977a) Differentialdiagnose der Mikroverkalkungen: Die verkalkte mastopathische Mikrocyste. Radiologe 17: 217

Lanyi M (1977b) Differentialdiagnose der Mikroverkalkungen: Röntgenbildanalyse von 60 intraductalen Carcinomen, das "Dreiecksprinzip". Radiologe 17: 213

Lanyi M (1982a) Formanalyse von 152 Mikroverkalkungsgruppen maligner Genese. Das "Dreiecksprinzip". Fortschr Röntgenstr 136: 77

Lanyi M (1982b) Formanalyse von 136 Mikroverkalkungsgruppen benigner Genese. Fortschr Röntgenstr 136: 182

Lanyi M (1983) Formanalyse von 5641 Mikroverkalkungen bei 100 Milchgangskarzinomen: Die Polymorphie. Fortschr Röntgenstr 139: 240

Lanyi M, Citoler P (1981) Differentialdiagnostik der Mikroverkalkungen: Die kleinzystische (blunt duct) Adenose. Fortschr Röntgenstr 134: 225

Lanyi M, Neufang KFR (1984) Möglichkeiten und Grenzen der Differentialdiagnostik gruppierter intramammärer Mikroverkalkungen. Fortschr Röntgenstr 141: 430

Leborgne R (1951) Diagnosis of tumors of the breast by simple roentgenography, calcifications in carcinomas. AJR 65: 1

Moskowitz M (1979) Screening is not diagnosis. Radiology 133: 265

Sickles EA, Abele JS (1981) Milk of calcium within tiny benign breast cysts. Radiology 141: 655

Urban J (1976) Changing patterns of breast cancer. Cancer 37: 111

Urban JA, Adair FE (1969) Sclerosing adenosis. Cancer 2: 625

Willemin A (1972) Les images mammographiques. Karger, Basel

Zippel HH, Hardt M, Citoler P (1981) Kriterien zur Abgrenzung von Frühfällen des Mammakarzinoms. Dtsch Med Wochenschr 106: 605

Diagnostic Value of Galactography in the Detection of Breast Cancer

G. Kindermann

Universitäts-Frauenklinik der Freien Universität Berlin,
Pulsstrasse 4, 1000 Berlin 19, Federal Republic of Germany

Introduction

Other than a lump, skin retraction, or pain in the breast, nipple discharge is the most common complaint of patients with breast problems. Nonpregnant patients with a serosanguinous, watery, or bloody discharge become alarmed as they think it may be due to cancer. The color of the discharge is of little value for the diagnosis. Cytology can be valuable but is not totally reliable. The method of choice is galactography (ductography, contrast mammography). Our experience with this method since 1964 is reported in this paper.

Method

In all cases of unilateral (or sometimes bilateral) pathologic discharge from the nipple galactography is performed. Patients found to have galactorrhea are excluded from the study. We no longer use cytology because of its lack of accuracy. The technique is simple. The patient is placed in a comfortable supine position on the X-ray table. The breast is gently stroked with radial movements toward the nipple to localize the area producing the discharge. Only patients with an actual discharge are eligible for this procedure. After the duct involved has been located the nipple, the areola, and the surrounding skin are cleaned with an antiseptic. A rounded smooth dilator is used to gently explore the nipple and widen the ostium. The duct is then cannulated with a blunt, thin needle. A water-soluble contrast medium (60% urografin) is used. In most cases 0.2–0.5 ml is sufficient to fill the duct. It is important to inject the correct amount of contrast fluid to avoid its escape into the breast tissue. When this happens, the evaluation of the X-ray may be impossible or very difficult. The patient may also experience pain.

Immediately after the injection the needle is withdrawn, and mammograms are made in the lateral and vertical views. The normal galactogram shows the typical milk ducts and their branches. A galactogram is considered pathologic in the presence of filling defects, complete or incomplete blockage, and/or dilatation with irregular outlines or caliber changes.

For the surgical procedure the X-ray pictures are placed on a bright screen in the operating theater. This enables us to direct the orientation during surgery. In most cases we have removed the involved milk duct area through a periareolar incision. The apex of the excised tissue near the nipple is marked with a suture for the pathologist. The wound is drained for 24–28 h with a redon drain.

After the operation the surgical specimen is fixed in its original shape on a cork board for the laboratory work. After a 24-h fixation the excised specimen is trimmed into several tissue blocks, so that most milk ducts are cut longitudinally for microscopic evaluation. Step sections of these blocks are necessary, since very small intraductal changes are generally encountered.

Early Breast Cancer
Edited by J. Zander and J. Baltzer
© Springer-Verlag Berlin Heidelberg 1985

Results

Between 1964 and 1982 (Universitätsfrauenklinik Erlangen/Nürnberg) and 1979 and 1982 (Universitätsfrauenklinik Charlottenburg/Berlin) galactography was performed on 1,694 women with pathologic discharge from the nipple. In 34.9% ductal segment biopsy was necessary secondary to pathologic findings on the X-rays (Table 1). In the majority (65.1%) pathologic X-ray findings in the milk duct system that could have caused the discharge were excluded. The histological results of the biopsied cases are shown in Table 2. No intraductal disease was found in 14 cases (2.3%). In 97.7% an anatomical cause for the discharge was detected microscopically. Most of the lesions were benign (70.1%). The lesions were premalignant or malignant in 27.6% of cases, being invasive carcinomas in 9.4%, carcinomata in situ in 3.0%, and premalignant lesions (i.e., extended intraductal proliferations: solid, adenomatous, or papillary) in 15.2%. Only 1 of the 55 patients with invasive ductal carcinoma had axillary lymph node metastases. This low frequency of axillary lymph node involvement (1.8%) provides a good prognosis for these patients found to have breast cancer.

Table 1. Results of galactography in patients[a] with pathologic discharge from the nipple

Galactography	Cases	Percent
No pathologic findings	1,105	65.1
Pathologic result indicating biopsy	589	34.9
Total	1,694	100.0

[a] Patients seen at the University Hospital for Women, Erlangen/ Nürnberg (1964–1982) and the University Hospital for Women, Charlottenburg, Berlin (1979–1982)

Table 2. Histological results in cases of pathologic galactograms[a]

Histological diagnosis	Cases	Percent
No pathologic findings	14	2.3
Cystic disease	155	26.3
Papilloma	258	43.8
Benign intraductal papillary, solid or adenomatous proliferation	89	15.2
Carcinoma in situ	18	3.0
Carcinoma	55	9.4
Total	589	100.0

[a] Patient from same series as in Table 1

Discussion

Pathologic discharge from the nipple may be the first sign of an underlying malignant intraductal lesion. Neither the color nor the cytology of the discharge can predict the nature of ductal disease with certainty (Barth et al. 1975; Kindermann et al. 1970; Leis 1975). Galactography (contrast mammography) is now the procedure of choice for examination of such cases. The advantage of contrast mammography is the exact localization of the involved ducts and the non-palpable intraductal lesions by X-rays in two planes. In cases of filling defect, dilatation, irregular contours, or blockage in the galactogram, biopsy, i.e., the excision of the involved duct system is necessary. The purpose of galactography is not to predict the nature or extent of the underlying breast disease, but to select and localize the area of surgery.

In our material, a biopsy was necessary in only one-third (34%) of the cases with pathologic discharge. Without any palpable findings the surgeon can only be guided by galactograms in appropriate removal of the breast tissue involved (Kindermann et al. 1970; Kindermann 1977). Good cooperation between radiology and surgery services is needed for success to be achieved in this field. In addition, the histology laboratory must have the capacity to perform the additional work. In our opinion, only extensive laboratory work allows discovery of the small intraductal changes generally encountered.

Conversely, the results show the nonspecificity for cancer: 70.1% of the lesions we found were benign. This diagnostic procedure is therefore not comparable to cytology and colposcopy for cervical cancer. However, since no better method is available, we must expend the extra effort necessary to screen out the 27.6% of premalignant or malignant changes in the duct system of patients with no other symptom than discharge. Since only one patient had lymph node involvement, a good prognosis is expected for those women with cancer, and the procedure may be considered as early detection of intraductal breast cancer.

In addition to the considerable number of occult invasive cancers and carcinomas in situ, many lesions with intraductal proliferations requiring further surgery (e.g., subcutaneous mastectomy) or at least a careful follow-up of the patients in this high-risk group were detected by this method.

Summary

Pathologic discharge from the nipple may be the only symptom of an early stage of carcinoma. Galactography is then the diagnostic method of choice to locate early intraductal, non palpable lesions. The technique of galactography, the adequate surgical approach in the case of pathologic galactograms (milk-duct segment resection), and the appropriate histological workup of the surgical specimen are demonstrated. We report our experience (1964–1982) in 1,694 patients with galactography. In 589 cases a milk-duct segment resection was necessary (34.9%). Histologically we found invasive intraductal cancer in 9.4% and ductal carcinomas in situ in 3.0%. Extensive intraductal solid papillary or adenomatous proliferations were found in 15.2% of the patients subjected to excision and in 43.8% of papillomas. In the case of papilloma this diagnostic procedure is an adequate treatment.

Acknowledgement. I am indebted to Dr. Paterok, (Erlangen) for his help in the evaluation of the material in 1980–1982.

References

Barth W, Müller R, Mayle M (1975) Die weibliche Brustdrüse im Galaktogramm. Dtsch Med Wochenschr 100: 1213

Kindermann G, Ober KG, Rummel W, Weishaar J (1970) Radiographic demonstration of milk duct (galactography) in pathological discharge from the nipple. Excision of milk ducts and an adopted histological work up. Int J Gynaecol Obstet 8: 273

Kindermann G, Rummel W, Weishaar J (1971) Der Wert einer kombinierten Diagnostik der Mammaerkrankungen − Mammographie, Galaktographie, Thermographie, Histologie. Arch Gynacol 211: 39

Kindermann G, Rummel W, Egger H, Weishaar J, Paterok EM, Willgeroth F, Ober KG (1978) Various methods of early detection of breast cancer. In: Grundmann E (ed) Early diagnosis of breast cancer. Fischer, New York

Kindermann G (1977) Über Definition, Diagnostik und Behandlung der sogenannten „Frühfälle" des Mammacarcinoms. Geburtshilfe Frauenheilk 37: 829

Leis HP (1975) Evaluation of nipple discharge. In: Gallager S (ed) Early breast cancer. Wiley, New York

Paulus DD (1975) Contrast mammography. In: Gallager S (ed) Early breast cancer. Wiley, New York

Rummel W, Kindermann G, Egger H. Weishaar J, Willgeroth F, Paterok EM (1976) Pathologische Absonderung aus der Mamma. Galaktographie und histologische Abklärung. Geburtshilfe Frauenheilk 36 : 1062

A Topical View of the Benefit-Risk Ratio in Mammography

Friedrich-Ernst Stieve

Gesellschaft für Strahlen- und Umweltforschung mbH,
Ingolstädter Landstrasse 1, 8042 Neuherberg, Federal Republic of Germany

Introduction

In 1977, the International Commission on Radiological Protection (ICRP) again recommended a system of dose limitation for activities involving human exposure to ionizing radiation. The main recommendations for this system are that (a) no practice shall be adopted unless its introduction produces a positive net benefit; (b) all exposures shall be kept as low as reasonably achievable, economic and social factors being taken into account; and (c) the dose equivalents administered to individuals shall not exceed the limits recommended by the Commission.

In other words, the three major objectives are as follows:

Justification,

Optimization,

Limitation of doses administered to human individuals.

In paragraph 92 of the above-mentioned recommendations the Commission explains the importance of the general recommendations in relation to the medical exposure of patients for diagnostic and therapeutic purposes:

(92) Medical exposure is, in general, subject to most of the Commission's system of dose limitation, that is: unnecessary exposures should be avoided, necessary exposures should be justifiable in terms of benefits that would not otherwise have been received and the doses actually administered should be limited to the minimum amount consistent with the medical benefit to the individual patient. The individual receiving the exposure is himself the direct recipient of the benefit resulting from the procedure. For this reason it is not appropriate to apply the quantitative values of the Commission's recommended dose-equivalent limits to medical exposures.

Similar recommendations or conclusions have been made by other international organizations or commissions, such as the World Health Organization (1980) and the United Nations Scientific Committee on the Effects of Atomic Radiation (UNSCEAR) (1977, 1982). It is, therefore, not surprising to find the same tenor in the report of the Government of the Federal Republic of Germany to the German Bundestag.

In mammography radiation-induced malignant disease is the most important potential late somatic effect of examining the female breast.

According to numerous measurements the genetic effects are negligible as the exposure to the ovary is very low, so that the calculated risk is probably of no importance. For risk evaluations it is therefore only necessary to compare the benefit due to the examination

Early Breast Cancer
Edited by J. Zander and J. Baltzer
© Springer-Verlag Berlin Heidelberg 1985

with the somatic detriment defined as the mathematical expectation of the harm incurred from the exposure of the breast tissue to radiation.

Basis of Risk Estimates for the Effects of Ionizing Radiation

This risk-benefit analysis is based on several assumptions, which should be mentioned first.

1) The *risk factor* for the development of breast cancer following exposure in women is based upon the observation that the female breast is one of the most sensitive organs for cancer induction by ionizing radiation (e.g., BEIR 1972, 1980; UNSCEAR 1977; Mole 1978). The mechanism of induction and promotion of malignant tumors has not yet been fully identified. Quite a number of theories have been proposed, but most have been gradually abandoned, since none could account for the large array of properties of the tumor cell. A critical review of the existing theories is given in the 1977 UNSCEAR Report. Nevertheless, it seems certain that the neoplastic transformation of the breast tissue is the final result of a complex chain of ethological and pathogenic events. Some of the main factors are specified in Fig. 1. The probability that those changes will induce a tumor is very low. Therefore it is characterized as stochastic event, whose probability rather than its severity is regarded as a function of dose.

2) *Typical data* on the estimation of carcinogenetic effects on human beings are collected at relatively high dose levels, e.g., 1 Gy and more. The region of low-level radiation (0.01−0.2 Gy) for x-rays and gamma rays (so-called low LET radiation) in which no reliable data exist is of principal interest in the evaluation of risk levels. Estimates of the effects with these dose ranges are mostly obtained indirectly by linear interpolation between the dose range of interest and the response and the data points at high doses. This relationship is referred to as the "linear, no threshold" relationship (Fig. 2). It contrasts with the curvilinear relationship derived from biological experiments, which is composed of a linear and a linear-quadratic component. This curve is probably the result of the interaction of a multiple event model for radiation carcinogenesis. The straight linear extrapolation of low doses from high doses therefore grossly overestimates the risk factor. It is not yet known, however, whether threshold values exist or not.

3) *Experimental data* are derived from laboratory animals. The incidence of mammary tumors in irradiated mammals varies markedly depending on the strain and the type of the

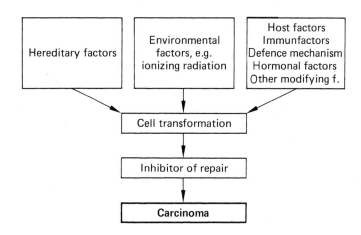

Fig. 1. Factors influencing the development of cell cancer as a sequential process from cell transformation to the neoplastic process

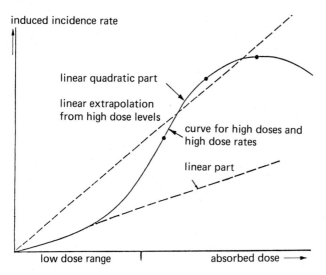

induced incidence rate

linear quadratic part

linear extrapolation
from high dose levels

curve for high doses and
high dose rates

linear part

low dose range | absorbed dose →

Fig. 2. Schematic dose-response relationship curves for radiation-induced cancers. The *curved solid line* is probably the realistic curve for low LET radiation. The *linear extrapolation* from epidemiological data at higher dose levels results in overestimation of risk at low dose levels

tumor (Shellaberger 1976; NCRP 1980). These experiments are performed in genetically homogeneous strains. In contrast, human beings are genetically inhomogeneous, as is shown by the different incidence of mammary tumors in different populations. Any risk estimate concerned with exposure of the breast for the purpose of radiodiagnosis must therefore be considered with caution and strong reservations.

Basis of Risk Calculation for Malignant Tumors of the Breast

For risk calculation it is usual to standardize epidemiological data. Usually the values derived from different studies with higher dose levels are linearly extrapolated to dose levels of 0.01 Gy per million exposed population. This is the only possible way of comparing the radiation risk from different exposures in different populations when the number of malignancies in the irradiated population is sufficient to give statistical significance of the amount by which the expected number of the same malignancies in the control population is exceeded. It is clear from the above-mentioned assumption that such estimates in breast cancer are only approximate, even for the comparison of benefit and risk in the sense of the ICRP recommendations.

Epidemiological Studies on the Incidence of Breast Cancer

Some epidemiological data collected in quite population groups are available. Human epidemiological data are available mainly for three categories of exposure:

Therapeutic Irradiation for Benign Diseases. Several studies estimated the incidence of additional breast tumors following the treatment of postpartum mastitis with x-rays (Mettler et al. 1969; Shore et al. 1977). The most extensive study is the Rochester study, which includes 606 women treated with x-rays, compared for breast cancer incidence with two control groups: one as a check on familial predisposition to cancer and the other to check the possible association of mastitis with breast cancer not treated with x-rays. The incidence rate of breast cancer/1000 per year

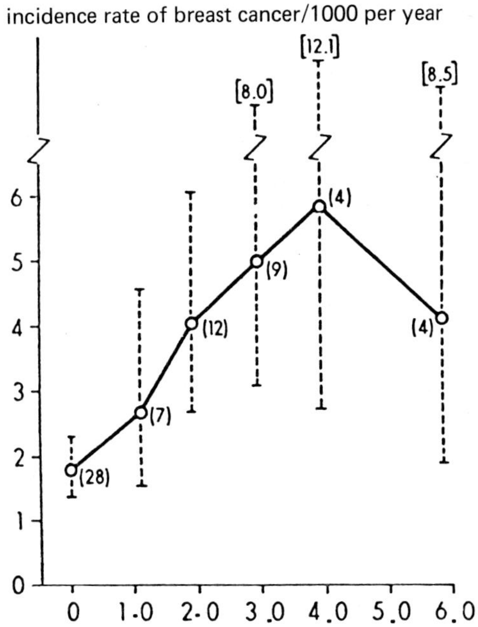

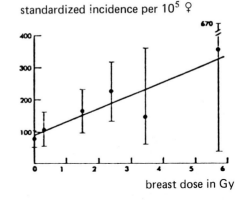

Fig. 3. Breast cancer incidence rate by average dose to both breasts in mastitis patients in the interval 10–34 years after irradiation. *Numbers in parentheses* are the numbers of breast cancer cases in each dose group; *error bars* show 80% confidence intervals. (After Shore et al. 1977)

standardized incidence per 10^5 ♀

Fig. 4. Standardized incidence rate of breast cancer per 100,000 woman-years at risk in pneumothorax patients subjected to fluoroscopy, as a function of estimated cumulative breast dose, with adjustment for age at explosure and duration of follow-up. *Bars* show 80% confidence intervals. (Boice 1979)

breast dose in Gy

incidence rate for breast cancer following an average radiation dose to both breasts in mastitis patients 10–34 years after treatment [taken from the study of Shore et al. (1977)] is given in Fig. 3 with the 80% confidence intervals and numbers of breast cancer cases in each dose group.

Exposure to Multiple Fluoroscopies. Two main epidemiological studies give estimates on the additional risk in women subjected to multiple fluoroscopic examinations during the treatment of tuberculosis with pneumothorax. These are the Nova Scotia study on breast cancer (MacKenzie 1965; Myrden and Hilz 1969, Myrden and Quilan 1974) and the follow-up study of Boice et al. (1977, 1979).

There are, of course, uncertainties affecting dose estimates based on many variables. The standardized incidence rate of breast cancer in fluoroscopic pneumothorax patients per 10,000 women-years (Wy) in women at risk, adjusting for age at exposure and duration of

age-adjusted* breast cancer incidence rates (cases/100.000 women per year)

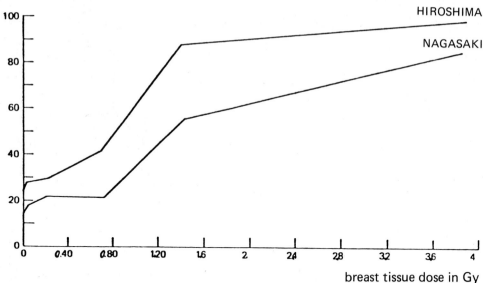

* adjusted to the total age ATB distribution for both cities

Fig. 5. Age-adjusted breast cancer rates versus radiation dose, by city. (After Tokunaga et al. 1979)

follow-up as a functin of estimated cumulative breast doses according to Boice (1979), are given in Fig. 4. The 80% confidence limits are also presented.

A-Bomb Explosions. Two main studies analyze breast cancer incidence as a function of dose among women survivors in Hiroshima and Nagasaki (McGregor et al. 1977; Tokunaga et al. 1979). The group of exposed women is compared with a group of nonirradiated women in Hiroshima and Nagasaki, who had essentially different rates of breast cancer. The age-adjusted dose-response relationship is presented in Fig. 5. The dose estimates for Hiroshima have been subjected to new calculations. But the incidence of additional tumors due to the exposure of ionizing radiation is considered reliable.

When the results are compared the assessment of dose appears generally less favorable for the fluoroscopy group and the A-bomb survivors than for mastitis patients.

To sum up, it can be said that the dose estimates for radiation therapy are more reliable than those for the group of fluoroscopy patients and the survivors of Hiroshima and Nagasaki. But the data as a whole are rather consistent.

The incidence of breast tumors − expressed with reference to a dose of 0.01 Gy and exposure of 1 million persons − is given in Table 1. The data are consistent with other risk estimates and can be used to calculate risk of induction of breast cancer in radiodiagnosis.

Age Dependence. Several epidemiological studies demonstrate that the risk of breast cancer depends on age. The estimates by Boice et al. (Boice and Stone 1978; Boice et al. 1978a, b; Boice 1979) demonstrate that the risk is highest between puberty and the age of 20. The average risk estimates for women exposed at ages between 20 and 40 are similar to those in the quoted studies. Figure 6 demonstrates the incidence of breast tumors as a function of age (data taken from Boice).

Table 1. Incidence of breast tumors per 0.01 Gy and per million persons (UNSCEAR 1977)

Exposure	Risk coefficient/ year (10^{-6})		Risk coefficient/ total (10^{-6})	
	Morbidity	Mortality	Morbidity	Mortality
Fluoroscopy	20–50	6.2	210	110
Therapy	30	8.3	210	60
Hiroshima + Nagasaki	1.5	0.6	30	10

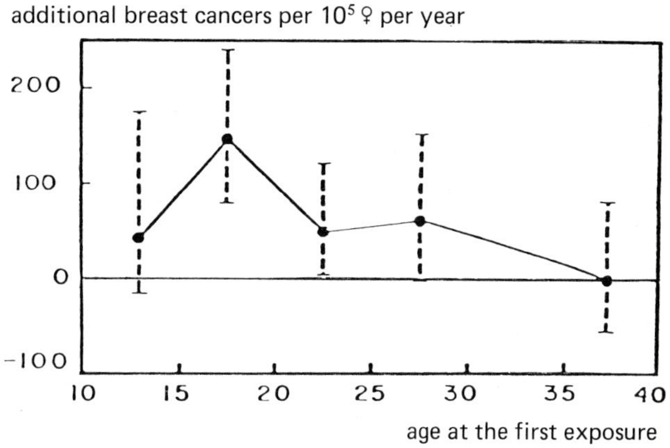

additional breast cancers per 10^5 ♀ per year

Fig. 6. Age-dependence of the incidence of female breast cancer induced by radiation exposure. [Statistical data from Boice (1979)]

age at the first exposure

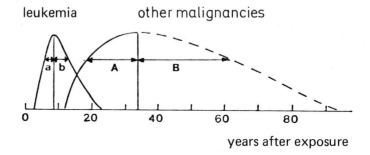

Fig. 7. Frequency distribution for incidence of leukemia and other cancers in a population with a constant survival rate

years after exposure

Latency Period. The time interval between radiation exposure and the diagnosis of breast cancer probably induced by radiation seems to be independent of dose, but it depends heavily on the age at exposure.

This can be concluded from data on breast cancer among high-dose and low-dose atomic bomb survivors (Kerr 1978; Land 1978) and the two medical series. The minimum latency period for women about 25 years of age and older seems to be 5 years. For girls and women between 15 and 25 the average latency period is about 22–25 years (Yoshizawa 1974; Boice et al. 1978a).

According to the risk estimates developed by Persson, using the model of Hashizume (Fig. 7), the maximum latency period will be longer than the observation time in the quoted

malignant significance factor

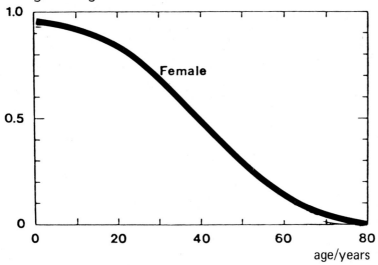

Fig. 8. Age-dependent malignancy significance factor for the calculation of breast tumor risk. (After Hashizume et al. 1981)

series. The existence of a maximum latency period cannot be determined on the basis of the available data, since it can be more than 30 years. According to Persson most data on the incidence of malignant tumors indicate that all malignancies, except leukemia, have similarly shaped incidence frequency curves. It might therefore be possible to transfer the data for leukemia incidence to other tumors and introduce two significance factors for malignancy incidence: one for leukemia and one for all other types of cancer. The malignancy significance factor would naturally be expected to be small in old people, as their life expectancy would also be shorter. The frequency distribution for incidence of malignant tumors used by Hashizume (1976, 1981) in the calculation of a malignant significance factor is given in Fig. 8.

Other Data for Risk Estimates of the x-Ray Exposure of the Female Breast

To calculate the risk factor for somatic effects it is necessary to compare the data on life expectancy in the average population of Germany with the occurrence of malignant tumors of the breast and the mean dose to the tissue at risk.

Figure 9 shows data on the mean life expectancy of females in the Federal Republic of Germany grouped by age. The mean life expectancy for women aged 30 years is 46 years; for women up to 40 years it is 37 years; and for women up to 50 years, 28 years.

The spontaneous rate of breast cancer incidence according to the epidemiological data published in the findings of the Ministry of Youth, Family and Health (1980) (Fig. 10) is 300 per million in the age group between 30 and 40 years; 1,150 per million in the age group between 40 and 50 years; and 2,000 per million age group over 50.

According to recent publications the number of persons dying from breast cancer has remained almost constant for the last 10 years (Fig. 11). The mean dose to the tissue at risk in the breast, according to measurements by Säbel et al. (1976, 1977, 1981, 1982) and other

completed year of age

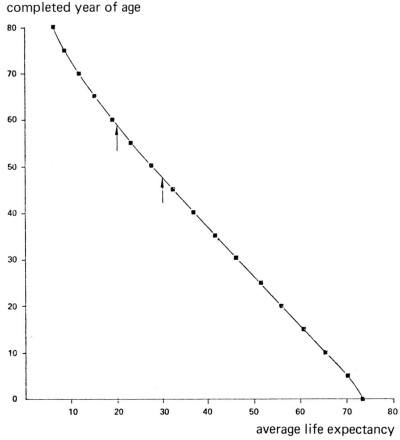

average life expectancy

Fig. 9. Mean life expectancy of females in the Federal Republic of Germany (1972–1974). (Data from the Bundesministerium für Jugend, Familie und Gesundheit 1980)

publications (e.g., UNSCEAR 1982), amounts to approximately 0.02 Gy when the so-called standard technique is used. With the screen-film technique the dose is about 10% of the above value, while with the recently introduced grid technique the dose is about 25% and in xeromammography ranges between 25% and 100% of the standard dose (Table 2).

Tumors Detectable Only by Mammography

Mammography is extremely useful in detecting tumors at a stage when it is not possible to diagnose them by palpation or other examination methods. A great many publications mention the number or percentage of tumors that cannot be detected except by mammography.

A mean value derived from several publications is given in Table 3. The tumors diagnosed by the mammographic technique only in a population similar to that of the Federal Republic of Germany account for 90 per 100,000 examinations in the age group of 30–40 years and for 580 per 100,000 examinations in the age group of 50–60 years. It is possible to

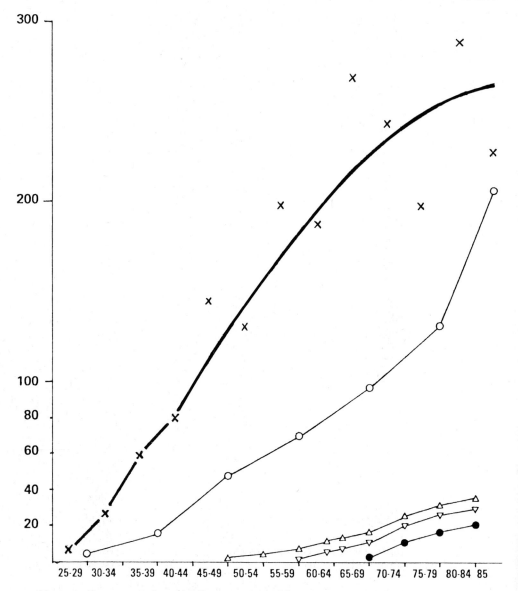

X mortality rate and morbidity rate per 10⁵ population (females)

○ mortality rate per 10⁵ population (females)

diseases per 10⁵ (females) (induced by examinations of the breast
△ examinations at the age of 30
▽ examinations at the age of 40
● examinations at the age of 50

Fig. 10. Morbidity and mortality rates for breast cancer per 10⁵ population (females) in the Federal Republic of Germany. Morbidity rate (1978) according to statistical data collected in keeping with the regulations of the World Health Organization; morbidity data according to the cancer registries of Baden-Württemberg

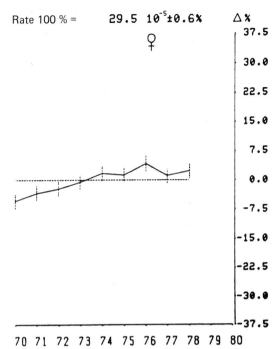

Rate 100 % = **29.5 10⁻⁵±0.6%** Δ**%**

Fig. 11. Mortality of breast cancer in the Federal Republic of Germany as a function of year. (Bundesminister des Innern 1983)

Table 2. Mean parenchymal dose per exposure of a medium-sized breast, parenchyma diameter 5 cm

Technique	Dose in Gy	Relative dose (%)
Standard technique	0.02	100
Screen film system	0.001−0.04	5− 20
Grid mammography	0.002−0.1	10− 50
Xeromammography	0.005−0.02	25−100

Table 3. Risk and benefit of x-ray examinations of the breast

Examination
  Beginning at the age of 30 with a mean survival time of 46 years $36 \cdot 10^{-5}$/year
  Beginning at the age of 40 with a mean survival time of 37 years $31 \cdot 10^{-5}$/year
  Beginning at the age of 50 with a mean survival time of 28 years $36 \cdot 10^{-5}$/year

Tumors diagnosed by mammography only
  Age group 31−40   90 per 10^5 examinations
  Age group 41−50   250 per 10^5 examinations
  Age group 51−60   580 per 10^5 examinations
  Age group > 60   450 per 10^5 examinations

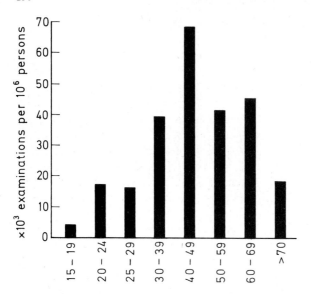

Fig. 12. Age distribution of x-ray examinations of the female breast in Berlin (West) during 1978. Statistical analysis of examination results recorded in clinics and private practices

conclude that the greatest benefit of the mammographic examination is to be found in the latter age group.

When the frequency of x-ray examinations of the female breast is analyzed with reference to the age of the patients (Fig. 12) it is found that the age group most at risk is not submitted to the examination necessary for early detection of mammary cancer. It therefore seems imperative to inform patients that particularly in this age group detection of breast cancer in a preclinical stage will result in a higher survival rate without significantly augmenting the risk of inducing a breast cancer.

Risk Resulting from x-Ray Examinations of the Female Breast

The calculated risk for the female population is about 36 per 100,000 examinations, assuming that the examinations are conducted every 5 years for the age group 30–40; every 2 years for the age group 40–50; and every year for the age group over 50. In the age group 40–50 the risk amounts to 31 per 100,000 and in the age group over 50 years about 21 per 100,000, without regard to reduction of the malignancy significance factor. The number of cancers actually induced will probably be much lower, mainly in the higher age group. The risk can also be reduced by a factor of 2 by introducing the grid technique.

Although the calculations applied here overestimate the risk it is not advisable to screen a population from the age of 30 onward, as the calculated risk is about 50% of the benefit of diagnosing the tumor and the incidence of the tumor in this age group is very low. According to health statistics the probability of detecting a cancer increases with advancing years. In the older age groups the morbidity rate increases from about 300 per million in the age group of 30–40 by a factor of 4–7, and the risk of cancer induction decreases by the same amount.

Implications of Risk-Benefit Analysis

Justification

Cancers of the breast are found by mammography at a stage when other examinations, especially physical examinations, are negative. It is therefore justified when clinical findings give rise to a significant suspicion of mammary tumors. Mammography should not be performed in women under the age of 30−40, unless there are clinical indications to justify it. In other words, only women with symptom, including those at greater than average risk, should be submitted to mammography. There is little evidence that high-risk patients or those with symptoms are more susceptible to the potential carcinogenic effects of low-level diagnostic radiation than women presumed to have normal breasts (Boice et al. 1978; Shore 1979; NCRP 1980).

A routine basic mammogram should be performed mainly in high-risk groups aged 30−40 years, as this mammogram helps to detect minor changes which are typical for incipient mammary cancers. In the age group of 40−50 years the women at risk should be routinely submitted to mammography in a screening program even if there are no clinical signs of a tumor. There are indications that some women have a higher risk of developing cancer than others (e.g., Holleb 1976; BRH 1976). Women with a family history or a reproductive history or who have themselves had prior breast cancer or other tumors belong to the high-risk groups. For symptom-free women over 50 a definite benefit of mammography has been demonstrated. In this age group mammography is indicated for all women as a part of a regular screening program.

Optimization

The World Health Organization emphasizes that quality assurance can reduce cost, by reducing film wastage; decrease radiation exposure by optimizing operational factors and the recording system; and improve medical imaging by visualizing small masses with low contrast against the surrounding tissue, which is important in the diagnosis.

As a consequence, the x-ray equipment used for mammography should meet the standards that are recognized as optimal. X-ray facilities should be subjected to regular quality assurance reviews to ensure radiographs that fulfil the diagnostic requirements while keeping patient exposure as low as possible (WHO 1982).

Limitation of Dose to the Individual

The examination should be performed with the aim of reducing radiation dose to the lowest level consistent with the recording of adequate diagnostic information. There are various circumstances in which higher dose levels are recorded than necessary. Dose measurements may help to introduce the technical modifications required to bring down the dose range to about 0.01 Gy and lower in the tissue at risk. The reduction of the dose will reduce the potential carcinogenic effect. Insistence on optimal quality in examinations of the breast with the lowest possible dose, and performance of the examination of patients in whom it is reasonable to expect that the examination is useful, will comply with the recommendations of the International Commission on Radiological Protection (1977, paragraph 205): A careful attention to techniques would, in many cases, result in a considerable reduction of dose due to medical procedure, without impairment of their value."

Summary

In order to fulfill the requirements of the International Commission on Radiological Protection for the exposure of patients to ionizing radiation in x-ray diagnosis it is necessary to demonstrate that mammography is justified and that it is conducted under optimal conditions and with as low a dose to the tissue at risk as possible.

Data available from epidemiological surveys show that the glandular tissue of the breast is one of the tissues most sensitive to radiation. In this connection the induction of malignant neoplasms is one of the most important late effects of radiation exposure.

It is probable that routine radiological examinations of the female breast lead to radiation-induced carcinoma. Therefore, an examination of the total female population is only recommended in the age group over 50 years, since in this age group the risk of not detecting a malignant tumor in time is far greater than the risk of producing radiation-induced cancer. In this age group the latency period is so long that a cancer is hardly likely to develop.

Females under 50 years of age should only be submitted to mammography if this is clinically indicated or if they belong to the risk group.

Optimization of the examination and quality control help both to reduce the dose to the lowest level consistent with the recording of adequate diagnostic information and to lower the risk due to radiation.

References

BEIR (1972) Report II. The effects on population of exposure to low-level of ionizing radiation. Report of the Advisory Committee on the Biological Effects of Ionizing Radiation. National Academy of Sciences, National Research Council, Washington D.C.

BEIR (1980) Report III. The effects on population of exposure to low-level of ionizing radiation, 1980. National Academy of Sciences, National Research Council, Washington D.C.

Boice J (1979) Carcinogenesis. Pergamon, Oxford

Boice JO, Monson RR (1977) Breast cancer in women after repeated fluoroscopic examinations of the chest. JNCI 59: 823–832

Boice JD, Stone BJ (1978) Interaction between radiation and other breast cancer risk associated with repeated fluoroscopic chest examinations of women with tuberculosis. Radiat Res 73: 373–390

Boice JD, Land CE, Shore RE et al. (1978a) Risk of breast cancer following low-dose radiation exposure. Radiology 131: 589–597

Boice JD, Rosenstein M, Trout ED (1978b) Estimation of breast doses and breast cancer risk associated with repeated fluoroscopic chest examinations of women with tuberculosis. Radiat Res 73: 373–390

Bond P v (1979) Quantitative risk in radiation protection standards. Radiat Environ Biophys 17: 1–25

BRH (Bureau of Radiological Health) Bulletin (1976) US Dept. of Health, Education and Welfare, Rockville, Maryland, vol X no 6, March 29

Bundesminister des Innern (1983) Die Krebssterblichkeit in der Bundesrepublik Deutschland 1970–1978. Ergebnisse des Informationssystems über Krebsmortalität und Krebscharakteristika, vol 1/2. TÜV, Rheinland

Bundesminister für Jugend, Familie und Gesundheit (1980) Daten des Gesundheitswesens vol 151. Kohlhammer, Stuttgart

Chiacchierini RP, Ludin FE, Scheidt PC (1976) A risk benefit analysis by life table modeling of an annual breast-cancer screening program which includes x-ray mammography. Proceedings of the Third International symposium on the detection and prevention of cancer. 26 April–1st May 1976, New York

Deutsche Krebshilfe, Bonn (1979) Empfehlungen zum Einsatz der Mammographie bei der Früherkennung des Brustkrebses. Deutsche Krebshilfe, Bonn, April

Fox StH, Moskowitz M, Saenger EL, Keriakes JG, Milbrath J, Goodman MW (1978) Benefit/risk analysis of aggressive mammographic screening. Radiology 128: 359–365

Friedrich M (1978) Neue Entwicklungstendenzen der Mammographietechnik: Die Raster-Mammographie. Fortschr Röntgenstr 128: 207–222

Hashizume T (1981) Medical irradiation in Japan; stochastic risk estimation and its reduction. Nippon Acta Radiol 41: 445–474

Hashizume T, Maruyama T, Kuamoto Y (1976) Estimation of population dose from diagnostic medical examinations in Japan 1974. 2. Estimation of genetically significant dose. Nippon Acta Radiol 36: 208–214

Haus AG, Doi K, Metz ChE, Bernstein J (1977) Image quality in mammography. Radiology 125: 77–85

Hempelmann LH, Hall WJ, Philips M, Cooper RA, Ames WR (1975) Neoplasmas in persons treated with X-rays in infancy: Fourth survey in 20 years. JNCI 55: 519–530

Holleb A (1976) Restoring confidence in mammography. Carcinoma 26: 374–378

International Commission on Radiological Protection (1977) Recommendations of the International Commission on Radiological Protection. ICRP Publication No 26. Pergamon, Oxford

International Commission on Radiological Protection (1982) Protection of the patient in diagnostic radiology. ICRR Publication No 34. Pergamon, Oxford

Kerr GD (1978) Organ doses estimates for Japanese atomic-bomb survivors. Report ORNL 5436 (Oak Ridge National Laboratory, Oak Ridge, Tennessee)

Land CE, Boice JD, Shore RE et al. (1980) Breast cancer risk from low-dose exposure to ionizing radiation: results of parallel analysis of three exposed populations of women. JNCI 65: 353–376

Land CH, McGregor DH (1979) Breast cancer incidence among atomic bomb survivors: implications for radiobiological risk at low doses. JNCI 62: 17–21

Land CE, Norman JE (1978) Latency periods of radiogenic cancers occuring among Japanese A-bomb survivors. In: Late biological effects of ionizing radiation vol. 1. International Atomic Energy Agency, Vienna, pp 29–47

Lester RG (1977) Risk versus benefit in mammography. Radiology 124: 1–6

MacKenzie I (1965) Breast cancer following multiple fluoroscopies. Br J Cancer 19: 1–8

McGregor DH, Land CE, Choi K (1977) Breast cancer incidence among atomic bomb survivors, Hiroshima and Nagasaki, 1950–1969. JNCI 59: 799–811

Mettler FA, Hempelmann LH, Dutton AM, Pfifer JW, Toyooka ET, Ames WR (1969) Breast neoplasms in women treated with X-rays for acute postpartum mastitis. A pilot study. JNCI 43: 803–811

Mole RH (1978) The sensitivity of the human breast to cancer induction by ionizing radiation. Br J Radiol 51: 401–405

Myrden JA, Hilz JE (1969) Breast cancer following multiple fluoroscopies during artificial pneumothorax treatment for pulmonary tuberculosis. Can Med Assoc J 100: 1032–1034

Myrden JA, Quilan JG (1974) Breast cancer following multiple fluoroscopies with pneumothorax treatment of pulmonary tuberculosis. Ann R Coll Phys Surg Can 7: 45

National Cancer Institute (1976) Guidelines for breast cancer detection. Department of Health, Education and Welfare, Bethesda

National Council on Radiation Protection and Measurements (1980) NCRP Report No 64: Influence of dose and its distribution in time on dose-response relationship for low-let radiation. Washington D.C.

Persson B (1981) Review of various weighted dose concepts used for estimation of risk from medical X-ray diagnosis. In: Drexler G, Eriskat H, Schibilla H (eds) Patient exposure to radiation in medical X-ray diagnosis. Possibilities for dose reduction. Commission of the European Communities EUR 7438

Richter B (1978) Zur Effizienz mammographischer Reihenuntersuchungen. Fortschr Röntgenstr 129: 494–500

Säbel M (1982) Strahlenexposition und Bildgüte der Xeromammographie. Röntgenpraxis 35: 463–468

Säbel M, Weishaar J, Willgeroth F (1976) Radiation exposure of the breast in film- and xeromammography. Strahlentherapie 151: 504–510

Säbel M, Paterok EM, Weishaar J, Willgeroth F (1977) Untersuchungen zur Bildgüte bei Film- und Xero-Mammographie. 1. Mitteilung: Wiedergabe kleiner Strahlenkontraste. Fortschr Röntgenstr 126: 529–536

Säbel M, Paterok EM, Willgeroth F, Weishaar J (1981) Dosissparende Aufnahmeverfahren bei der Mammographie. In: Sauer R (ed) Neue Aspekte der Diagnostik und Therapie des Mammakarzinoms. Zuckschwerdt, München, pp 22–59

Shellaberger CJ (1976) Modifying factors in rat mammary gland carcinogenesis. In: Yuhas JM, Tennat RW, Regan JB (eds) Biology of radiation carcinogenesis. Ravens, New York

Shore RE (1978) Dose-response relationships in radiogenic breast cancer. JNCI 60: 728

Shore RE, Hempelmann LH, Kowaluk E et al. (1977) Breast neoplasms in women treated with X-rays for acute postpartum mastitis. JNCI 59: 813–822

Stieve F-E (1982) Strahlenexposition von Patienten bei Röntgendiagnostischen Maßnahmen. In: Strahlenschutz in Forschung und Praxis, vol 23. Thieme, Stuttgart, pp 37–78

Taylor LS (1980) Some non-scientific influences on radiation protection standards and practice. The 1980 Sievert Lecture. Health Phys 39: 851–874

Tokunga M, Norman JE, Asano M, Tokuoka S, Ezaki H, Nishimori I, Tsuji Y (1979) Malignant breast tumors among atomic bomb survivors. JNCI 62: 1347–1359

United Nations Scientific Committee (1977) The effects of atomic radiation sources and effects of ionizing radiation. Report to the General Assembly, with annexes. United Nations, New York

United Nations Scientific Committee (1982) The effects of atomic radiation: Ionizing radiation: sources and biological effects. 1982 Report to the General Assembly, with annexes. United Nations, New York

Upton AC, Beebe GW, Brown JM, Quimby JM, Shellaberger C (1977) 1977 Report of NCI Ad Hoc Working Group on the risks associated with mammography in mass screening for detection of breast cancer. JNCI 59: 480–493

Watson P (1977) A survey of radiation doses to patients in mammography. Br J Radiol 50: 745–750

Willgeroth F, Paterok EM, Säbel M, Weishaar J (1980) Untersuchungen zur Bildgüte bei Film- und Xero-Mammographie. 2. Mitteilung. Wiedergabe mittlerer Strahlenkontraste. Fortschr Röntgenstr 132: 433–437

World Health Organisation (1980) Efficacy and efficiency of diagnostic application of radiation and radionuclides. Report of a Meeting organised by the World Health Organisation and the Government of the Federal Republic of Germany. Neuherberg, 5–7 December 1979, RAD/80.4 WHO Genf

World Health Organisation (1982) Quality assurance in diagnostic radiology. World Health Organisation, Geneva

Würthner K (1978) Kritische Bemerkungen zu Risikoberechnungen bei der Mammographie. Röntgenblätter 31: 318–322

Yoshizawa Y, Kusama T (1975) Search for the lowest irradiation dose from literatures on radiation induced breast cancer. Nippon Acta Radiol 35: 1125–1130

Recent Progress in the Ultrasonic Detection of Breast Cancer

M. Friedrich

Klinikum Steglitz, Röntgendiagnostik,
Hindenburgdamm 30, 1000 Berlin 45, Federal Republic of Germany

Introduction

Attempts to use ultrasound for diagnosis of diseases of the breast are approximately as old as the development of mammography. Since mammography has been criticized with reference to radiation hygiene, breast sonography has recently shifted to the center of public and scientific interest. In press reports, breast sonography has already been prematurely described as a time-tested and reliable alternative to mammography. Only the newest technological development and the presently beginning worldwide scientific activity in the field of breast sonography can contribute towards defining and consolidating the position of ultrasound in the spectrum of breast diagnostics.

Methodological Aspects of Breast Sonography

No generally recognized and accepted examination plan yet exists. This is due on the one hand to the fundamental difficulties, and on the other to the different expectations connected with breast sonography. Among the principal difficulties is the nonuniform and variable tissue structure of the breast, composed as it is of fat as well as glandular and connective tissue, and the lack of a homogeneous basic echographic pattern for detection of small focal lesions.
Secondly, sound coupling to the easily deformable organ is difficult.
Thirdly, detection of the smallest lesion requires an extremely high resolving power and, at the same time, an easily surveyable sound-image field.
Fourthly, it was a long time before the problems of complete volume recording and sound-image documentation for the screening approach were solved.
Also, entirely different apparatus concepts are derived from the different applications of breast sonography to supplement other examination procedures by clarification of unclear findings or as a basic examination to reveal completely occult, impalpable findings.

Manual Scan Procedures

Mention should first be made of the oldest procedure, which is the conventional slow B-image compound scan, which achieves considerable resolving power with small-aper-

Early Breast Cancer
Edited by J. Zander and J. Baltzer
© Springer-Verlag Berlin Heidelberg 1985

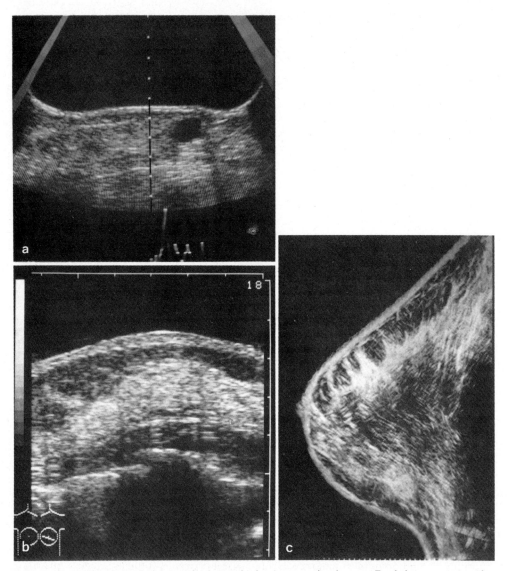

Fig. 1a–c. Different techniques of ultrasonic breast examination. **a** Real-time sector probe (Combison 100 W, Kretz Technik), 3.5 MHz, integrated water coupling, A-mode analysis; **b** electronic linear-array probe (LS 3000, Picker/Hitachi), 5 MHz, external water bag coupling, diagram of probe position at *lower left;* **c** immersion breast sonogram, (Octoson, Ausonics), 3.5 MHz, compound scan in free breast immersion

ture, short-focus high-frequency transducers. In particular, Gros et al. (1978) acquired a great deal of clinical experience with this procedure. However, the examination is usually slow and tedious and only suitable for specific differentiation of palpable or otherwise localized processes. It cannot be used to reveal breast alterations not yet known to be present.

All other manual scan procedures presently work according to the real-time principle. Attention should be called here to the mechanical real-time scanners with an integrated water path, e.g., the short-range scanner to Combison-100 R (Kretz Co., Fig. 1a), the real-time ultrasonic "Lupe" Biosound (Biodynamics Co., Fig. 6a–c), and the higher-frequency, dynamically focused transducers presently coming onto the market for all electronic linear-array scanners (Fig. 1b). While the ultrasonic Lupe Biosound with a working frequency of 8–10 MHz offers a resolving power of less than 1 mm, though only over a very narrow image field, we think the presently available 5-MHz linear-array scanners represent a good compromise from the point of view of resolution, sound-image field range, and financial considerations.

Manual scan procedures have the following advantages:
1) Direct coordination of palpation findings and sonogram.
2) Same positioning of the patient for sonography and operation.
3) As a rule, better physical resolving power than automatic immersion procedures as a result of higher acoustic frequencies.
4) Easily read sonophysical criteria.
5) Possibility of assessing the consistency of tumors.

The following disadvantages should be mentioned; the last four all follow from the first:
1) Lack of a general anatomical view of the entire organ.
2) Usually incomplete coverage of the entire organ.
3) Inadequate sound-image documentation.
4) Poor reproducibility.
5) Limited possibility of delegating the examination.

Automatic Scan Procedures

These include scanners with an external water path and immersion scanners. The two main representatives of the first category are the Sonolayergraph, SSL 25a (Toshiba Co.) and the EUE 2b breast scanner from Hitachi Co. Both are slow-working arc or linear scanners with 5-MHz transducers. The weight of the water bag leads to considerable compression of the breast, which is largely advantageous. Both devices have remarkable resolving power and produce an arcuate or linear automatic scan over an image field about 15 cm wide and at scanning intervals of 2–4 mm. Japanese authors (Kobayashi 1979) and Pluygers and Rombaut (1980) in Europe have gathered particularly extensive clinical experience with these devices.

The following immersion scanners should be mentioned: (1) the Octoson (Ausonics Co.); (2) the Life-Instruments breast scanner (Senomatic 3D in Europe); and (3) the SMV 120 immersion scanner from the Technicare Corp.

These devices were designed according to the examination concept of free breast immersion or breast compression in a water bath with the patient lying in a prone position. They permit an automatic linear-sector or compound scan of the breast in programmable layer intervals and directions. An important advantage is the good anatomical overview of the entire organ (Fig. 1c); the principal disadvantage is the absence of coordination of palpation findings and ultrasonic image, particularly with a view to subsequent surgery. A further advantage of the immersion scanner lies in the fact that sound coupling is generally unproblematic; the length of time necessary for complete volume coverage of the organ (at least 30 min) is a drawback. The SMV 120 scanner attempts to compensate for the disadvantage of lacking coordination of palpation findings and ultrasonic image by means of a built-in TV camera with a scan-level indicator.

A recent addition to the rather expensive immersion scanners mentioned so far has been made in the form of real-time devices with special breast attachments for automatic and rapid sonographic breast imaging. Mention should be made of the breast attachment developed at the German Clinic for Diagnostics (Bielke et al. 1980), which uses the transducer of the Combison 100 R (Kretz Co.). Other attachments are based on the principle we suggested years ago, namely that of rotational breast scanning, in which circular scanning of the breast is done by a real-time probe in a breast attachment. All these devices lead to breast compression, which is sonophysically favorable for a number of reasons (Gros et al. 1978). They unite the advantage of a relatively high resolving power with that of the real-time principle, with a short examination period and complete volume coverage of the breast. A disadvantage is the difficulty in correlating palpation findings and ultrasonic image. The problem of sound-image documentation has doubtless been solved in the form of videotape recordings.

Further Methodological Aspects of Breast Sonography

Gros et al. in 1978 first pointed out the advantages of breast compression in manual compound scanning procedures. The main advantage of breast compression lies in an increased reflexivity of breast tissue due to increased vertical alignment of interstitial acoustic boundary surfaces to the transducer. The second advantage is the reduction of the necessary penetration depth, and a further one, the possibility of assessing the consistency of breast tissue, either in the form of a time-motion recording in the compound scan or directly by compression and decompression in the real-time scan. The increased reflexivity of the compressed glandular tissue facilitates the recognition of acoustic shadow zones behind scirrhous tissue configurations. Even with immersion scanners we have found breast compression to be more advantageous than free immersion (Friedrich et al. 1981). Due to the often considerable tissue thickness in free immersion, almost all immersion scanners provide incomplete penetration of the central breast areas, with formation of a central structureless shadow. The phase relations of sound waves and the focusing of the sound beam are strongly impaired after a few centimeters, because of the extremely nonuniform structure of the breast tissue, so that the sonophysical criteria − of a cyst, for example − are more clearly recognizable with compression than in free immersion. In addition, the enhanced reflexivity of the surrounding breast tissue leads to enhanced echographic contrast between hyporeflexive tumor and hyperreflexive parenchyma. As a disadvantage of breast compression, it must be admitted that discrete retraction phenomena only evident in free immersion may escape detection and that breast compression may result in distortion of anatomical structures and displacement of palpation findings.

Advantages and disadvantages also arise from the opposing conceptions of single scan and compound scan. The single scan leads to clearer definition of echographic criteria, e.g., subsequent sound amplification behind a cyst or an acoustic shadow zone behind a carcinoma; it usually also permits better assessment of the echo texture. On the other hand, the compound scan leads to a better contour delineation of round objects, a better delimitation of multidirectional boundary surfaces and stellate figures, and a greater density of information (better sound-image implementation) through ultrasound exposure from different directions (see below, reflection computer tomography).

The statements of Pluygers and Rombaut (1980) concerning A-image analysis of solid breast lesions have received little attention and no verification. The authors regard a divergence of the declining side of the A-image curve in a tumor with differing overall amplification as a sign of malignancy and parallel decline as a sign of benignity. At least this statement should be taken as an indication that, as far as possible, ultrasonic devices for breast diagnostics should also furnish an A-image.

More Recent Developments in Reflection Ultrasound of the Breast (Reflection Ultrasound Computed Tomography)

Robinson and Knight, in 1981, were the first to report on various postprocessing computer reconstruction techniques as an extension of the conventional compound scan with digital scan converters. They first discussed the mechanism of improving resolution, specifically for spot reflectors, by circular scanning from many different directions and coordinate-related superposition (Fig. 2a). Carson et al. (1981, personal communication) also described the surprisingly clear visualization of breast architecture yielded by compound scanning of the breast in coronal layers.

The principle consists in a linear or sector-shaped scanning of the object from many different directions in coronal orientation and computerized superposition of these images on the basis of exact coordinate correction. While, with the simple linear scan (Fig. 2b), the spongy polygonal lobular structure of the breast is virtually unrecognizable, it is almost inconveivable that precise computation from 12 single linear scans of the quality of Fig. 2b should yield a very life-like ultrasonic image of the interstitial septation of the breast. With this procedure, the resolving power is isotropically distributed over the entire image area and is in the order of magnitude of 1 mm. There is a surprising correspondence between the mammographic and the sonographic image in the reflection computer tomogram. There has not yet been any clinical experience with this method.

Diagnostic Information Yielded by Breast Sonography

Differentiation of Solid/Cystic and Malignancy/Benignity Criteria

Like mammography, ultrasound can yield information about the tissue composition of the breast: postmenopausal breasts with predominantly fatty infiltration show a hyporeflexive echo pattern, whereas the parenchyma of younger women, consisting of a mixture of connective, fatty, and glandular tissue, generally shows a hyperreflexive structure.

The important differential-diagnostic information provided by breast sonography in connection with a palpable or non-palpable process is whether it is solid or cystic. Detection of cysts (Fig. 3) has always been one of the domains of ultrasound and is possible in the breast with almost 100% sensitivity and specificity. Depending on the type of apparatus, breast cysts ranging down to pinhead size can be traced. Breast cysts are always characterized by a reflex-free zone with smooth inner walls, occasionally with septations or inner ridge-like projections and a subsequent hyperreflexive zone behind the cyst due to lacking sound attenuation in the cyst fluid. As a rule, palpable breast cysts present no diagnostic problem, even without ultrasound, since they can be aspirated and filled with air (pneumocystography). Sonographic detection of impalpable or unsuspected breast cysts can of course be helpful for interpretation of dense glandular areas poorly visualized in the mammogram and for clarification of mammographically unclear focal shadows. In addition, to a limited degree, sonography can differentiate between simple uncomplicated

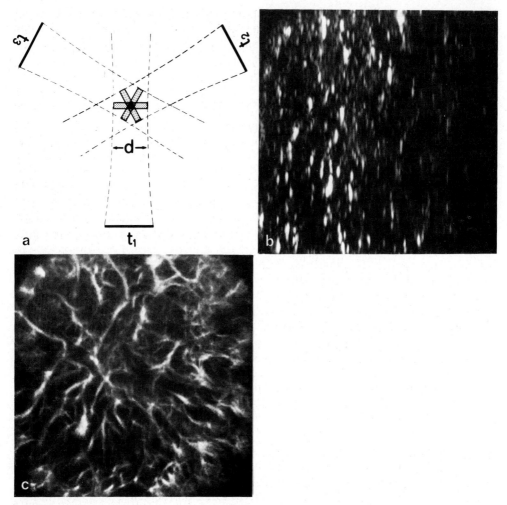

Fig. 2. a Principle of image refinement through computer compound scan, demonstrated for a point target. *t1, t2, t3* different scanning positions; *d* beam width of the transducer. *Black central intersecting point* of beam widths corresponds to the pulse duration or axial resolution. **b** Linear vertical scan of fat-infiltrated postoperative breast specimen in coronal section. Scanning step size: 0.6 mm; image area: 12 × 12 cm; image matrix: 200 × 200 picture elements; 2-MHz transducer; (Friedrich et al. 1982) **c** Large-area high-resolution reflection ultrasound computer tomogram of breast specimen shown in **b**. Compound scan of 12 single linear scans with 30° increments; scanning step size: 0.6 mm; image area: 12 cm × 12 cm; image matrix: 200 × 200 picture elements; image resolution: approx. 1 mm. (Friedrich et al. 1982)

cysts and so-called complicated cysts (Fig. 4). "Complicated" cysts are those with intracystic vegetations or irregular wall contours, or in whose immediate proximity such abnormalities as solid extensions, thickened ductal structures can be detected. In any case, even a cyst which appears to be sonographically uncomplicated should, for diagnostic and therapeutic reasons, be punctured with subsequent pneumocystography. In addition, a short-term follow-up is necessary, since otherwise causal or concomitant malignant processes may be overlooked.

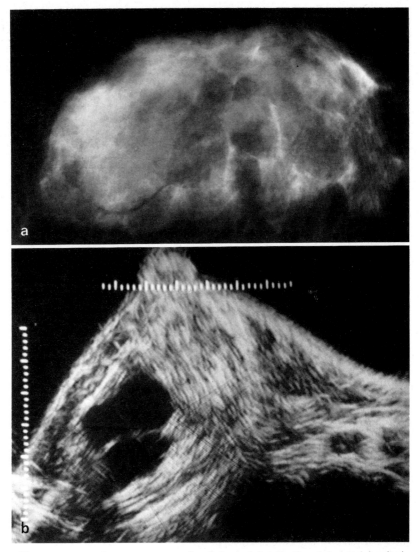

Fig. 3a, b. Septated breast cyst seen in **a** mammogram (cephalocaudal projection, lobulated density in outer quadrant) and **b** immersion sonogram (Octoson, Ausonics; free immersion technique, anechoic lobulated region with internal septation and smooth outlines)

Secondly, breast sonography provides evidence of reflex-containing, i.e., solid circumscribed focal lesions. The sonographic tumor criteria are the shape, the contour, the boundary echo and inner echo structure, the reflex behavior behind the tumor, and the bilateral shadow zones. The following criteria of benignity are idealized in the literature: a round shape, a smooth outer contour, a homogeneous, moderately strong inner echo structure with uniform distribution, a well-defined posterior wall echo and an indifferent reflex zone behind the tumor (Fig. 5). Only the more recent and more comprehensive morphological studies (Cole-Beuglet et al. 1982, 1983; Harper and Kelly-Fry 1980; Kasumi et al. 1982) have shown that even with fibroadenomas, these ideal criteria of benignity are

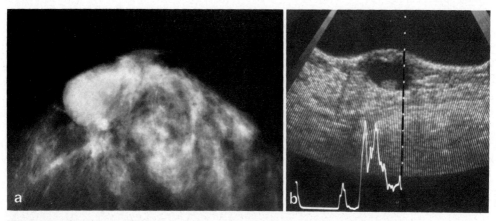

Fig. 4a, b. "Complicated" breast cyst, 3 months after biopsy in the supra-areolar region, seen in **a** mammogram (cephalocaudal projection, round density in the retroareolar region) and **b** real-time sonogram [3.5-MHz sector probe (Combison 100, Kretz Technik), anechoic region with irregular internal outline and round echogenic internal lesion, histologically intracystic papilloma]

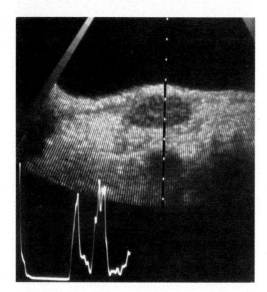

Fig. 5. Real-time sonogram of fibroadenoma. Sector real-time probe, 3.5 MHz, with integrated water coupling (Combison 100 W, Kretz Technik). Circumscribed hyporeflective region with smooth outlines, weak and uniform internal echo pattern, and well-defined posterior echo

not present in any considerable percentage, but that there is clear overlapping of the sonographic appearance of benign and circumscribed malignant tumors.

The following have been described as criteria of malignancy: an irregular shape and outer contour, an inhomogeneous inner reflex pattern that is partially weak and partially strong, a strong entrance echo with a weak or absent exit echo, and different degrees of sound attenuation, recognizable by an acoustic shadow zone behind the tumor. Figure 6 shows such a circumscribed breast tumor of the "intermediate" type according to Kasumi (Kasumi et al. 1982). The morphological analysis of these circumscribed breast tumors is dealt with below. First the more simple and generally accepted sonophysical criteria of the stellate, infiltrative scirrhous carcinoma with infiltrating growth (Fig. 7) are discussed. The star shape causes a strong refraction and absorption of the sound in the tumor; this

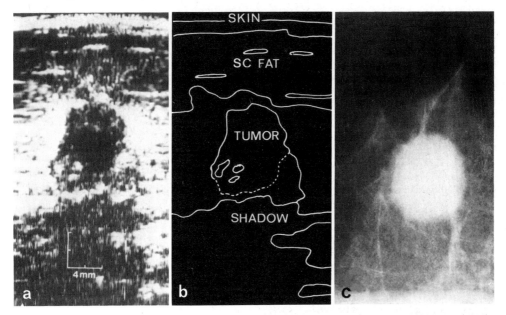

Fig. 6a—c. "Circumscribed" breast carcinoma, intermediate type according to Kasumi et al. (1982).
a Real-time sonogram mechanical linear-array probe, 8 MHz, Biosound, Biodynamics, circumscribed hyporeflective area with inhomogeneous internal echoes, irregular outline, and weak posterior echo; **b** schematic diagram of sonogram shown in **a**; **c** mammogram of circumscribed breast carcinoma approx. 1 cm in diameter

manifests itself in the sonogram as a hyporeflexive, mostly irregularly bordered zone with an intensified entrance echo and absent posterior-wall echo and with an acoustic shadow. Only in exceptional cases do some scirrhous carcinomas show only the hyperreflexive star figure of the entrance echo without a shadow zone. Kobayashi (1979) related the occurrence of acoustic shadow zones to the high connective-tissue content and the irregular structure of the productive fibrosis of these infiltrating carcinomas. Though the occurrence of an acoustic shadow zone behind infiltrating carcinomas is very sensitive, it is not specific for a carcinoma, since it can also occur behind any other scirrhous tissue configuration, such as hyaline scars, and also radially hyalinized fibroadenomas and normal scars. Acoustic shadow zones can also occur behind calcifications or oblique interlobar septa and lead to misinterpretations.

Considerably greater interpretation difficulties arise with circumscribed carcinomas, which according to Kasumi (Kasumi et al. 1982), constitute at least 17% alone and, together with the so-called intermediary type, about 30% of all carcinomas. Kasumi classifies the circumscribed carcinomas into the larger group of the so-called distinct type, which shows great similarity with benign structure patterns but has an irregular outer contour and a coarse inner echo pattern; the shadow type, which largely corresponds to the scirrhous carcinoma with macroscopically infiltrative growth; and the intermediary type between the two. Of a total of 864 sonographically classified carcinomas, 147 (17%) were of the circumscribed type. Of these 147 carcinomas, 102 (70%) were of the distinct type and 16 tumors (11%) evidenced criteria of a benign tumor. Thus 80% of circumscribed carcinomas and a total of about 14% of all carcinomas have a sonomorphologically ambiguous appearance.

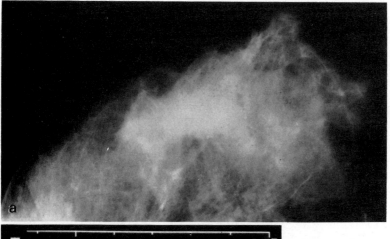

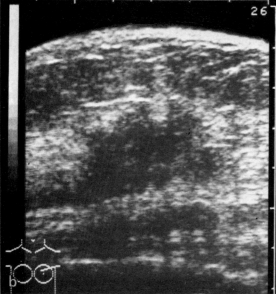

Fig. 7a, b. Infiltrating breast carcinoma, scirrhous type. **a** Mammogram, cephalocaudal projection, stellate tumor density, and retraction of breast parenchyma; **b** real-time sonogram, 5-MHz linear-array probe with water coupling, upper outer quadrant, radial section; 3-cm hyporeflective area with shadow and jagged outline

Analysis of the sonographic criteria of a smaller collective of our own also showed the broad overlapping of sonographic benignity/malignancy criteria for circumscribed tumors (Fig. 8). The basis is the selective value of a positive test, which is defined from the relation of the correct responses of all that are positive to the prior probability of the disease in the collective. This parameter among others was put forward by Moskowitz (1982) as a grading criterion for a screening test. It becomes evident that, even with application of all sonomorphological criteria in the described frequency distribution (Fig. 8), the group of carcinomas cannot be divided much better than by the pure age distribution of fibroadenoma and carcinoma. For purposes of comparison, Fig. 9a shows a solid carcinoma and Fig. 9b, a lobular fibroadenoma with a largely isomorphous sonographic appearance. The published collectives of other authors (Schmidt et al. 1981; Igl et al. 1982; Thiel and Schweikhart 1982) also do not permit derivation of any better selective sonographic values

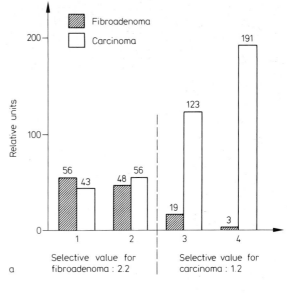

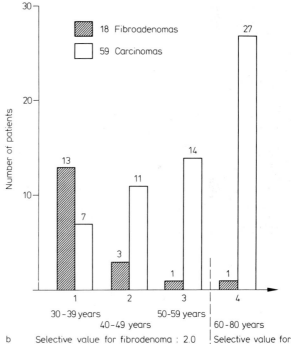

Fig. 8a, b. Selective values found in 18 fibroadenomas and 59 carcinomas for the combination of age distribution and all sonographic tumor criteria (**a**) and for age distribution alone (**b**)

for carcinoma diagnosis when there is a high prior probability of carcinoma in the collective. In practice, this can mean that, at least in the extreme cases, i.e., at the extremes of the age scale and also at the extremes of the epidemiological risk scale, these clinical factors, being of greater informational value, must be given priority over the sonographic picture alone in deciding to seek real diagnostic clarification, i.e., biopsy.

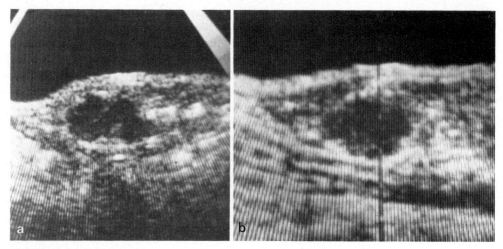

Fig. 9a, b. Isomorphological aspect of malignant and benign "circumscribed" breast tumors: **a** circumscribed breast carcinoma, histologically solid carcinoma; **b** circumscribed benign breast tumor, histologically fibroadenoma

Doppler Sonography

In the case of palpable solid alterations, Dopper sonography may offer a possible solution to this diagnostic dilemma. Wells et al. in 1977, were among the first to conduct Doppler ultrasonic examinations of palpable breast tumors with a continuous-wave device. The procedure consists in manual scanning of the breast with an 8-MHz Doppler transducer and a scanning frequency of 3.5 kHz and channel-separation of 22 db. After amplification, demodulation, and low-pass filtering, these signals are either monitored via headphones or registered on a tape recorder for subsequent spectral analysis. Decisive importance attaches to comparison of the recording over the tumor with that over the corresponding contralateral site, the malignancy criteria in ascending order being: (a) increased volume; (b) increased volume and increased frequency; and (c) the so-called characteristic sound, i.e., a continuous flow in the diastole (cf. Fig. 10a). According to Minasian and Bamber (1982), the Doppler frequency distortion in relation to the tumor size is clearly greater in small tumors, probably because of increased microcirculation in the tumor periphery, than in large tumors with necrotic centers. The data from a larger collective, reported on by Wells et al. in October 1979 in Philadelphia at the First Congress on the Ultrasonic Examination of the Breast, show that with Doppler sonography in palpable breast tumors differentiation of the carcinoma from other nodes is possible, with a selective value of the positive test of 6.6. With a prior probability of the carcinoma of $39/332 = 12\%$ this is a surprisingly good result, which nevertheless is not sufficient from the clinical point of view to justify omission of a biopsy.

The current status of ultrasonic Doppler breast sonography can be summarized as follows:

1) The important Doppler signals probably arise from vessels outside small tumors.
2) The absolute measurements alone may be misleading; comparison with the contra-lateral site seems to be essential.
3) The required sensitivity is at the limit of the capability of contemporary instruments.
4) Future work will involve studies of total signal energy and frequency spectral distribution.

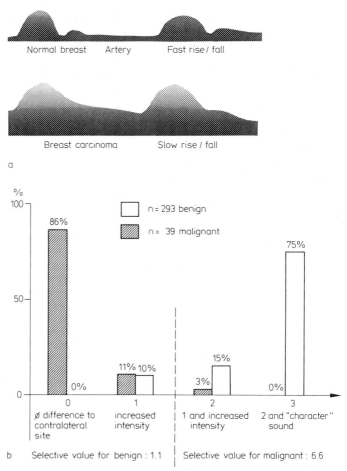

Fig. 10. a Doppler flow curves of normal breast artery and breast carcinoma; **b** results of Doppler ultrasound examinations of 332 palpable breast tumors. (Modified from Wells et al. 1979)

Transmission Ultrasonic Computed Tomography of the Breast

As described above, fibroadenomas and circumscribed carcinomas have a relatively weak inner echogenicity. As a result, they are often overlooked in the hyporeflexive pattern of fatty breasts. These conditions provide a fundamental argument against the use of the reflection ultrasonic procedure as a screening method for breast tumors, particularly in older patients. It may be possible in the future to eliminate this fault through transmission ultrasonic computed tomography. Basically, with this procedure, sectorial or transla-tion-rotation scanning of a breast immersed in a water bath is performed in coronal sections, two measurement parameters being obtained: (a) the time of flight in the tissue; and (b) the attenuation of sound. One such device, developed by Greenleaf and Bahn in 1981, is a scanner of this type that scans four coronal layer levels simultaneously. According to the same reconstruction algorithm as is used in x-ray computed tomography, cross-sectional breast images are obtained, which are composed of the local values for sound velocity or attenuation in the tissue. Measurements by Greenleaf and Bahn over 187

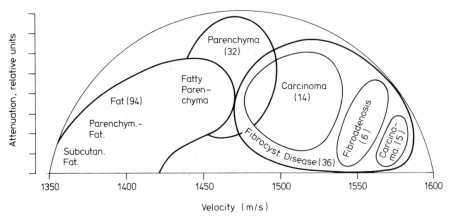

Fig. 11. Distribution of means of ultrasonic attenuation and velocity in transmission ultrasound computed tomography of 187 regions in 18 patients aged 29–68 years. (Modified from Greenleaf and Bahn 1981)

tissue regions in 18 patients yielded the following sonophysical features of breast tissue (Fig. 11):

1) Subcutaneous fatty tissue is characterized by relatively low sound velocity and attenuation, in contrast to fatty parenchyma, which has higher velocity and attenuation.

2) Average glandular tissue shows sound velocities between 1,450 and 1,500 m/s and a wide range of variation in sound attenuation. In general, it is practically impossible to differentiate between fatty tissue, normal glandular tissue, and cancer tissue by the parameter of sound attenuation.

3) However, any tissue-containing solid breast nodule can be distinguished from the surrounding fatty tissue on the basis of its higher sound velocity. This is a definite advantage over the reflection ultrasonic procedure alone.

4) Unfortunately, further overlapping between the sound velocities in cancer tissue and mastopathic tissue results from the fact that the more compact cancer tissue of older women has a higher sound velocity than the looser cancer tissue of younger women.

According to these measurement values, it seems in any case rather improbable that cancer nodules would be discovered in diffuse mastopathic tissue, since the velocity range of the latter encompasses that of the cancer tissue. Moreover, the resolution of current ultrasound transmission CT images is still relatively poor.

Diagnostic Value of Breast Sonography

The most enthusiastic statements concerning the value of breast sonography are found in publications by Pluygers and Rombaut (1980). In contrast to all other authors (Cole-Beuglet et al. 1981, 1982; Friedrich 1982; Harper and Kelly-Fry 1980; Igl et al. 1980; Rosner et al. 1980; Schmidt et al. 1981; Thiel and Schweikhart 1982; Weiss et al. 1978), these workers assert the all-round superiority of breast sonography over mammography, even for early tumor stages. Most authors concur in their reports that differentiation of benign breast alterations with ultrasound is as good as or superior to that afforded by

Table 1. Sensitivity of sonography and mammography for the detection of breast carcinoma (review of literature)

Author(s)	(No of Patients) year	Sonography			Mammography/ xerography		Sonography + mammography	
Teixidor and Kazam	(19) 1977		26/33	(79%)	31/33	(94%)	32/33	(97%)
Gros et al.	(6) 1978	T0	5/13	(38%)	–		–	
		T1	18/26	(69%)				
		T2	138/160	(86%)				
Kobayashi	(11) 1978	T1	31/40	(78%)	28/37	(76%)		
		T2	52/58	(90%)	49/56	(88%)		
Pluygers et al.	(17) 1980	T0	7/12	(58%)	4/12	(33%)	8/12	(66%)
		T1	43/52	(82%)	42/50	(81%)	48/52	(92%)
Cole-Beuglet et al.	(2) 1981	T1	7/24	(29%)	13/20	(65%)	20/20	(100%)
			7/19	(36%)				
		T2	49/53	(92%)	29/36	(80%)		
Igl et al.	(10) 1980	T0 (13) \} T2 (13) \}	29/31	(94%)	29/31	(94%)	31/31	(100%)
Rosner et al.	(18) 1980		16/24	(67%)	22/24	(92%)	24/24	(100%)

mammography. This can be attributed on the one hand to the nearly 100% differentiation of solid and cystic breast alterations, and on the other to the more sensitive sonographic detection of circumscribed lesions in glandular parenchyma with high connective-tissue content. With solid circumscribed breast lesions, however, the value of breast sonography is generally seen in the actual detection of such lesions as a supplement to mammography, and not in the differentiation of their fine tissue structure. A critical evaluation, particularly a comparison with mammography, is rendered difficult by the fact that most authors mention solely the detection sensitivity for the carcinomas, and give no figures for false-positive or correct-negative diagnoses. Moreover, the success rates depend, of course, on whether the carcinoma was actually discovered by the examination or, for example, only visualized with the examination modality.

With these reservations, most authors put the detection sensitivity of sonography for breast carcinoma on the same level as that of mammography (Table 1). Only Pluygers and Rombaut (1981) and Kobayashi (1978) consider ultrasound to be markedly superior, even for smaller carcinomas; on the one hand, the mammographic success rates are far below average in the collective of Pluygers and Rombaut, and on the other hand, the breasts are generally smaller in the collective of the Japanese authors, which is favorable for sonography but unfavorable for mammography.

In a more recent study by Cole-Beuglet et al. (1981) with the Octoson immersion scanner, breast sonography in tumors less than 2 cm in size evidences a far lower sensitivity (29% or 30%) than xeroradiography (65%). Since very different physical factors and diagnostic criteria are involved, it does not seem appropriate, in our opinion, to compare ultrasound and mammography as competitive procedures. On the contrary, they are complementary

Table 2. Selective value of tests in groups with different prevalence rates of carcinoma

Authors	Number n	True-positive	False-positive	Predictive value of positive test	Prevalence of carcinoma	Selective value for carcinoma
High prevalence of carcinoma						
Schmidt et al. 1981	143	46/53	28/78	62%	40.4%	1.54×
Igl et al. 1982	170	70/78	17/92	80.4%	45.9%	1.7×
Thiel and Schweickhart 1982	493 (212)	84/92	16/212	84%	43.4%	1.9× sonography
	493 (212)	82/87	60/209	57.7%	41.6%	1.4× mammography
Medium prevalence of carcinoma						
Cole-Beuglet et al. 1982	1,003	54/71	29/83	65%	7%	9.3×
Wells et al. 1979	332	35/39	9/293	79%	11.7%	6.8× Doppler-sonography

in the evidence they provide, which is clearly illustrated by the higher success rates with combined application. The results of Rosner et al. (1980) are interesting in this connection: of the 8 cases not sonographically discovered in a collective of 24 carcinomas, 6 were clinically occult and only recognizable by microcalcifications in the xeromammogram. When sonography and mammography were combined the success rate increased from 67% with sonography alone and 92% with mammography alone to 100%.

If the above-mentioned selective value of the positive test are considered as an assessment criterion for a screening procedure, the collectives reported in the literature must be subdivided into those with high, low, and medium prevalence of carcinoma (Table 2). It becomes clear that in collectives with a high carcinoma prevalence, i.e., in the examination of women with symptoms, the diagnostic evidence of a carcinoma has a high predictive value but the test has a relatively low selection value. This applies in the same way to both mammography and sonography. It is only in collectives with low carcinoma prevalence, i.e., in true screening collectives of women with no symptoms, that the selective value of a screening modality can become apparent. In the collective of Cole-Beuglet et al. (1982), breast sonography evidenced a selective value of the positive test for carcinoma of 9.3 at a carcinoma prevalence of 7%. For comparison, Moskowitz (1982) reports a selective value of the positive test for carcinoma between 20 and 50 for mammography in true screening collectives.

Summary

The following methodological assertions can be made:
1) Expensive immersion scanners of contemporary design offer no significant advantages over less costly alternatives. In the future, these will mainly comprise high-frequency dynamically focused real-time probes which can be used both manually for specific

clarification of palpation findings and in breast attachments presently being developed for automatic, rapid, and complete volume coverage of the breast.

2) The problems of sound-image documentation have largely been solved.

3) The diagnostic value of Doppler ultrasonic examination of the breast must be further defined.

4) Advanced procedures for reflection ultrasonic image calculation are being developed; their future importance is difficult to assess at present. The same applies for transmission ultrasonic computer tomography.

The following can be said about the diagnostic value:

5) With reference to *screening,* i.e., early diagnosis of impalpable tumors, sonography lacks the great advantage of mammography, defined as the possibility of detecting microcalcifications, allowing early diagnosis. Moreover, in the epidemiologically more important screening collective of older women with a fatty glandular parenchyma, it also lacks the advantage of high tumor contrast between solid nodules and fatty tissue afforded by mammography. On the contrary, it is charged with the disadvantage of poor tumor contrast or none at all in these cases. Some day it may be possible to eliminate this disadvantage through transmission ultrasonic CT. To counterbalance the disadvantage of mammography, i.e., lack of tumor contrast in the breasts of younger women, which have a high content of connective tissue, sonography offers the advantage of revealing circumscribed breast lesions in these cases.

6) For the so-called clarification of palpable breast tumors, a great advantage of sonography is the immediate differentiation between cystic and solid. In numerous cases this leads to immediate extensive clarification by puncture and pneumocystography and cytology. Particularly in its rapid availability for clinical practice, this sonographic information is also very valuable for areas not clearly visualized by mammography in nonassessable focal opacities. Mammography, on the other hand, is only useful for a fatty parenchyma which can be clearly visualized, e.g., for detection of a lipoma or fatty cyst in the area of a palpable resistance.

7) The value of both procedures for clarification is very limited in all other cases, i.e., when a focal density is detected in the mammogram or when is not seen in poorly visualized tissue, or in the case of sonographic detection of a circumscribed solid breast lesion. The value of the procedures lies mainly in the detection of the alteration in addition to the clinical examination. As a rule, both the mammographic and the sonographic tumor criteria are too uncertain to make a biopsy superfluous. It must be emphasized again and again that there is considerable overlapping of the mammographic and sonographic malignancy/benignity criteria, that both procedures have their "blind" areas, and that clinical factors, such as the patient's individual risk, case history, and even age, often permit a more probable assessment of the nature of a lump than all imaging procedures.

8) The recommendations for application of ultrasonic mammography can presently be defined as follows:

   a) As a supplementary procedure to mammography, sonography improves diagnostic accuracy in numerous cases.

   b) Sonography is useful for differentiation of cystic, solid, or complex breast alterations.

   c) In radiologically dense breasts sonography is a valuable examination sometimes yielding information indicating the diagnosis.

   d) In cases of fibrocystic mastopathy, sonography provides clear evidence and permits follow-up without radiation exposure.

e) In young patients, sonography can be used for the first examination of palpable breast nodules.

f) Sonography is useful when new nodules occur in pregnant women, since mammography is usually inconclusive.

g) When breast prostheses are involved sonography provides a valuable aid to assessment of the glandular tissue surrounding the silicon implant, since in contrast to roentgen rays, sound waves are able to pass through the silicon prosthesis.

References

Bielke G, Nieswandt Z, Wessels G, Schmarsow R, Kiefer H (1980) Echtzeit-Mammasonographie mit Hilfe eines speziellen Applikators. Tumor Diagnostik 5: 255−259

Burns PN, Halliwell M, Wells PNT, Webb AJ (1982) Ultrasonic doppler studies of the breast. Ultrasound Med Biol 8: 127−143

Carson PL, Scherzinger AL, Oughton TV, Kubitschek JE, Lambert PA, Moore GE, Dunn MG, Dick DE (1979) Progress in ultrasonic computed tomography (CT) of the breast. Spie 173: 372−391. Application of Optical Instrumentation in Medicine VII by the Society of Photo-Optical Instrumentation Engineers, Box 10, Bellingham, WA 98225, USA

Cole-Beuglet C, Goldberg BB, Kurtz AB, Rubin CS, Patchefsky AS, Shaber GS (1981) Ultrasound mammography: a comparison with radiographic mammography. Radiology 139: 693−698

Cole-Beuglet C, Goldberg BB, Kurtz AB, Patchefsky AS, Shaber GS, Rubin CS (1982) Clinical experience with a prototype real-time dedicated breast scanner. AJR 139: 905−911

Cole-Beuglet C, Soriano RZ, Kurtz AB, Goldberg BB (1983) Fibroadenoma of the breast: sonomammography correlated with pathology in 122 patients. AJR 140: 369−375

Friedrich M (1980) Ultraschalluntersuchung der Brust. Erfahrungen mit einem hochauflösenden "Real-Time"-Gerät. Radiologe 20: 209−225

Friedrich M (1981) Neue technische Entwicklungen der Röntgen- und Ultraschalluntersuchung der Mamma. Röntgenpraxis 34: 181−195

Friedrich M (1982) Was leistet die Mamma-Sonographie? Gynäkol Prax 6: 393−414

Friedrich M, Claussen CC, Felix R (1981) Methodische Aspekte der Mammasonographie. Fortschr Röntgenstr 135/6: 704−713

Friedrich M, Hundt E, Maderlechner G (1982) Computerized ultrasound echo tomography of the breast. Eur J Radiol 2: 78−87

Greenleaf JF, Bahn RC (1981) Clinical imaging with transmissive ultrasonic computerized tomography. J.E.E.E. Trans Biomed Eng BME 28/2: 177−185

Gros CHM, Dale G, Gairard B (1977) Echographie mammaire: critères de malignité. Sénologia 4: 47−57

Gros CHM, Dale G, Gairard B (1978) La compression en échographie mammaire. Senologie 3/2: 3−12

Harper P, Kelly-Fry E (1980) Ultrasound visualization of the breast in symptomatic patinets. Radiology 137/2: 465−469

Igl W, Lohe K, Eiermann W, Bassermann R, Lissner J (1980) Sonographische Carcinomdiagnostik der weiblichen Brust im Vergleich zur Mammographie. Tumor Diagnostik 5: 247−253

Kasumi F, Fukami A, Kuno K, Kakitani T (1982) Characteristic echographic features of circumscribed cancer. Ultrasound Med Biol 8/4: 369−375

Kobayashi T (1978) Clinical ultrasound of the breast. Plenum, New York

Kobayashi T (1979) Diagnostic ultrasound in breast cancer: analysis of retrotumorous echo patterns correlated with sonic attenuation by cancerous connective tissue. J Clin Ultrasound 7: 471−479

Minasian H, Bamber JC (1982) A preliminary assessment of an ultrasonic doppler method for the study of blood flow in human breast cancer. Ultrasound Med Biol 8/4: 357−364

Moskowitz M (1982) Reihenuntersuchungen zur Diagnostik des Mammakarzinoms: Wie wirksam sind unsere Untersuchungsmethoden? In: Frischbier HJ (ed) Die Erkrankungen der weiblichen Brustdrüse. Thieme, Stuttgart

Norton SJ, Linzer M (1979) Ultrasonic reflectivity tomography: Reconstruction with circular transducer arrays. Ultrasonic Imaging 1: 154–184

Pluygers E, Rombaut M (1980) Ultrasonic diagnosis of breast diseases. Tumor Diagnostik 4: 187–194

Robinson DE, Knight PC (1981) Computer reconstruction techniques in compound scan pulse-echo imaging. Ultrasonic Imaging 3: 217–234

Rosner D, Weiss L, Norman M (1980) Ultrasonography in the diagnosis of breast disease. J Surg Oncology 14: 83–96

Schmidt W, Teubner J, van Kaick G, von Fournier E, Kubli F (1981) Ultrasonographische Untersuchungsergebnisse bei der Mammadiagnostik. Geburtshilfe Frauenheilkd 41: 533–539

Teixidor HS, Kazam E (1977) Combined mammographic-sonographic evaluation of breast masses. AJR 128: 409–417

Teubner J, van Kaick G, Pickenhan L, Schmidt W (1982) Vergleichende Untersuchungen mit verschiedenen echomammographischen Verfahren. Ultraschall 3: 109–118

Teubner J, Müller A, van Kaick G (1983) Echomorphologie der Brustdrüse. Vergleichende sonographische, radiologische, anatomische und histologische Untersuchungen von Mammapräparaten. Radiologe 23: 97–107

Thiel CH, Schweikhart G (1982) Ultraschallmammographie: Ihre Bedeutung im Rahmen einer integrierten Mammadiagnostik. Fortschr Röntgenstr 137/1: 1–12

van Kaick G, Schmidt W, Teubner J, Lorenz D, Lorenz A, Müller A (1980) Echomammographie mit verschiedenen Gerätetypen bei herdförmigen Läsionen. Tumor Diagnostik 4: 179–186

Wade G, Elliott S, Khogeer I, Flesher G, Eisler J, Mensa D, Ramesh NS, Heidbreder G (1980) Acoustic echo computer tomography. In: Metherell AF (ed) Acoustical imaging, vol 8. Plenum, New York, pp 565–576

Weiss L, Rosner D, Glenn WE (1978) Visualization of breast lesions with an advanced ultrasonic device: results of a pilot study. J Surg Oncology 10: 251–271

Wells PNT, Halliwell M, Skidmore B, Webb AJ, Woodcock JP (1977) Tumour detection by ultrasonic Doppler blood flow signals. Ultrasonics 15: 231–232

Wells PNT, Burns PN, Cole SE, Halliwell M, Turner GM, Webb AJ (1979) Ultrasonic doppler studies of the breast. I. Inter. Congress on the ultrasonic examination of the breast, Philadelphia

Ultrasound Mammography:
Possibilities and Limitations in the Detection of Early Breast Cancer

G. Lauth, V. Duda, and B. J. Hackelöer

Zentrum für Frauenheilkunde und Geburtshilfe der Philipps-Universität Marburg, Pilgrimstein 3, 3550 Marburg/Lahn, Federal Republic of Germany

Introduction

From September 1979 to September 1982 a series of 221 women with pathologically confirmed breast cancer underwent an extended diagnostic procedure at the Medical Center for Gynecology and Obstetrics in Marburg. All 221 cases were examined sonographically with the U.I. Octoson system (Ausonics/immersional scanning system with eight 3-MHz transducers) and radiologically with the Senographe 500 t system (CGR Koch & Sterzel/screen film mammography). The possibilities and limitations in the detection of early breast cancer by ultrasound and its diagnostic differentiation from other lesions, e.g., fibrocystic disease, will be illustrated with reference to 30 cases of breast carcinoma with a pathohistological diameter of 1 cm or less (= 13.6% of all carcinomas examined).

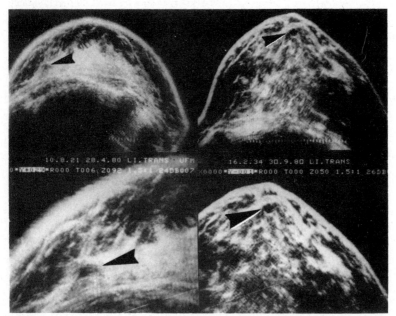

Fig. 1. Two examples of early breast cancer with different ultrasonic appearances: *left*, small structural discontinuity; *right*, relatively well-defined mass

Early Breast Cancer
Edited by J. Zander and J. Baltzer
© Springer-Verlag Berlin Heidelberg 1985

Results

The smallest carcinoma we detected by ultrasound had a diameter of up to 5 mm by morphological investigation. This compares very well with the reports of Fields (1980): 5 mm, Harper and Kelly-Fry (1980): 7 mm, and Jellins et al. (1975): 5 mm. In principle, small breast cancers have the same ultrasonic appearance as larger ones. They may vary from hyporeflective and poorly defined discontinuities of breast architecture to relatively well-defined hyporeflective masses (Fig. 1).

An acoustic middle shadow is not a definitive sign for malignancy, nor is it an obligatory diagnostic tool for carcinoma. Nevertheless, in our experience it can furnish helpful clues in the investigation of carcinoma, especially when it is well defined and can be produced from different angles or in different planes (Figs. 2 and 3).

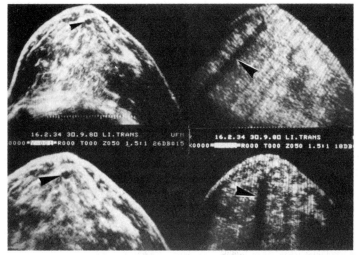

Fig. 2. Small carcinoma with well-defined acoustic middle shadow sign produced from different angles

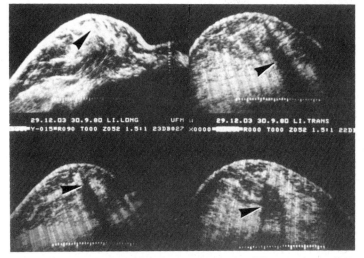

Fig. 3. Small carcinoma with acoustic middle shadow sign produced in different planes (*left*, longitudinal plane; *right*, transverse plane) and from different angles

Table 1. Correlation between sonographic and radiologic diagnosis of 30 small carcinomas with a diameter of less than or equal to 1 cm on morphological investigation

Carcinoma up to 1 cm in diameter 30 = 100%	Sonography positive 23 = 76%	Sonography negative 7 = 23%
x-Ray positive 28 = 93%	22 = 73%	6 = 20%
x-Ray negative 2 = 6%	1 = 3%	1 = 3%

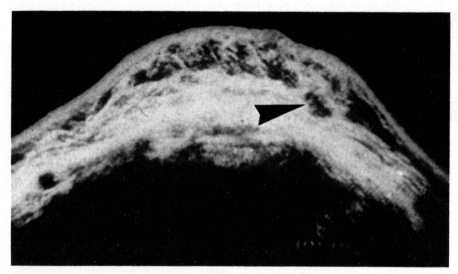

Fig. 4. The presence of microcalcifications would not be suspected in the mass shown in this sonogram

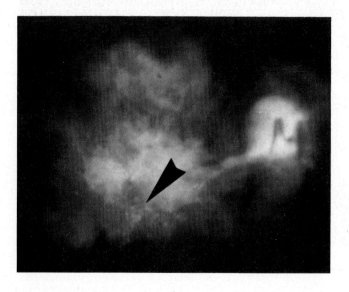

Fig. 5. Same mass as in Fig. 4, x-ray of the surgical specimen clearly showing many clustered microcalcifications

The correlation shown in Table 1 was obtained between ultrasonographic and radiologic diagnosis of 30 small carcinomas, 23 of which were diagnosed by ultrasonography and 28 by radiology as being suggestive of malignancy.

Table 1 classes seven cases as „x-ray positive", in which clustered microcalcifications only had been seen. It must be admitted that detection of microcalcifications by sonography is not yet possible (Fig. 4). An x-ray investigation of surgical specimens is certainly the best way of checking for successful removal of microcalcifications (Fig. 5). Although it would be possible to examine surgical specimens by ultrasound, such an investigation could only provide ineffective clues.

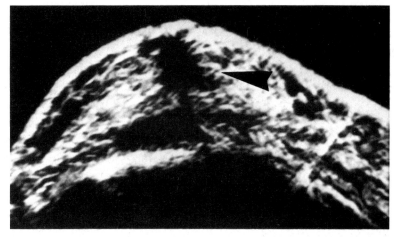

Fig. 6. Sonogram of a 2-cm mass, later found to contain a 5-mm mass of scirrhous carcinoma

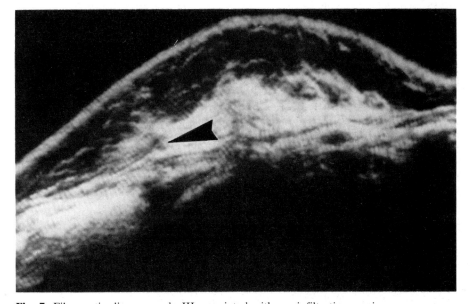

Fig. 7. Fibrocystic disease grade III associated with noninfiltrating carcinoma

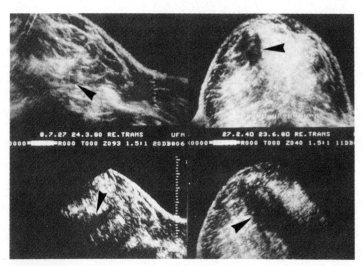

Fig. 8. Fibrocystic disease (*left,* grade III; *right,* grade II) with suggestive ultrasonic appearance

The 23 cases classed under "Sonography positive" in Table 1 include 7 cases in whom sonography showed fibrocystic changes more clearly than the carcinoma itself (Fig. 6).

In four cases sonography showed a mass suspected to be malignant, when a fibrocystic disease of a very high degree (grade III according to Prechtel) was associated with a noninfiltrating carcinoma (Fig. 7).

It must be stated, however, that of 29 cases with fibrocystic disease grade III (without any changes suggesting incipient malignancy) and 61 cases with fibrocystic disease grade I or II, 83% and 69%, respectively, were suspected to be malignant (Fig. 8).

Such counts, limiting the usefulness of ultrasonic diagnostic techniques for early breast cancer, must by no means be discouraging. The method certainly is not suitable for definition of the degree of fibrocystic changes. It is also not informative about changes of fibrocystic disease into malignant growth or about infiltrating growth of carcinoma at all. The chance of detecting any fibrocystic changes by sonography opens up the possibility of keeping patients at risk under observation, however.

References

Fields SI (1980) Ultrasound mammographic-histopathologic correlation. Ultrasonic Imaging 2: 150–161

Hackelöer BJ, Lauth G, Duda V, Hüneke B, Buchholz R (1980) Neue Möglichkeiten der Ultraschallmammographie. Geburtshilfe Frauenheilkd 40: 301–312

Hackelöer BJ, Hüneke B, Duda V, Eulenburg R, Lauth G, Buchholz R (1981) Sonographische Differentialdiagnose der Mammakarzinome. Ultraschall in der Medizin 2: 129–134

Harper P, Kelly-Fry E (1980) Ultrasound visualization of the breast in symptomatic patients. Radiology 137: 465–469

Jellins J, Kossoff G, Reeve TS, Barraclough BH (1975) Ultrasonic grey scale visualization of breast disease. Ultrasound Med Biol 1: 393–404

Lauth G, Duda V, Hackelöer BJ, Eulenburg R, Hüneke B (1982) Vergleichende Untersuchungen mit der Ultraschall- und Röntgen-Mammographie bei 200 Patientinnen mit Mammakarzinom. 2. wissenschaftliche Tagung der Deutschen Gesellschaft für Senologie, Köln, June 1982

Prechtel K (1972) Beziehungen der Mastopathie zum Mammakarzinom. Fortschr Med 90: 41–45

Ultrasonic Findings in Early Breast Cancer and Diagnostic Problems

D. Mulz[1], D. Land[2], S. Gluth[2], A. Knüpfer[1]

[1] University Hospital of Erlangen/Nürnberg, Department of Gynecology and Obstetrics, 8520 Erlangen, Federal Republic of Germany
[2] Institute of Statistics and Documentation, University of Erlangen/Nürnberg, 8520 Erlangen, Federal Republic of Germany

Sonography is a controversial method for the diagnosis of early breast cancer, particularly in doubtful cases. Many investigators question its value altogether. Mammography is undoubtedly the diagnostic method of choice. However, there are many processes that are not amenable to diagnosis at all, or only marginally, unless certain criteria are met. The difficulties of diagnosis are further compounded by palpable lesions not seen on mammograms and nonpalpable lesions that are seen on mammograms.

Since 1977 we have been working on the basis of a research program coordinated by the Deutsche Forschungsgemeinschaft (German Research Foundation), at the University Hospital of Erlangen, dealing with the combination of sonogram and low-dose mammogram. The results of this program will be shown briefly. Obviously, statements about the value of a method only become convincing when clear statistics are available. Statistical details are not the target of this paper. Suffice it to say that we investigated 3431 patients up to October 1982. Statistical analysis with clean data was achieved in 1974 patients (Fig. 1).

In the case of benign lesions, direct breast sonography solved the problem of the nonpalpable cystic breast lesion and also that of the occult cystic lesion that does not show up on the mammogram.

The reliability of the method in any cystic lesion, no matter what size, was 98%. We aspirated more than 1700 cysts and did not encounter any problems. Also, we think we solved the problem of the nonpalpable round shadow on the mammogram which is postulated in the world literature to account for up to 10% of occult cancers.

We did not encounter problems with localization since we conducted examinations with the patients in the same position as on the operating table.

We diagnosed 536 fibroadenomas among the solid lesions. This initial diagnosis was confirmed by the pathology report in 77% of cases. Solid and cystic lesions cannot be differentiated by mammography. Radiologists have great difficulty in differentiating or even seeing a lesion, because of all the overlying structures within the breast. The acoustic properties of the tissue are no help to the radiologist, but they are essential for the sonographer in differentiation of cystic and solid lesions. Most breast lesions are either cysts or fibroadenomas.

We also examined 411 cancers. In an earlier paper we documented almost 100% accuracy with tumors of above 1.5 cm vertical depth. These are obviously palpable tumors, with only rare exceptions. In these tumors mammography is not essential, since they are biopsied anyway.

Early Breast Cancer
Edited by J. Zander and J. Baltzer
© Springer-Verlag Berlin Heidelberg 1985

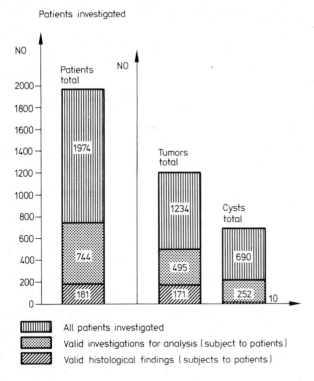

Patients investigated

Fig. 1. Overview for statistical analysis. Patients investigated in 30 consecutive months

More importantly, we can say that if we consider tumors of all sizes, including the subclinical tumors, we still achieved 76% accuracy in preoperative diagnosis of malignancy. In other words, one can depend on correct primary diagnosis of malignancy in over three-quarters of all cases.

Since statistical analysis demonstrated high reliability for sonography, we have gradually changed the indications for its use in Erlangen. We do not use it when the diagnosis is obvious, but have recourse to it when the diagnosis is uncertain using other methods. We have documented increased precision in these cases.

λ-Correlation documents the accuracy of the method used in terms of the final diagnosis (Table 1). In our material it doubled the accuracy of mammography in cases where diagnosis was difficult.

The value of sonography can be demonstrated in differentiation of dysplasia of various grades, carcinoma in situ, fibroadenoma, and cancer (Fig. 2). Clear statistical data could be given in every case. Simultaneously with the changes in the tissue revealed by histological examination, there was an increase in the sonographic diagnosis of malignancy. In the cases of carcinoma in situ, the investigator estimated the area to be malignant or at least suggestive of malignancy in almost every case.

All these results were obtained with a machine produced in 1977. For high diagnostic accuracy, high resolution is needed. How can dysplasia be depicted in the mammogram? The pictures in Fig. 3 show cancer and normal milk duct structures. The marker beside the tumor indicates the depth of 1 cm. This demonstrates the accuracy of the method.

In the case of borderline tumors or carcinoma in situ an irregularity or heterogeneity is frequently noticed on the screen. This is not easily demonstrated on a slide, because the

Table 1. λ-Correlation for final histological diagnosis

Ultrasound diagnosis	Histological diagnosis				
	Benign	Benign tumor	Dysplasia	Malignant tumor	Total
O.K.	0	2	2	0	4
Benign	4	48	9	4	65
Doubtful	5	7	6	10	28
Malignant	8	6	11	42	67
Total	17	63	28	56	164

$\lambda = 38.6\%$

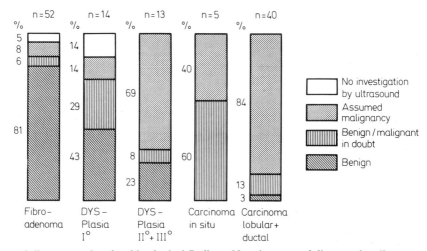

Fig. 2. Ultrasound diagnoses related to histological findings. Note increase of diagnosed malignancy in dysplasia and carcinoma in situ. Obvious correlation with changes in tissue according to pathology

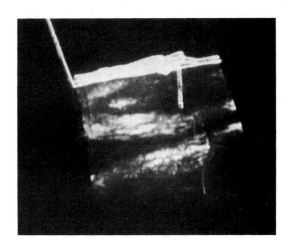

Fig. 3. Small cancerous area in the breast. Marker height 1 cm. Combined-plane technique

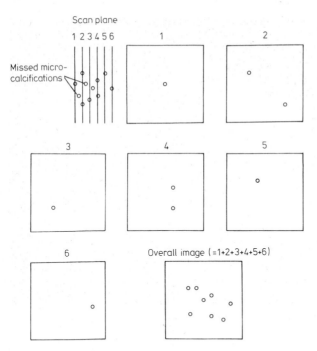

Fig. 4. Several single images must be combined to give one combined-plane picture

changes are very subtle. By the same token, no tumor shadow can be demonstrated in such cases.

All statements as to the volume of a tumor have to be treated with great caution. Its size in the ultrasonic image is dependent on the plane of the scan. Similarly, on a pathology slide the size of a lesion can also be misjudged depending on the plane of a cut.

Our findings were questioned many times with reference to visualization of microcalcifications. We have never claimed to see microcalcifications directly.

We needed to remember that the sonogram is always dependent on echoreflections. Hard particles give higher impedance-type reflections than soft tissue. Therefore, the apparatus needs a high dynamic range for visualization of these differences in impedance. Moreover, several scan planes together are needed for accurate assessment of the area investigated. This is demonstrated in Fig. 4. If the single scan planes are considered together, the microcalcification pattern is clearly obvious (Figs. 4, 6).

The two pictures obtained of a carcinoma with adjacent microcalcifications with the simple-scan technique (Fig. 5) and with the combined-plane technique (Fig. 6) give added confirmation. On the basis of this, we decided to designate our findings as benign, equivocal, or malignant. Finally, ultrasonic diagnosis is highly dependent on the expertise of the investigator, who has to decide how to interpret the echoes.

In summary, our statistical analysis proves that 97% of all malignant processes can be detected, but only at the expense of a false-positive rate of 33%. In other words, a diagnosis of malignancy is correct in three of four cases. Considering the three diagnostic groups of malignant, equivocal, and suggestive of microcalcification, we were able to document very high overall accuracy.

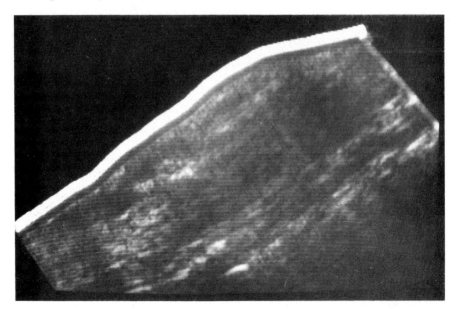

Fig. 5. Breast cancer with microcalcifications. Simple-scan technique

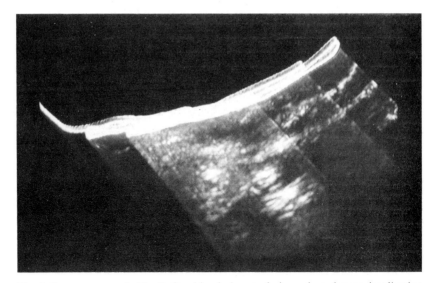

Fig. 6. Same cancer as in Fig. 5. Combined-plane technique gives clearer visualization of microcalcifications

Reliability of Ultrasound of the Breast with Automated and Manual Scanning Compared with x-Ray Mammography

M. Kessler[1], W. Igl[1], R. Bassermann[2], H. Bohmert[3], W. Eiermann[4], and K. J. Lohe[5]

[1] Radiologische Klinik und Poliklinik, [2] Pathologisches Institut, [3] Chirurgische Klinik,
[4] II. Frauenklinik, Klinikum Großhadern, Ludwig-Maximilians-Universität München,
 Marchioninistr. 15, 8000 München 70, Federal Republic of Germany
[5] I. Frauenklinik und Hebammenschule,
 Maistrasse 1, 8000 München 2, Federal Republic of Germany

The constant discussion about the radiation risk in mammography and its limited value in dense breasts and in the differential diagnosis of microcalcifications has repeatedly prompted clinical investigation of alternative diagnostic procedures.

Wild's first publication about ultrasonic examination of the breast dates back to the year 1951 (Wild and Neal 1951). Wider application of the method, however, was made possible only by the technical advances in recent years. The present level of sophistication in equipment allows two new features of diagnostic evaluation: complete morphological representation of the breast, comparable to that given by mammography, with automated water-path scanners; and differentiation of palpable or mammographically proven lesions with manually operated compound or real-time apparatus.

However, early detection of breast carcinoma has so far not been possible with either of these methods.

In our hospital, ultrasound has been used in breast diagnostics since 1978 (Igl et al. 1980, to be published; Kessler et al. 1983).

Studies have been conducted in 1,000 randomly selected patients examined with an automated water-path scanner SMV 50 E, 4.2 transducer from the Technicare Company. The apparatus supplies 120 sagittal sector scans of the female breast in 2 minutes, at slice intervals of 1.7 mm.

In addition, 201 selected patients have been examined preoperatively with a Picker Compound Echoview 80 LDI, 5 MHz, with a water bag.

In 50 cases, again preoperatively, the compound scan was compared with a real-time scan. For this purpose a Siemens Diasonics RA-1, 7.5 MHz with oil coupling was used.

Morphologically, the corresponding sonographic findings can be set against the parenchymal patterns of the mammogram.

A sonographically fatty breast, for instance, shows weak echoes (Fig. 1a). In contrast, a dense breast is echogenic with a small subcutaneous fat layer (Fig. 1b).

The sonograms were evaluated according to the criteria described in the literature (Cole-Beuglet et al. 1980; Kobayashi 1980; Kobayashi et al. 1974).

The analysis of contour, form, internal echoes, boundaries, attenuation, or enhancement allows differentiation of cystic, solid benign, and solid malignant masses. In addition, there are indirect sonographic criteria, such as alteration of breast form, retraction and thickening of the cutis or the nipple, dilated ducts, destruction of the structures close to the chest wall, and lymph node enlargement.

Early Breast Cancer
Edited by J. Zander and J. Baltzer
© Springer-Verlag Berlin Heidelberg 1985

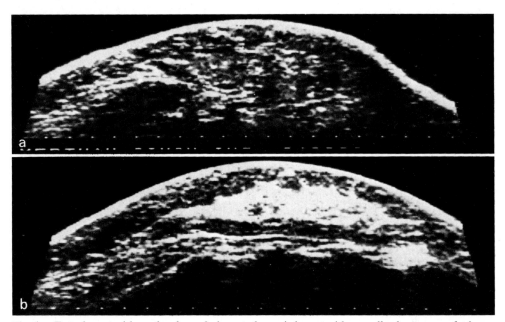

Fig. 1. a Fatty breast with weak echoes; **b** dense echogenic breast with a small subcutaneous fat layer

Table 1. Diagnostic accuracy of x-ray mammography and automated
ultrasound in detection of cysts ($n = 76$)

	x-Ray mammography		Ultrasound	
	n	%	n	%
True positive	42	55	75	99
False negative	34	45	1	1

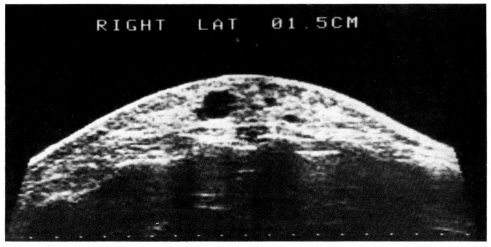

Fig. 2. Multiple cysts in a dense parenchyma – echo-free, well-defined lesions with distal
enhancement

Table 2. Diagnostic accuracy of x-ray mammography and automated
ultrasound in detection of fibroadenoma ($n = 78$)

	x-Ray mammography		Ultrasound	
	n	%	n	%
True positive	75	96	40	51
False negative	3	4	38	49

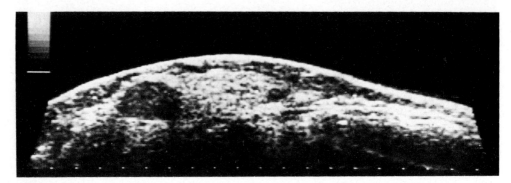

Fig. 3. Smooth round lesion with weak homogeneous internal echoes: fibroadenoma of the breast

The results are as follows: In a comparison we detected and correctly classified 165 masses in a total sample of 204 masses by mammography, but only 149 with automated ultrasound.

When cystic and solid masses are considered separately, sonography is clearly superior in the detection and differential diagnosis of cysts. Sonography allowed differentiation of cysts down to a size of 0.4 cm, even in dense parenchyma (Table 1 and Fig. 2).

For the study of solid lesions, mammography is clearly more accurate. Adenomas smaller than 1 cm could normally not be detected with the automated scan. When larger than 1 cm they were detected in young, dense breasts better than in weakly echogenic postmenopausal breasts (Table 2 and Fig. 3).

Carcinoma was confirmed in 50 cases in 104 biopsies. In two patients the carcinoma could not be diagnosed either by mammography or by ultrasound. But a total of 16 carcinomas was missed with ultrasound.

A classification by tumor size shows that the sonographically negative findings consisted mainly of small tumors with a good prognosis, which were in stage T1 and smaller than 1 cm (Tables 3 and 4).

In an automated scan these carcinomas were not detectable even when the examination was repeated with prior knowledge of the site of the pathologic findings. The subsequent manual sonography, however, was clearly positive, showing seven carcinomas smaller than 1 cm, including even the ductal carcinoma in situ illustrated in Fig. 4.

Apart from the poor resolution of the automated scan, it was noted that in 12% of 1,000 examinations there was shadowing behind the nipple despite compression. Furthermore, in 14% of predominantly dysplastic breasts, the evaluation was limited because of diffuse

Table 3. Diagnostic accuracy of x-ray mammography and automated ultrasound in 104 biopsies (50 carcinomas)

	x-Ray mammography		Ultrasound	
	n	%	n	%
True positive	48	46	34	33
True negative	42	40	35	34
False positive	12	12	19	18
False negative	2	2	16	15

Table 4. Diagnostic accuracy of x-ray mammography and automated ultrasound in relation to tumor size (n = 50 carcinomas)

	TIS	T1 < 1 cm	T1 > 1 cm	T2	T3	T4
Total number	2	10	14	12	11	1
x-Ray mammography	2	9	14	12	10	1
Ultrasound	–	2	11	11	9	1

shadowing due to the fixed geometry of a tangential beam, and in many cases the upper outer quadrant could not be visualized with beam angles of approximately 60°.

These phenomena are avoidable with the manual method because the beam angles can be varied.

With the compound technique, 201 patients were examined preoperatively. In 94 a carcinoma was histologically verified; in 83 cases the result of manual scanning was true positive and in 11, false negative.

When 78 carcinomas were subdivided by size, tumors in stages T2 to T4 were reliably verified. However, in stage T1, of 18 neoplasms smaller than 1 cm only 12 were correctly diagnosed (Tables 5 and 6).

The poor diagnostic accuracy in automated ultrasound and the time-consuming nature of the compound method motivated us to undertake a third study, in which 50 patients were examined preoperatively, each with the compound technique and with the speedy real-time technique. This examination was carried out with the prior knowledge of mammographic localization of masses but not of their x-ray classification (Friedrich 1980; Friedrich et al. 1981; Teubner et al. 1982).

In 89 (85%) of the cases studied neoplastic lesions were confirmed, the results thus being relatively highly consistent with those of mammography; but a lower degree of consistency was achieved when only suggestive calcifications were visible (Tables 7 and 8).

On four occasions the classification of findings recorded with the real-time apparatus was hampered by the fact that sonographic criteria such as irregular boundaries or central shadowing could not be accurately identified.

Classification was better with the compound technique, but in spite of the best axial and lateral resolution, even with the prior knowledge of exact localization, three carcinomas 5 mm in size could not be made visible due to unsophisticated equipment, but were seen in the real-time technique.

Generally, however, no significant difference in resolution between the two systems could be detected on a phantom breast with simulated cystic defects.

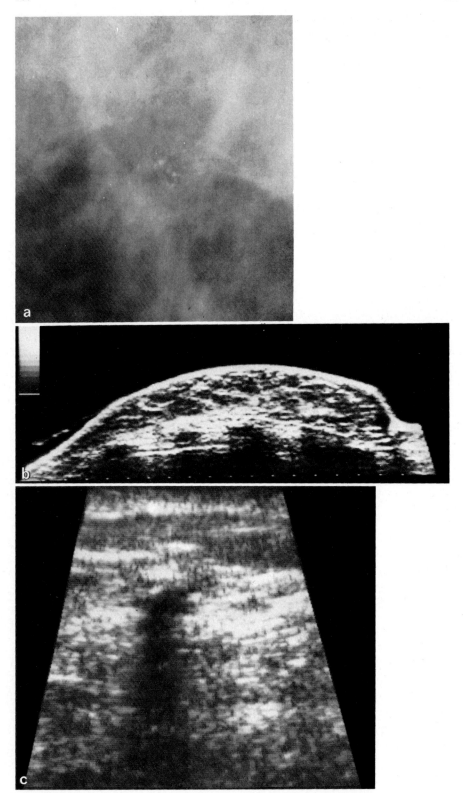

Table 5. Diagnostic accuracy of manual scanning in 201 biopsies and 94 histologically proven carcinomas

	n	%
True positive	83	41
True negative	70	35
False positive	37	18
False negative	11	6

Table 6. Diagnostic accuracy of manual scanning in relation to the tumor's size ($n = 78$) (Picker Compound Echoview 80L DI, 5 MHz)

	T1 < 1 cm	T1 > 1 cm	T2	T3	T4
Total	18	26	28	4	2
True positive	12	24	28	4	2
False negative	6	2	28	4	2

Table 7. Diagnostic accuracy of manual ultrasound compared with x-ray mammography and histology ($n = 50$, malignant $n = 27$, benign $n = 23$)

	Detection		Classification	
	n	%	n	%
x-Ray mammography	50	100	48	96
Compound	48	96	45	90
Real-time	46	92	43	86

Table 8. Detection of carcinomas by manual ultrasound compared with x-Ray mammography ($n = 27$)

	Carcinomas ($n = 27$)		T1 < 1 cm ($n = 11$)		In situ ($n = 4$)
	n	%	n	%	n
x-Ray mammography	27	100	11	100	4
Compound	24	89	9	82	3
Real-time	23	85	9	82	2

◄

Fig. 4a–c. Clustered microcalcifications in a ductal carcinoma in situ. The automated scan (**a**) shows no pathologic findings. Weakly echogenic lesion with central shadowing in the real-time scan (**c**)

Table 9. Percentage distribution of ultrasound criteria in 67 cysts

	n	%
Smooth	63	94
Round, oval	64	96
Echo-free	59	88
Distal enhancement	56	84
Bilateral wall shadowing	25	37

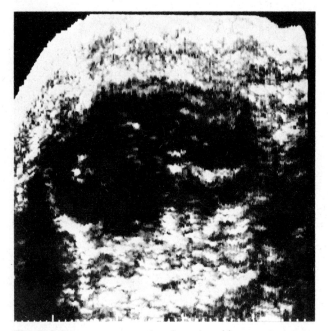

Fig. 5. Inhomogeneous weak echoes in a biopsy-proven cyst

The resolution in the automated apparatus was clearly lower, however (Madsen et al. 1982; Teubner et al. 1982).

Besides the technical limitations misinterpretations arose from the fact that the aforementioned sonographic criteria are not always valid. These criteria were best fulfilled with cysts. As a rule, they are smoothly marginated, round or oval, and echo-free. Distal enhancement and bilateral shadowing are present (Jellius et al. 1977).

In cysts smaller than 1 cm the distal enhancement may be absent. In larger cysts or hematocysts or in the presence of cell detritus, internal echoes can also be found; enhancement is not detectable (Table 9 and Fig. 5).

The criteria for solid lesions were even more markedly atypical. Adenomas are smoothly marginated, and homogeneous with intermediate to strong echo density, the distal enhancement being moderate or absent (Cole-Beuglet et al. 1980).

However, 22% of the adenomas evaluated showed a central shadowing and it was not possible to differentiate them clearly from a carcinoma (Table 10 and Fig. 6).

Table 10. Percentage distribution of ultrasound criteria in 46 fibroadenomas

	n	%
Smooth	33	72
Round, oval	36	78
Homogeneous	35	76
Central shadowing	10	22

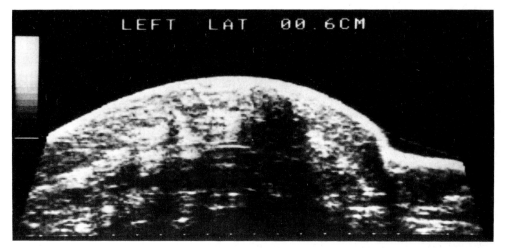

Fig. 6. Biopsy-proven fibroadenoma, irregular and lobulated with central shadowing

In their classic form, carcinomas are irregularly marginated and inhomogeneous, and the contours are not sharply defined. Depending on the stroma-to-epithelium ratio, a distal central shadowing can be found with increasing collagen content. This shadowing is most typical for scirrhous carcinoma (Hackelöer et al. 1981).

Of the carcinomas in this study however, 17% were smoothly marginated and rather homogeneous; in 34% there was an absence of shadowing; there can even be enhancement. For medullary and mucinous carcinoma in particular, therefore, the differential diagnosis against adenoma and also against cyst can be impossible (Table 11 and Fig. 7).

Microcalcifications lie below the resolution capability of sonography. The large number of biopsies recommended following mammography will not be reduced by sonography, however, since fibrocystic disease can actually yield sonographic images suggestive of a malignant tumor.

In 35% of 31 histologically verified cases of calcifying fibrocystic disease a weakly echogenic lesion was found. In 35% central shadowing was even demonstrated (Table 12 and Fig. 8).

A carcinoma can be best diagnosed by mammography when it is 3–5 mm in size. The resolution appropriate for this can of course also be obtained by sonography. Nevertheless, from experience with various modes of equipment we think it unrealistic to abandon mammography at present. It is true that automated scanners may allow complete visualization of the breast and that manual apparatus allows reliable representation of

Table 11. Percentage distribution of ultrasound criteria in 35 carcinomas

	n	%
Irregular	29	83
Lobulated	30	85
Inhomogeneous	29	83
Central shadowing	23	66

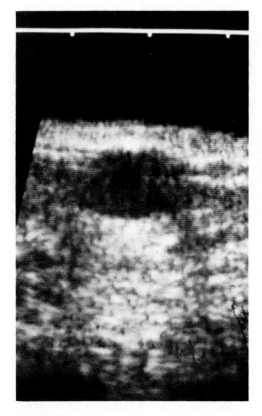

Fig. 7. Medullary carcinoma of the breast: smooth oval lesion with homogeneous weak internal echoes and distal enhancement

pathological lesions smaller than 1 cm. As a rule, however, verification requires palpation or mammography. A selection of sick patients from a symptom-free collective is not possible at present (Friedrich et al. 1981).

In our opinion, sonography today is not a method competing with mammography but rather a complementary one. It provides additional information concerning the genesis of pathologic lesions in the female breast.

Therefore, for patients under 30 years of age, with a palpable mass, we recommend sonography first. If there is a solid tumor, further mammographic or histological evaluation will be necessary if there are any doubts as to the nature of the lesion or if a high-risk patient is concerned.

For patients over 30 years, sonography is recommended in addition to mammography, since there will be dense breast tissue in which evaluation can be difficult. Moreover,

Table 12. Ultrasound criteria in 31 biopsy proven cases of fibrocystic diseases of the breast

	n	%
Irregular	13	42
Lobulated	11	35
Weak internal echoes	16	52
Inhomogeneous	5	16
Central shadowing	11	35

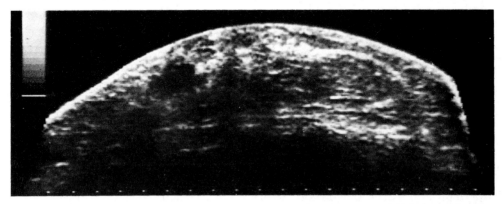

Fig. 8. Biopsy-proven benign fibrocystic disease: irregular and lobulated mass of the breast with weak internal echoes

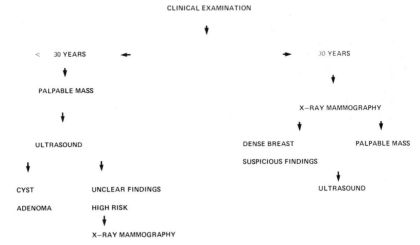

Fig. 9. Schematic diagram of x-ray mammography and ultrasound in the diagnosis of breast diseases

sonography is useful for the differentiation between cystic and solid masses. Neither sonography nor mammography allows reliable classification of a smoothly marginated, solid mass or even clustered calcifications into benign and malignant groups. Even in future the pathologist will have to decide this (Fig. 9).

Acknowledgement. This work was supported by the grant no Li 85-19-2 from the Deutsche Forschungsgemeinschaft.

References

Cole-Beuglet CM, Goldberg BB, Patchefsky AS, Rubin CS, Schneck CD, Soriano RZ (1980) Atlas of breast ultrasound. Telles, Philadelphia

Friedrich M (1980) Ultraschalluntersuchung der Brust. Erfahrungen mit einem hochauflösenden "Real-time" Gerät. Radiologe 20: 209

Friedrich M, Claussen CC, Felix R (1981) Methodische Aspekte der Mammasonographie. Erfahrungen mit einem Immersionsscanner. Fortschr Röntgenstr 135: 704

Igl W, Lohe K, Eiermann W, Bassermann R, Lissner J (1980) Sonographische Karzinomdiagnostik der weiblichen Brust im Vergleich zur Mammographie. Tumor Diagnostik 5: 247

Igl W, Kessler M, Bassermann R (to be published) In: Schildberg H (ed) Echomammographie. Perimed, Erlangen

Jellius J, Kossoff E, Reeve TS (1977) Detection and classification of liquid-filled masses in the breast by gray-scale echography. Radiology 125: 205

Hackelöer BJ, Hüncke B, Duda V, Eulenburg R, Lauth E, Buchholz R (1981) Sonographische Differentialdiagnose der Mammakarzinome. Ultraschall 2: 129

Kessler M, Igl W, Krauss B, Bassermann R, Bohmert DH, Eiermann W, Lohe KJ, Lissner J (1983) Vergleich von Mammographie und automatisierter Sonographie an 700 Patientinnen. Fortschr Röntgenstr 138: 331

Kobayashi T (1980) Current status of breast ultrasonography and ultrasound tissue characterization of breast cancer. In: Lindberg DAB, Kaihara S (eds) Medinfo 80. North Holland, Amsterdam

Kobayashi T, Takatani O, Hattori N, Kimura K (1974) Differential diagnosis of breast tumors. The sensitivity graded method of ultrasonotomography and clinical evluation of its diagnostic accuracy. Cancer 33: 940

Madsen EL, Zagzebski JA, Frank GR (1982) An anthropomorphic ultrasound breast phantom containing intermediate-sized scatters. Ultrasound Med Biol 8: 381

Teubner J, van Kaick G, Pickenhahn L, Schmidt W (1982) Vergleichende Untersuchungen mit verschiedenen echomammographischen Verfahren. Ultraschall 3: 109

Wild J, Neal D (1951) Use of high-frequency ultrasonic waves for detecting changes of texture in living tissues. Lancet 1: 655

A Topical View of the Value of Infrared Thermography in Breast Cancer

R. Amalric and J. M. Spitalier

Cancer Institute, 232 Boulevard de Sainte Marguerite, 13273 Marseille Cedex 09, France

Introduction

Infrared thermography (IRT) is still not well-known or as much used as it deserves, because its purpose is generally misunderstood. It is a method of functional investigation, and does not give anatomical static images but yields unique data on the dynamic behavior of breast cancers.

When used in a multidisciplinary unit (physicians, radiologists, surgeons, and pathologists) on a large scale, IRT provides immediate or deferred information (sometimes with prognostic significance). It yields unique data in four precise fields:

Early detection for small cancers (TO nonpalpable and T1 in the UICC classification).

Prognosis and therapeutic decision.

Follow-up after treatment.

Breast cancer screening, since high-risk patients can be identified.

Study Material

In 13 years of practice we have examined 46,000 patients by means of IRT, 11,500 of whom had palpable tumors. All these patients were submitted to physical examination and mammography. In 8,021 confirmation by pathology (cytology and/or biopsy) was obtained. These last examinations revealed 3,305 benign breast lesions and 4,716 carcinomas (Table 1).

Most of these cancers have been treated by the same staff members and have been followed-up for many years, with periodic combined screening with IRT. Thus, 18,000 thermograms have been performed during the same period for follow-up of 4,000 breast cancers treated by surgery and/or radiotherapy (most often by breast-conserving therapy).

Table 1. Study material

46,000 Breast examinations with IRT
11,500 Palpable tumors
8,021 Verified by microscopic examination
– 3,305 Benign tissue changes
– 4,716 Carcinomas

Early Breast Cancer
Edited by J. Zander and J. Baltzer
© Springer-Verlag Berlin Heidelberg 1985

Table 2. Thermographic grading of breast cancer

Thermographic grade	Type of thermogram
TH 1	Normal infrared thermogram
TH 2	Benign type of infrared thermogram
TH 3	One sign leading to suspicion of malignancy
TH 4	One sign of malignancy or several signs leading to suspicion of malignancy
TH 5	Several sign of malignancy

Table 3. Cancer significance of grades TH 3, TH 4, and TH 5

Thermographic grade	Cancer (n)	TH 3, TH 4, or TH 5 (n)	% Cancer
TH 3	1,060	1,906	56
TH 4	1,502	1,836	82
TH 5	1,575	1,678	94

Methods

We have classified mammary thermograms into five categories (Amalric et al. 1978) according to the presence or absence of suggestive or malignant signs, to allow the best possible comparison with the other methods of diagnosis. *Suggestive signs* include: asymmetrical hypervascularization, hot spot of 2.5° C, full hyperthermia of 2° C, and limited edge sign.

Signs of malignancy include: anarchic hypervascularization, hot spot of 3° C or more, full hyperthermia of more than 2° C, extended edge sign.

The five categories have an increasing significance for cancer probability, with a grading from TH1 to TH5 (Table 2).

Table 3 shows that categories TH3 to TH5 indicate a significant probability of cancer; in the case of palpable tumor, the cancer probability is 56% for suggestive TH3 images, while category TH5 is positive with a reliability of up to 94%.

Detection of Small Cancers and IRT

If we consider all the breast cancers examined, of whatever size, the reliability appears satisfactory, with 88% abnormal thermograms (TH3, TH4, and TH5).

Other methods also seem to be acceptably reliable, with an overall reliability of 87% – 95% (Table 4).

Nevertheless, the reality is quite different in the special case of small cancers in category T1 according to UICC (palpable only if the diameter is more than 5 mm in diameter and never growing to more than 20 mm) and very small cancers (not palpable at all and falling in the T0 category, i.e., the very ones we are most anxious to discover).

The positive reliability of IRT is thus only 72%, and that of other methods ranges from 60% to 83%. As a matter of fact a study of 680 small cancers (515 T1 and 165 T0) has shown that false-negative rates were 40% for physical examination, 28% for IRT, 25% for mammography, and 17% for ultrasonography (Table 5).

Table 4. Total positive reliability of four examination methods (any size of breast tumor)

	True positive + suggestive (*n*)	Cancers (*n*)	%
Clinical examination	4,121	4,716	87
Mammography	4,147	4,424	94
Infrared thermography	4,138	4,716	88
Ultrasonography	614	646	95

Table 5. False-negative results with different examination methods in 680 small breast cancers (165 T0 and 515 T1; UICC)

Clinical examination alone	272/680	= 40%
Infrared thermography alone	193/680	= 28%
Mammography alone	164/669	= 25%
Ultrasonography alone	20/118	= 17%

Table 6. False-negative results in 680 T0 and T1 cancers by examination methodcombination

	False negatives (*n*)	Cancers (*n*)	% False negatives
Clinical examination alone	272	680	40
Clinical + mammography	136	677	20
Clinical + radio + IRT	21	677	3

It is surprising to find that mammography is no more reliable than the other methods for very small cancers, which it is obviously important to detect in a systematic mass screening program. It appears, then that no method is infallible. Each involves very significant rates of defective errors. It is useless to support any against any of the others. Fortunately, these different methods are based on different principles (palpable consistency, thermal emission, photographic effect, acoustical impedance). It is unusual for them all to give wrong results at the same time for a particular cancer. The combination of these different diagnostic modalities thus allows mutual correction of errors (Table 6).

Two essential features emerge from our statistics for small carcinomas: The association of clinical examination and mammography led to 20% of false negatives.

Their combination with IRT reduces this rate to only 3%, i.e., a detection rate of 17% for small cancers (136 cases out of 680 T0 and T1), solely thanks to IRT examination.

In the cases of occult cancer that is masked by a benign tumor or tissue changes (dense breast of young women), IRT can be considered to be superior to mammography, which is often inadequate.

Finally, in subclinical cancers, Table 7 shows that the first alarm has been sound in more than half the cases screened out by IRT.

Thus, with reference to detection we conclude that IRT must not be used alone for a mass screening method, because of the 28% false-negative results for small cancers; and the

Table 7. First alarm in 165 subclinical, nonpalpable cancers
(T0: UICC)

Thermography alone	88 cases	= 53%
Thermography + mammography	52 cases	= 32%
Mammography alone	25 cases	= 15%

Mammogram abnormal in 47% of cases
Thermogram abnormal in 85% of cases

radioclinical investigation involves 20% false negatives, but with IRT in addition the false-negative rate falls to 3%.

This triple examination is recommended for high-risk women and for every patient presenting with mammary symptoms including benign mastopathy.

IRT and Breast Cancer Prognosis

The specific thermal emission of breast cancers is directly linked with their doubling times by Gautherie and Gros (1977). The long-term prognosis following curative treatment of breast cancer is a function of this rate of growth.

According to this, it appears consistent that the initial level of the thermal gradient of a defined cancer will have a prognostic significance. In fact, this has been verified by several investigators, including Loyd Williams (1969).

We have followed up more than 1,000 cases of operable breast cancers according to the first thermogram; 432 were treated 5 years ago.

More than half these cancers were treated by breast-preserving surgery (lumpectomy and limited axillary dissection) prior to curative radiotherapy. This led us to study the thermal gradients according to the SBR histoprognostic classification of Scarff (1968) and Bloom and Richardson (1957), and the involvement of axillary nodes.

Table 8 shows a striking parallel between grading according to the prognostic SBR classification and the thermal gradient rise. Grade III cancers (with the poorest prognosis) are found in six out of ten cases with a thermal gradient higher than 3° C, as against one out of ten with a thermal gradient of 2° C.

Similarly, there is a clear correlation between the axillary node involvement rate (number of positive nodes) and the thermal gradient rise of the initial IRT (Table 9).

The node involvement rate is only 10% for 2° C, and it reaches 70% for 3° C and more.

The practical implication of these data is a clear decrease in 3- and 5-year the survival: the disease-free survival rate at 5 years is reduced by half with a thermal gradient of 4° C and more (Table 10).

The survival difference is still more significant when related to the existence of thermographic signs of fast growth on the initial thermogram.[1]

Table 11 shows that in cases with such signs the survival at 5 years is decreased by a factor of 3 (from 61% to 19%).

---

1 Thermographic signs of fast growth are described by Amalric et al. (1978)

Table 8. Thermal gradients and histoprognosis[a]

Gradient ≤ 2° C	11%
Gradient = 2.5° C	27%
Gradient ≥ 3° C	62%

[a] Distribution of 120 grade III, SBR classification

Table 9. Axillary pathologic stage according to mammary temperature gradient

Mammary gradient	Axillary nodes + ve.	%
≤ 2° C	70	10
= 2.5° C	134	20
≥ 3° C	473	70

[a] Distribution of 677 positive axillary nodes

Table 10. Survival rates according to temperature gradient[a]

Gradient	3 Years	5 Years
< 4° C	58%	42%
≥ 4° C	37%	21%

[a] 504 operable breast cancers (T3/N0−N1; UICC)

Table 11. Disease-free survival and fast growth thermographic type[a]

	Cases (n)	Fast-growing IRT type	Not fast-growing IRT type
3 Years	823	40%	86%
5 Years	432	19%	61%

[a] Operable breast cancers T1−T2−T3/N0−N1; UICC)

Thus, with reference to prognosis we conclude that IRT supplements the results of other investigations (clinical staging, histological grade, axillary staging, determination of hormone receptor status) in indicating whether or not the risk of treatment failure should be considered high in a particular patient. Thus IRT helps to determine the therapeutic strategy, particularly regarding the indications for adjuvant medical therapy to complement the definitive local and regional treatment.

IRT and Posttreatment Follow-Up

The treatment of operable cancer with breast-preserving techniques, i.e., curative radiotherapy with or without limited surgery, involves particular problems in long-term follow-up of the treated breasts. Here again, IRT complements physical examination, mammography, and echotomography. Thermography helps greatly in evaluating the viability of posttreatment residual lesions, which may appear suggestive on either clinical or mammographic examination. This allows types of errors to be avoided: delaying an urgent salvage operation and incurring surgical disfigurement when a cure has been attained by other means but not been recognized (Amalric 1979).

The addition of IRT to conventional radioclinical examination increases diagnostic reliability by a factor of 4 (Table 12).

Table 12. Combined follow-up after conservative management of breast cancer[a]

	False positives	False negatives
Physical/radiological follow-up	21/220 = 10%	9/220 − 4%
Physical/radiological follow-up + IRT	6/220 = 2.5%	2/220 = 1%

[a] IRT correction of false results of physical and radiological examination

On the other hand, systematic follow-up after the treatment of breast cancer, requiring at least one IRT each year, allows early detection of cancer in the opposite breast (true screening). During 10 years of regular posttherapeutic follow-up, we have observed a 7% incidence of new cancer in the contralateral breast, 20% of these cases being subclinical, and nonpalpable.

Finally, IRT is also useful to monitor the response to palliative systemic therapy in patients having foci of disease which are sufficiently superficial. In general, thermographic regression precedes any clinical evidence of response to hormonal therapy, chemotherapy, or local radiotherapy. Serial thermograms are also of value for objective documentation of the patient's response in her clinical record.

Thus, with reference to systematic follow-up we conclude that IRT is useful in early detection of nonsterilization or of a local recurrence after conservative treatment for breast cancer. It also allows the detection of cancer in the other breast cancer while it is still not apparent on clinical and/or radiologic examination.

IRT and Forecasting of Cancer Risk

"False-positive" results of IRT, i.e, isolated abnormal thermograms with no clinical and radiographic signs, are often considered as misleading results. But if one takes the trouble to follow up patients showing such anomalies for a long enough time, further development of new cancers is observed in many cases.

This "advance view" of cancer risk is perhaps the most surprising oncological aspect of IRT. In our series, a computerized investigation has been completed on 1,416 isolated abnormal thermograms followed up for 1−8 years, with an average surveillance period of 32 months: 89 cancers have been reported, i.e., a total rate of 6.3% (Amalric et al. 1981).

Depending on whether or not normalization of the thermogram subsequently occurs, this cancer rate ranges from 0.5% to 12%. In cases with persistent thermal anomalies there are 22 times as many cancers as in those with normalized thermograms (Table 13).

The rate of development of breast cancer in persistent abnormal thermograms rises progressively with the passage of time (Table 14). The actuarial rate of cancer development in the breast is *26%* in our series in the 5th year.

This very significant rate of cancer development has been confirmed by studies by Gautherie and Gros (1980): by following up patients with benign mastopathy for 1−12 years after an abnormal IRT, they found cancers in 44%.

Thus a persistent abnormal breast thermogram represent the *highest known risk factor* for the future development of breast cancer. This is probably the most unexpected and the most important contribution of IRT in the field of oncology.

Table 13. Cancer development rates in isolated abnormal thermograms by evolution over time

Abnormal IRT	Normalization	Persistency
Number of cases	714	702
Average age	40 Years	44 Years
Average log before development	30 Months	45 Months
Number of cancers developed	4	85
Percentage of cancer development	0.56%	12.1%

Table 14. Isolated persistently abnormal thermogram as predictor of cancer risk[a]

Number of years following the first isolated IRT	Percentage of expected breast carcinomas
0−1	7.5%
0−2	11%
0−3	15%
0−4	19%
0−5	26%

[a] Actuarial calculation: 702 patients, 85 breast cancers, 1- to 8-year follow-up, average age 44

Conclusions

After 13 years of study, IRT is more useful to us than ever, both in day-to-day practice and in clinical research and our evolving understanding of breast cancer.

We must emphasize that some cancers become apparent first thermally, then radiographically, and finally clinically, IRT revealing them on average 2 years earlier than clinical examination.

This anticipatory significance of IRT makes it essential in breast disease, not only for early detection of small cancers, but also for determination of prognosis, for follow-up of known cancers, and for anticipation of further cancers.

References

Amalric R, Giraud D, Altschuler C, Deschanel J, Spitalier JM (1978) Analytical, synthetical and dynamic classification of mammary thermograms. Acta Thermographica 3: 5−17

Amalric F, Giraud D, Altschuler C, Amalric R, Spitalier JM (1979) Infra-red thermographic follow-up after breast cancer curative radiotherapy. Acta Thermographica 4: 54−59

Amalric R, Gautherie M, Hobbins WB, Stark A, Thierrée RA (1981) Avenir des femmes à thermogramme infra-rouge anormal isolé. Nouv Presse Med 10: 3153−3155

Amalric R, Giraud D, Altschuler C, Amalric F, Spitalier JM, Brandone H, Ayme Y, Alvarez-Gardiol A (1982) Does infra-red thermography truly have a role in present-day breast cancer management? Progr Clin Biol Res 117: 269−278

Bloom JIG, Richardson WW (1957) Histological grading and prognosis in breast cancer. Br J Cancer
11: 359−377

Gautherie M, Gros C (1977) Thermologie mammaire: diagnostic, prognostic, surveillance. Concours
Médical 99: 2297−2310

Gautherie M, Gros C (1980) Breast thermography and cancer risk prediction. Cancer
45: 51−56

Lloyd Williams K (1969) Thermography in the prognosis of breast cancer. In: Heerma Van Voss SFC,
Thomas P (eds) Medical thermography. Bibliotheca Radiologica vol 5. Karger, Basel,
pp 62−67

Scarff RW, Torloni H (1968) Types histologiques des tumeurs du sein. In: Classification histologique
internationale des tumeurs. OMS ed, Genève, 2

Spitalier JM, Clerc S, Levraud J, Pollet JF, Medina M, Amalric R (1978) Thermography and future of
operable breast cancers. Acta Thermographica 3: 100−106

A Topical View of the Reliability of Fine-Needle Aspiration Biopsy in the Early Detection and Biological Characterization of Breast Cancer

Gert Auer and Michael Kronenwett

Karolinska Hospital and Institute, Department of Tumor Pathology, 104 01 Stockholm, Sweden

Introduction

At the Karolinska Hospital in Stockholm fine-needle aspiration biopsy of palpable breast lesions has been performed for more than 30 years. Pioneers like Zajicek and Franzén (Franzén and Zajicek 1968, Franzén 1974) brought about valuable methodological and clinical improvements to this biopsy technique. Because of its simplicity and patient acceptibility, fine-needle aspiration biopsy is the primary biopsy method for morphological diagnosis of breast lesions in Sweden today. The cytological diagnosis is conclusive and determines the therapeutic management. Only in cases in which fine-needle aspiration biopsy does not produce a clear diagnosis is a surgical biopsy performed. The needling of palpable breast lesions is simple but nevertheless requires an adequately trained and experienced investigator. There is no doubt that by far the best results are obtained by specialists who are able to examine the patient, perform the fine-needle aspiration biopsy, evaluate the aspirated cell sample, and make the microscopical diagnosis. Excellent results can be obtained when aspiration biopsy and diagnostic cytology are performed by different persons, as is the case at many places outside Sweden. This, however, requires the same high quality of work as mentioned above, and also close contact between the various specialists.

Sampling Techniques

In palpable breast lesions the cell material is obtained by using the Cameco instrument (Cameco, Enebyberg, Sweden) (Fig. 1). The fine-needle aspiration technique consists of inserting a thin needle (0.6−0.7 mm outside diameter) into the tumor mass and aspirating cellular material into the lumen of the needle by negative pressure produced by drawing back the plunger of a 10-ml syringe attached to the needle. During sampling, the needle is moved back and forth several times through the tumor mass, usually at different angles to the original angle of insertion. The aspirated cellular material consists of single cells or clumps of cells and has been proved to be a representative sample of the entire tumor cell population (Azavedo et al. 1982). In carcinomas, generally more than 90% of the aspirated cells are tumor cells. Small numbers of nontumor cells, especially leukocytes, benign mammary epithelial cells, fibroblasts, and fat cells, are usually mixed with the tumor cells. The aspirated cellular material is smeared onto a glass slide and generally air-dried and

Early Breast Cancer
Edited by J. Zander and J. Baltzer
© Springer-Verlag Berlin Heidelberg 1985

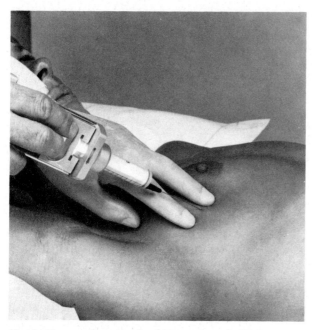

Fig. 1. Fine-needle aspiration biopsy of a palpable mammary lesion using the Cameco instrument (Cameco, Enebyberg, Sweden)

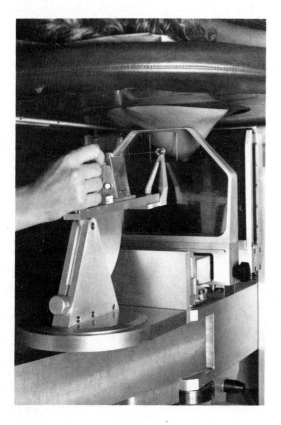

Fig. 2. Positioning for stereotactic biopsy (Nordenström 1977)

stained according to May-Grünwald-Giemsa or fixed with methanol and stained according to Papanicolaou.

Nonpalpable, mammographically demonstrated lesions can be needled by means of a stereotactic device. In our institute we use the Mammotest instrument developed by Björn Nordenström in Stockholm (1977, 1980). Figure 2 shows the general arrangement of the stereotactic instrument. The breast is fixed between two compression plates, and the position of the lesion is determined with the help of two stereoradiographs from which the coordinates are calculated. The biopsy instrument, consisting of a cannula 0.8 mm thick and an inner screw needle 0.55 mm thick, is then moved into the breast to the calculated position of the tumor. The screw needle is rotated into the tumor, and two stereoradiographs are again exposed to control its position. The cannula is then rotated over the screw needle, after which both are removed. The cell material retained in the grooves of the screw needle is handled according to the procedures mentioned above. The stereotactic technique used in Stockholm since 1977 makes it possible to obtain diagnostic material from nonpalpable, mammographically demonstrated lesions down to a size of 2–3 mm diameter. Thus, the fine-needle aspiration technique and the stereotactic technique make it possible to obtain diagnostic cellular material from both palpable and nonpalpable breast lesions without surgery.

Diagnostic Accuracy

The main goal of fine-needle aspiration biopsy is to differentiate between benign and malignant lesions. Concerning benign lesions the technique allows the diagnosis of pathologic processes such as mastitis, fat necrosis, benign mammary dysplasia, fibroadenomas, duct papillomas, etc.

The most important question is, naturally, the diagnostic accuracy in malignant lesions. Table 1 illustrates a comparison of cytological and histological material in 2,111 palpable mammary lesions studied by Zajicek (1974) at the Karolinska Hospital during the period 1955–1964. Since this period, the diagnostic accuracy of fine-needle aspiration biopsy has significantly improved. This may in part be due to the increased use of mammography.

Table 1. Comparison of cytological and histological reports in 2,111 palpable mammary lesions studied during the period 1955–1964 (figures in parentheses from 1964). (Zajicek 1974)

Cytological findings	Histological findings						Total
	Benign lesions		Precancerous lesions		Carcinoma		
	n	$\%$	n	$\%$	n	$\%$	
Negative for cancer	980	97.1	25	73.5	106	9.9 (6.1)	1,111
Suspected carcinoma	28	2.8	5	14.7	139	13.0 (11.3)	172
Carcinoma	1	0.1	4	11.8	823	77.1 (82.6)	828
Total	1,009		34		1,068		2,111

Table 2. Comparison of cytological and histological reports in 5,383 palpable mammary lesions studied during the period 1977−1983

Cytological findings	Histological findings			
	Benign lesions		Carcinoma	
	n	%	n	%
Negative for cancer	2,779	98.76	82	3.2
Suspected carcinoma	34	1.2	239	9.3
Carcinoma	1	0.04	2,248	87.5
Total	2,814	100	2,569	100

Table 3. Diagnostic accuracy of fine-needle aspiration biopsies from palpable mammary lesions studied during various periods between 1955 and 1982

	Histologically proven carcinoma	Aspiration biopsy False negative		Histologically proven benign lesions	Aspiration biopsy False positive	
	n	n	%	n	n	%
Zajicek 1955−1963	873	94	10.8	1,009	1	0.1
Zajicek 1964	195	12	6.1	202	0	0
Auer 1977−1982	2,569	82	3.2	2,814	1	0.04

Mammography is performed in all patients with palpable lesions and regularly precedes aspiration cytology. It is extremely useful in localizing lesions when palpation findings are doubtful. Positive or suggestive results of mammography may also motivate repeated and more intensive aspiration biopsies, which in turn increases the diagnostic accuracy. Table 2 shows a comparison of cytological and histological material from 5,383 palpable mammary lesions studied at the Karolinska Hospital during the period 1977−1982. Comparison of the results of Zajicek (1974) and the present authors (Table 3) clearly reveals the improvement of diagnostic accuracy in the Karolinska Hospital.

The diagnostic accuracy of the stereotactic fine-needle biopsy technique has recently been investigated and summarized by Svane (1983) for our hospital. This study comprised 120 consecutive cases with mammographically detected nonpalpable lesions. The lesions were stereotactically needled, surgically removed, and submitted to histological examination. Of the 120 lesions, 58 were found to be benign, whereas 62 were carcinomas.

The results show that in the 120 mammographically demonstrated nonpalpable breast lesions, about 80% of the cases in which the cellular material was quantitatively adequate yielded malignant or suspected malignant epithelial cells at needle biopsy. None of the 58 cases with benign lesions gave rise to a false-positive cytological report. One lesion was cytologically suggestive and another lesion was reported as atypical. This means that 56 of the histologically benign lesions, i.e., 97%, were cytologically correctly reported as benign. There was no false-positive cytological diagnosis.

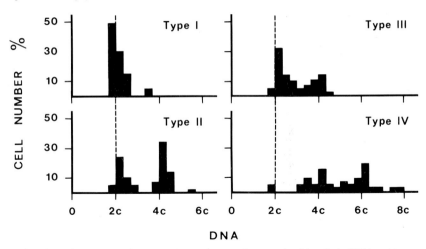

Fig. 3. DNA profiles from four types of mammary carcinoma characterized by their DNA patterns. The *broken lines* denote the mean 2c value of normal mammary epithelial cells (control cells)

Malignancy Grading

In contrast to the high degree of diagnostic accuracy of the fine-needle biopsy technique, there is at present no cytological method allowing satisfactory malignancy grading of the aspirated cellular material. Zajicek (1974) tried without success to find cytomorphological criteria allowing a reliable judgement of tumor malignancy. In recent years we have found that the nuclear DNA content of the tumor cells correlates extremely well with tumor malignancy (Auer et al. 1980). Breast carcinomas with tumor cells exhibiting diploid or diploid-tetraploid Feulgen DNA profiles (DNA histogram types I and II; Fig. 3) were found to be associated with long patient survival, whereas those with aneuploid DNA profiles (DNA histogram types III and IV; Fig. 3) were found to correlate with short patient survival, in spite of similarity in clinical stage, histomorphological type, grade of malignancy, and treatment. These studies were performed in archival May-Grün-wald-Giemsa- or Papanicolaou-stained smear preparations. Slides up to 20 years old were destained in acetic methanol, restained according to a modified Feulgen staining procedure (Gaub et al. 1975), and analyzed in a rapid scanning microspectrophotometer (Caspersson and Lomakka 1970); Caspersson and Kudynowski 1980). Figure 4 illustrates the relative frequency of types I–IV of DNA histograms in a group of patients who died within 2 years after diagnosis of a primary breast carcinoma and a group of patients who survived at least 10 years. These data indicate that DNA determinations in fine-needle aspirates can give prognostic information in individual cases, over and above that furnished by clinical staging and morphologic criteria.

Earlier work in model systems has shown that cells in the G0 phase, i.e., growth-arrested cells, can be discriminated from those in phases G1, S, and G2, i.e., proliferating cells, by measuring the total amount of proteins in the cell nucleus (Auer 1972; Auer and Zetterberg 1972; Auer et al. 1973; 1983a, b). Figure 5 shows the DNA and nuclear protein content in human G0 lymphocytes. These cells are characterized by a DNA amount of approximately 6×10^{-12} g, corresponding to 46 chromosomes and a total nuclear protein amount of 30×10^{-12} g. When these cells are growth activated, e.g., by addition of a mitogenic

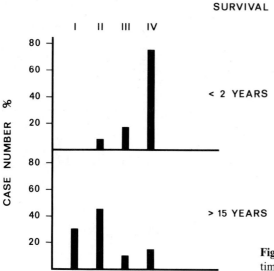

Fig. 4. Relationship between patient survival time and DNA profile type

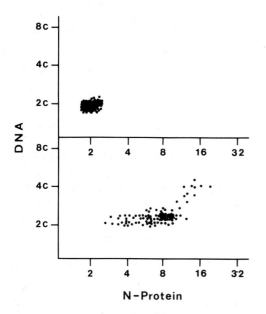

Fig. 5. Amount of Feulgen DNA (DNA, relative units) in individual quiescent (*top*) and growth-activated (*bottom*) human lymphocytes, plotted against the amount of nuclear protein (N-protein, relative units) in the same cells. Each *point* represents one cell ($n = 100$)

substance, a significant increase of the nuclear protein content occurs without a change in the amount of DNA. When the cells start to synthesize DNA, nuclear DNA and nuclear protein content increases simultaneously (Fig. 5). By measuring both DNA and nuclear protein content the growth activity in single, morphologically defined tumor cells can be determined. Figure 6 shows tumor cells from a diploid, i.e., type I, breast carcinoma. A large fraction of the breast carcinoma cells have cytochemical characteristics of growth-arrested G0 cells. The lower part of Fig. 6 shows a breast carcinoma with an aneuploid DNA distribution pattern, i.e., type IV carcinoma. In this tumor population all

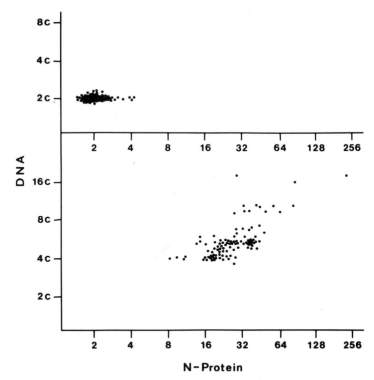

Fig. 6. Amount of Feulgen DNA (DNA, relative units) in individual mammary carcinoma cells from a DNA histogram type I tumor (*top*) and a DNA histogram type IV tumor (*bottom*), plotted against the amount of nuclear protein (N-protein, relative units) in the same cells. Each *point* represents one cell (*n* = 100)

cells exhibit cytochemical characteristics of growth-activated cells. These data are in line with the clinical observation that type I tumors have an extremely slow growth rate and a very low thymidine incorporation rate, whereas type IV tumors in general have a fast growth rate and an elevated thymidine incorporation rate (Auer et al. 1980a). Analyses of the proliferative state of a tumor cell population have been found to be of great importance for the therapeutic management of breast carcinomas.

Steroid Receptors

Estrogen and progesterone receptor amounts are quantitative parameters, which can be measured in cytological aspiration material and are important for the judgement of prognosis and therapy sensitivity. Silfverswärd (1979) in our hospital has shown that steroid receptor analyses can be performed in aspiration material with the same accuracy as in histological material. At the Karolinska Hospital, estrogen receptor determination is routinely performed for all breast cancer patients. We have also found that mammary carcinomas in which the DNA amounts in the tumor cells do not deviate conspicuously from diploid or tetraploid DNA values of normal mammary epithelium are characterized by high levels of estrogen receptor. On the other hand, mammary carcinomas containing a sizable number of cells with high degrees of aneuploidy are distinguished by low or even

Table 4. Median values of estrogen receptor (fmol/ug DNA) in primary mammary carcinoma (n = 147) exhibiting different DNA histogram types (I–IV; cf. Fig. 3)

DNA histogram type	No.	Median values (fmol ER/µg DNA)
I	48	1.30
II	43	1.00
III	35	0.21
IV	21	0.21

unmeasurable estrogen receptor levels (Table 4). These results strongly indicate a correlation between nuclear DNA distribution patterns and estrogen receptor levels in primary breast carcinomas. This correlation is of great practical value, especially for patients in whom the results of estrogen receptor analyses are difficult to interpret, i.e., breast cancer patients with high levels of estradiol in the plasma or with a high conversion of estrogen precursors to estradiol within the tumors.

Summary

The fine-needle aspiration biopsy technique is a simple and rapid method for the diagnosis of palpable breast lesions. The diagnostic accuracy is excellent provided that cell sampling and microscopy are performed by experienced investigators. Nonpalpable, mammographically demonstrated lesions can be needled by a stereotactic device allowing the cytologic examination of lesions down to a diameter of 2–3 mm.
Fine-needle biopsy material has been found to be suitable for quantitative cytochemical single-cell analysis. Retrospective DNA measurements in archival smear preparations have demonstrated a close correlation between the nuclear DNA content in breast carcinoma cells and patient survival time. It has also been found that the total amount of proteins in the cell nucleus reflects tumor cell growth potential. These data indicate that DNA and nuclear protein analyses in fine-needle smear preparations can contribute valuable prognostic information over and above that furnished by clinical staging and morphological criteria. Furthermore, analysis of steroid receptors in fine-needle biopsy material makes it possible to determine estrogen and progesterone receptor levels without the necessity of surgery.

References

Auer G (1972) Nuclear protein content and DNA-histone interaction. Exp Cell Res 75: 231–236
Auer G, Zetterberg A (1972) The role of nuclear protein in RNA synthesis. Exp Cell Res 75: 245–253
Auer G, Moore G, Ringertz NR, Zetterberg A (1973) DNA-dependent RNA synthesis in nuclear chromatin of fixed cells. Exp Cell Res 76: 229–233
Auer G, Caspersson T, Gustafsson S, Humla S, Ljung B, Nordenskjöld B, Silfverswärd C, Wallgren A (1980a) Relationship between nuclear DNA distribution and estrogen receptors in human mammary carcinomas. Anal Quant Cytol 2: 280–284

Auer G, Caspersson T, Wallgren A (1980b) DNA content and survival in mammary carcinomas. Anal Quant Cytol 2: 161–165

Auer G, Ono J, Caspersson T (1983a) Cytochemical identification of quiescent and growth-activated tumor cells. Anal Quant Cytol 5: 5–8

Auer G, Ono J, Caspersson T (1983b) Determination of the fraction of G_0-cells in cytologic samples by means of simultaneous DNA and nuclear protein analyses. Anal Quant Cytol 5: 1–4

Azavedo E, Tribukait B, Konaka C, Auer G (1982) Reproducibility of the cellular DNA distribution patterns in multiple fine needle aspirates from human malignant tumors. Acta Pathol Microbiol Immunol Scand [A] 90: 79–83

Caspersson T, Lomakka G (1970) Recent progress in quantitative cytochemistry: Instrumentation and results. In: Wied GL, Bahr GF (eds) Introduction to quantitative cytochemistry II. Academic, New York, pp 27–56

Caspersson T, Kudynowski J (1980) Cytochemical instrumentation for pathological work. Int Rev Exp Pathol 21: 1–54

Franzén S, Zajicek J (1968) Aspiration biopsy in diagnosis of palpable lesions of the breast. Acta Radiol (Stockh) 7: 241–262

Franzén S (1974) Thin needle aspiration biopsy in clinical oncology. Front Radiat Ther Oncol 9: 42–51

Gaub J, Auer G, Zetterberg A (1975) Quantitative cytochemical aspects of a combined Feulgen napthol yellow S staining procedure for the simultaneous determination of the nuclear and cytoplasmic proteins and DNA in mammalian cells. Exp Cell Res 92: 323–332

Nordenström B (1977) Stereotaxic screw needle biopsy of non-palpable breast lesions. In: Westinghouse W, Logan M (eds) Breast carcinoma: The radiologist's expanded role. Wiley, New York, pp 313–318

Nordenström B, Rydén H, Svane G (1980) Stereotaxic breast biopsy. In: Zornosa J (ed) Percutaneous needle biopsies: A radiological approach. Williams and Wilkins, Baltimore, pp 43–51

Silfverswärd C (1979) Estrogen receptors in human breast cancer. Thesis, Stockholm

Svane G (1983) Stereotaxic needle biopsy of non-palpable breast lesions. Thesis, Stockholm

Zajicek J (1974) Aspiration biopsy cytology: Part I. Cytology of supradiaphragmatic organs. In: Wied GL (ed) Monographs in clinical cytology. Karger, Basel, pp 136–196

Stereotactic Tru-Cut Biopsy of Nonpalpable Lesions in Mammography

W. Hoeffken[1] and W. Vaillant[2]

[1] Strahleninstitut für Diagnostik und Therapie,
  Machabäerstrasse 19–27, 5000 Köln 1, Federal Republic of Germany
[2] Einheit für Frühdiagnostik von Erkrankungen der Brust,
  I. Universitätsfrauenklinik, Maistrasse 11, 8000 München 2, Federal Republic of Germany

Introduction

In West Germany about 150,000 breast biopsies are carried out annually. As about 25,000 new cases of breast cancer appear per year, this means a relatively high biopsy rate of 125,000 biopsies in benign alterations. Some of these are necessary for prophylactic reasons in order to avoid later malignant development, but in a significant proportion of cases biopsy could be replaced by a reliable noninvasive technique for the confirmation of diagnosis.

Confirmation of Diagnosis in Palpable Lesions of the Breast

When a palpable lesion is detected further diagnosis is easily attained by
  Mammography
  Thermography
  Sonography
  Aspiration cytology
  Histology of material obtained by needle biopsy, drill biopsy or surgical biopsy.

Confirmation of Diagnosis in Nonpalpable Lesions Detected by Mammography

The detection of a problematic finding in the mammogram demands further confirmation of the diagnosis when benignity is not absolutely certain or malignancy is suspected. Confirmation of the diagnosis in such preclinical mammographic findings is especially important for the early detection of breast cancer.

The following methods are available to check the diagnosis in problematic mammographical findings:

Thermography. Sensitivity and specificity are relatively low for the detection of microcarcinomas.

Sonography. This method is appropriate for solid lesions with a diameter over 10 mm, but not for microcalcifications.

Early Breast Cancer
Edited by J. Zander and J. Baltzer
© Springer-Verlag Berlin Heidelberg 1985

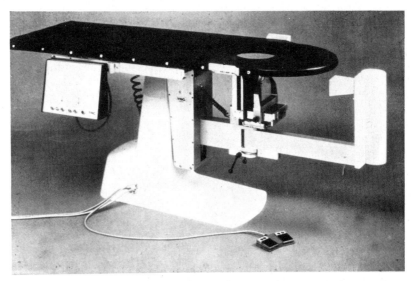

Fig. 1. TRC equipment developed by Nordenström fro stereotactic puncture

Control Mammography and Control Palpation. These methods cause problems because of the psychological stress and the risk of delayed diagnosis.

Exstirpation after Marking. Geometrical marking; cannula marking; hook marking; and dye/contrast agent marking are all possible. The *disadvantage* of exploratory excision is the high number of unnecessary biopsies.

Cytology Following Stereotactic Puncture. The TRC equipment developed by Nordenström (Fig. 1) is used for this procedure. The geometrical accuracy of the system is ± 1 mm, but in dense tissue the correct diagnosis can be prevented by "bending" of the cannula or dislocation of the area to be examined throughout the puncture. Furthermore, with the Nordenström-cannula, mainly stroma and little cell material is obtained. There is another disadvantage, in that the material is taken from a very small area, corresponding to the cannula diameter of 0.8 mm. For this reason a cannula with a diameter of 1.5 mm was developed, with which the "bending" is reduced and the material sampling is more effective.

Histology Following Drill Biopsy. Under stereotactic conditions a tissue cylinder can be taken for histological investigation by drill biopsy from a suspect area (Hauber 1981 a,b; Hollinger 1980, 1981). The disadvantage of the drill biopsy with a rotating hollow cannula lies in the fact that the retraction of the rotating cannula does not always guarantee a complete yield of the tissue cylinder. The Hollinger-cannula yields better results than the Hauber-cannula.
A special cannula was developed by K. F. Reich, whereby a tiny knife at the tip of the cannula cuts off the tissue cylinder. The diameter of this system is 2.5 mm.

Histology Following Punch Biopsy. Under stereotactic conditions a punch biopsy of the breast tissue can be obtained with the long-approved Tru-Cut cannula (Travenol), when the tissue concerned is correctly reached. This is reliably possible only in palpable, and thus externally fixable nodes, and not in stereotactic conditions, when deflection either of the tissue or of the cannula occurs. Accordingly a representative tissue cylinder cannot be obtained.

New Method. To avoid deflection of tissue and cannula it is necessary to take the punch biopsy at a shot-like velocity. Thus, a double-shot instrument with spring tension has been developed by Vaillant, Hoeffken, and Wimmer (Fig. 2).

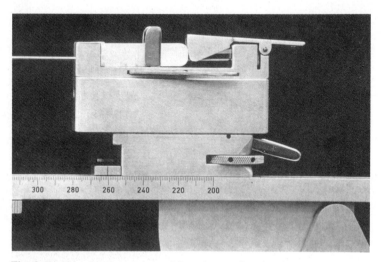

Fig. 2. Double-shot instrument with spring tension developed by Vaillant, Hoeffken, and Wimmer for punch biopsy sampling

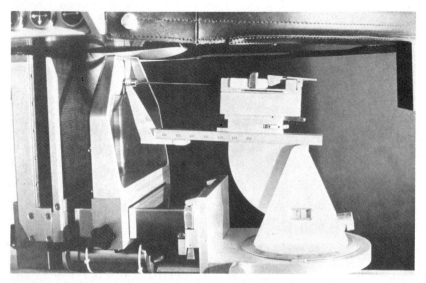

Fig. 3. Position of the breast in the double-shot instrument

Procedure for Double-Shot Biopsy

1) The patient is placed on the examination table in a prone position with the breast hanging down through the aperture. The breast is fixed between the compression plates (Fig. 3). Based on a radiogram in +15° and −15° the displacement of the suspect area is measured and calculated exactly with a special computer program.

2) After local anesthesia and incision of the cutis the Tru-Cut cannula, which has been fixed in a holding device, is manually pushed forward right up to the suspect tissue (Fig. 4a).

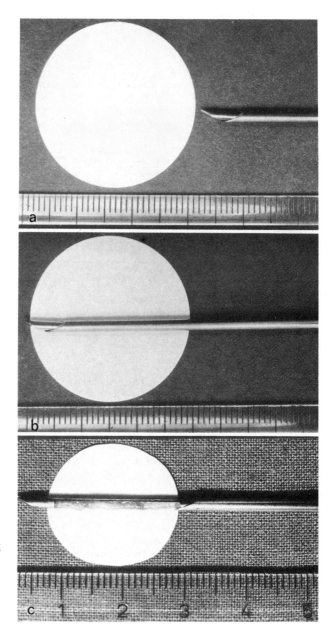

Fig. 4a–c. Scheme: **a** Positioning of the cannula preparatory to double-shot biopsy; **b** release of the first shot with the entire cannula; **c** before removal of the tissue cylinder

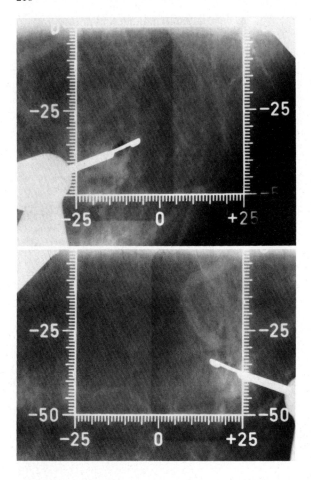

Fig. 5. Mammographic picture of the cannula during penetration of the tissue

3) Subsequently the holding block is fixed with the double-spring system to the sliding carriage of the targeting mechanism, followed by release of the first 'shot' with the entire cannula (Fig. 4b).
4) Retraction of the cannula sleeve exposes the downward pointing excavation of the inner cannula part.
5) While the breast is held up to press the tissue into the excavation the second shot is released: the cannula sleeve is pushed forward and cuts off the tissue cylinder.
6) The procedure is terminated by withdrawal of the cannula and removal of the tissue cylinder (Fig. 4c).

The advantage of this system lies in the high penetration speed obtained by the spring mechanism, which makes deflection of either the cannula or the suspect area impossible (Fig. 5).

Thus, reliable achievement of a representative tissue cylinder is guaranteed. It is 20 mm long and 2 mm in diameter. The biopsy material is fixed in Stieve's solution. The histological investigation it is now possible with complete tissue cross-cuts. The size of the cylinder allows differentiated histological diagnosis and thus ensures improved early detection of breast cancer (Fig. 6).

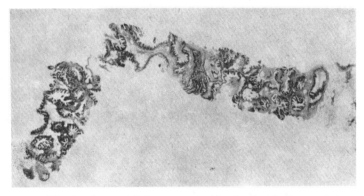

Fig. 6. Histology smear of tissue removed by the double-shot technique

Table 1. Results of examination of tissue removed by stereotactic puncture following suggestive appearance in mammogram (n = 120)

Benign	
Final diagnosis obtained (control investigation confirmed)	89
Biopsy arranged (histological investigation confirmed)	15
Malignant	
Result of cytology/histology confirmed	14
Not verified	2

Table 2. Diagnosis of breast cancer in tissue gained by stereotactic puncture ($n = 16$)

Cytology	Cannula 0.8	Cannula 1.5
Correct positive	4	4
False negative	2	0
Histology	Travenol cannula	Drill biopsy
Correct positive	3	3
False negative	0	0

Results

The results are shown in Tables 1 and 2.

Conclusions

The double-shot cut biopsy makes it possible to examine mammographically suggestive findings by histological investigation of a tissue cylinder taken by a stereotactic method, without the disadvantageous delay caused by control examinations after several months.

Benign alterations can subsequently be controlled by mammography, while malignant findings are surgically treated. The double-shot biopsy reduces the number of unnecessary surgical excisions and avoids delays in diagnosis.

References

Hauber KP (1981a) Gynäkol Praxis 5 (1981) 83–88, Die Mammabohrbiopsie – Eine wertvolle Erweiterung in der Diagnostik von Mammaerkrankungen.
Hauber KP (1981b) Gynäkol Praxis 5 (1981) 515–519, Die Mammabohrbiopsie – Kommentar und Schlusswort
Hollinger A (1980) Schweiz Rundsch Med 49 : 1823
Hollinger A (1981) Helv Chir Acta 48 : 171

Histology and Cytology Following Stereotactic Needle Biopsy

P. Citoler

Institut für Pathologie, Pferdmengesstrasse 10, 5000 Köln 51, Federal Republic of Germany

Introduction

With the agreement of clinical, mammographic, and cytological findings, the preoperative accuracy of "triple diagnosis" of palpable breast changes is almost 100%. However, clear agreement, i.e., unequivocally benign or malignant findings with all three methods, is observed in about 50% of cases (Table 1). In the remaining patients, the question of histological clarification has to be discussed.

In *nonpalpable* breast changes (mostly revealed by a mammographic finding), e.g., grouped microcalcifications, these three diagnostic methods cannot be combined. By definition, a palpatory finding cannot be established in these cases. It is also not possible to carry out a conventional aspiration cytology, for the same reason. The morphological substrate of these nonpalpable lesions could then only be demonstrated by means of an exploratory excision. Pinpointed biopsy and the histological identification may be very elaborate.

Pinpointed biopsy under stereotactic conditions (Nordenström and Zajicek 1977; Vaillant et al. 1982), has made it possible to come closer to demonstrating the morphological substrate of nonpalpable lesions, avoiding a biopsy in some cases.

Information on the morphological substrate of nonpalpable lesions can be obtained under stereotactic conditions by means of aspiration cytology and of punch biopsy with histological examination. The technique and the clinical problems of stereotactic puncture are described elsewhere in this monograph by Hoeffken and Vaillant. In this chapter the results of 62 histological investigations of punch biopsies and 97 aspiration cytologies

Table 1. Preoperative triple diagnosis in 445 mammary lesions investigated histologically (personal cases)

	Clinical examination + mammography + cytology		
	Agreement positive/suspect	Agreement negative	No agreement
Histology	$n = 179$	$n = 48$	$n = 218$ (49%)
Carcinomas ($n = 243$)	179	0	64 (14%)
Benign lesions ($n = 202$)	0	48	154 (35%)

Early Breast Cancer
Edited by J. Zander and J. Baltzer
© Springer-Verlag Berlin Heidelberg 1985

obtained stereotactically are compared and contrasted, and also analyzed with regard to their diagnostic relevance.

Nature and Diagnostic Information Supplied by the Material

The tissue cylinders obtained with the Tru-Cut cannula are 10−20 mm long and about 1 mm thick. They should be immediately fixed with a high-penetration fixative, so that if necessary they can be worked up histologically on the same day.

Especially in lesions with a bulky, tough, elastic consistency (e.g., fibroadenomas), the quality of the tissue cylinders is excellent. The *histological examination* of a cylinder from a homogeneous lesion provides largely the same information as can be obtained in an exploratory excision, with the limitation that a small area is investigated. The kind of growth, the degree of cell proliferation, and the presence of any cell atypias can be demonstrated. Similarly differentiated appraisals can be made in favorably situated cases with mastopathic lesions.

The material aspirated under stereotactic conditions to prepare *cytological smears* was generally scanter than that obtained by conventional puncture of larger palpable lesions. The latter is usually carried out freehand at several contiguous sites. In contrast, a single circumscribed small pinpointed site is punctured in the stereotactic procedure.

The *diagnostic information* accuracy provided by the material was subdivided into three groups. The following were considered as criteria: the size of the tissue cylinders; the amount of aspirated material; and the possibility of making a diagnosis that was unequivocally consistent with the mammographic findings. Thus the diagnostic information provided was designated as satisfactory when a carcinoma or carcinoma cells or a fibroadenoma were unequivocally demonstrated. The same applied when the histological or cytological investigation clearly supplied a morphological foundation for the mammographic finding (e.g., cystic adenosis in grouped microcalcifications, cells of cyst content with suspected cysts, etc.). When the material was very scant and uncharacteristic, the diagnostic information provided was designated unsatisfactory. Finally, in a number of cases the material obtained was not definitely representative for the lesion thought to be most likely on the basis of the mammograph (e.g., unremarkable histological or cytological findings despite suspicion of comedocarcinoma with calcification).

Table 2 shows the classification. In 67% of the tissue cylinders investigated histologically, it was possible to demonstrate with certainty the morphological background to the mammographic finding. On the other hand, this was only possible in 46% of the cytological cell smears after stereotactic cell aspiration. Accordingly, the percentage proportion of cytological smears which did not permit any or any definite appraisal was higher than that of the tissue cylinders investigated histologically. This superiority of the histological over

Table 2. Accuracy of stereotactic biopsy in diagnosis of nonpalpable mammary lesions

	Satisfactory	Dubious	Unsatisfactory
Histology			
Tru-Cut biopsy ($n = 62$)	67%	19%	14%
Cytology			
Needle biopsy ($n = 97$)	46%	24%	30%

the cytological investigation is understandable if, for example, the nature of the nonpalpable lesions concerned is considered. However, it requires more precise description.

Indications for Histological or Cytological Examination of the Material

The most frequent mammographic finding in the nonpalpable lesions investigated here were small round foci arousing the suspicion of fibroadenoma or cysts. Next in order of frequency were stellate opacities, most of mainly which proved to be caused by fibrosis or carcinoma of the scirrhous type, which had to be differentially diagnosed. Finally, foci of group calcifications of differing kinds were investigated. The question arises as to whether the proportion of verified diagnoses in the same mammographic finding is correlated with the nature of the investigation (histology or cytology).
As shown by Table 3, the best results (87% verified diagnoses) were obtained in stellate opacities with histological investigation of tissue cylinders after Tru-Cut biopsy. Even with the putative diagnosis of fibroadenoma, histological investigation could definitely confirm this diagnosis in 70% of cases, whereas only 30% could be detected cytologically. In grouped calcifications, the results were roughly the same. On the other hand, the cytological smears definitely provided more information than the tissue cylinders in the clarification of cysts.
The decision as to whether a histological or cytological method of investigation should be applied should thus be made with reference to the mammographic findings. Apart from the diagnosis of cysts, however, histology appears to provide better results.

Clinical Significance of Stereotactic Punctures of the Breast

The goal of this method is to detect the morphological substrate of nonpalpable breast lesions, while avoiding a surgical exploratory excision. The present results show that this objective was achieved in about 60% of the cases. It is to be expected that this proportion will rise with increasing experience.
However, its clinical application presupposes a very critical attitude on the part of the pathologist and optimal communication with the radiologist. Only when an unequivocal basis has been found for the mammographic findings can the objective of the investigation

Table 3. Diagnostic accuracy of histology and cytology in correlation with mammographic findings

Mammographic + findings	n	Satisfactory diagnosis in %	
		Histology (Tru-Cut)	Cytology (Aspiration)
Fibrosis?/Scirrhous?	48	87%	53%
Fibroadenoma?	53	70%	30%
Calcifications	32	50%	42%
Cysts?	26	33%	71%

[a] 159 stereotactic biopsies of nonpalpable mammary lesions

be regarded as achieved. If this does not apply, an exploratory excision is unavoidable.

A consecutive conventional surgical clarification was undertaken in the present group: (a) when carcinoma had been detected or was suspected; (b) when the morphological basis of the stereotactically punctured breast lesion could not be demonstrated unequivocally; and (c) at the beginning of the series of investigations, for our own check on the diagnostic reliability of the method. The remaining patients continue to be checked by clinical mammography. A surgical biopsy would have been meaningless in any case in a number of these patients, for example in the search for calcifications which had already been removed by punch biopsy and which had been detected histologically.

References

Nordenström B, Zajicek J (1977) Stereotaxic needle biopsy and preoperative indication of nonpalpable mammary lesions. Acta Cytol 21: 350–351

Vaillant W, Bohmert H, Remberger H (1982) Stereotaktische, präoperative Kennzeichnung von Mammaläsionen. MMW 124: 577–578

Surgical Aspects and Diagnosis of Nonpalpable Breast Lesions

K. G. Ober and F. Willgeroth

Universitäts-Frauenklinik, Universitätsstrasse 21/23, 8520 Erlangen, Federal Republic of Germany

In our department preoperative localization of a nonpalpable pathological change in the breast is based on mammographic examination in two planes. On this basis, we estimate the site of the lesion. We know that some aids, such as the use of powder or a lotion as a lubricant during palpation, improve diagnostic information. Experience has taught us that, when the skin is divided a number of lesions that were previously not palpable, can also be palpated. The most important diagnostic phenomena, however, are groups of microcalcifications (Kindermann et al. 1978; Rummel et al. 1976). In the final instance, assurance of their complete removal is possible only when they can be demonstrated in the x-ray film of the removed tissue.

Some figures might be of interest here: During the course of a year, we see about 190 women with breast cancer, and 90% of the lesions can be readily localized by palpation. In some 30% of the women presenting with palpable lesions adequate diagnosis is possible with the aid of ultrasound and subsequent mammocystography, so that there is no need to obtain an excision biopsy (Weishaar et al. 1977).

A separate report has been given on the discharging breast, the visualization of the lactiferous ducts, and the excision of the involved duct segment (Kindermann, this volume).

There remain about 150 patients a year in whom, on the basis of the mammographic findings, our radiologists recommend selective excision. When identifying our "target area," we rely exclusively on the mammograms obtained in two planes, which indicate with a high degree of reliability where the pathological lesions probably lie.

We do not make use of preoperative marking by the injection of a dye, nor do we use the technique of advancing the tip of a needle into the putative center of the lesions (Barth et al. 1977; Bolmgren et al. 1977; Frischbier and Lohbeck 1973; Hoeffken and Lanyi 1973). We have tried the first of these two procedures, but did not find it particularly convincing. In common with the second, it has the disadvantage that the time interval between the injection and the removal of tissue is relatively limited, which in a hospital with a very full surgical load, represents a difficult organizational problem. A further point is the radiation exposure to the patient, which we feel is not necessary. In our opinion, similar objections also apply to the technique described by Nordenström (Nordenström and Zajicek 1977).

Having detected − over the last 10 years − a number of minute infiltrative cancers with the aid of a painstakingly thorough histological examination technique, we are well aware of the limitations of mammography. The lesions concerned were found after histological

Early Breast Cancer
Edited by J. Zander and J. Baltzer
© Springer-Verlag Berlin Heidelberg 1985

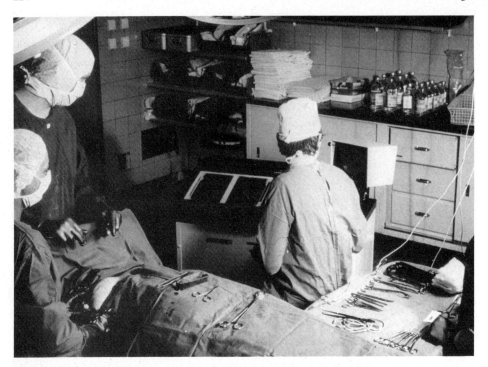

Fig. 1. Fluoroscopic examination of excised tissue at the operating table

work-up of breast tissue after bilateral subcutaneous mastectomy in patients in whom initially a diagnosis of lobular carcinoma in situ was recorded. All the resected tissue was cut into slices. Prior to embedding each slice was subjected to a radiological examination. Even so, no radiologic substrate was detected. We must, therefore, be conscious of the fact that even with the use of meticulously painstaking "research" examination techniques, only a certain percentage of the lesions present will be detected.

In recent years, in our hands, the fluoroscopic examination of the excised tissue and its inspection on the image intensifier screen at four-fold magnification at the operating table (Figs. 1−5) has proved highly successful (Willgeroth et al. 1978; Willgeroth and Paterok 1982). At this point, I shall not try to show you any microcalcifications, since, as every expert knows, decisive findings can be recognized only with the aid of a magnifying glass and halogen illumination or − if xerography is used − sometimes only by viewing the image at a certain angle.

Table 1 shows the indications in 512 excision biopsies. Groups of microcalcifications were the indication for excision in 357 cases, and tumours or opacities in 76 cases. There are more biopsies than patients because in some patients tissue was removed from both breasts, and in others multiple biopsies were taken.

A total of 512 biopsy specimens were examined fluoroscopically at the operating table. An exact breakdown of the number of biopsies in the individual patient, however, is available only for the last 332 patients, in whom 405 biopsies were obtained (Table 2). In 270 cases the lesion was detected in the first biopsy specimen (81.3%), while in 55 cases a second biopsy was required. In only 3 cases were 3 biopsy specimens needed, and in 4 patients, 4 biopsies. Thus, in almost 98% of the cases, the lesion was detected in the first or second biopsy specimen.

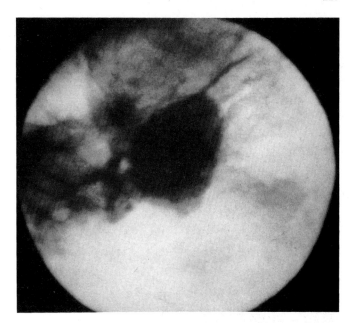

Fig. 2. Fluorsocopic examination of a small nonpalpable mass in excised breast tissue

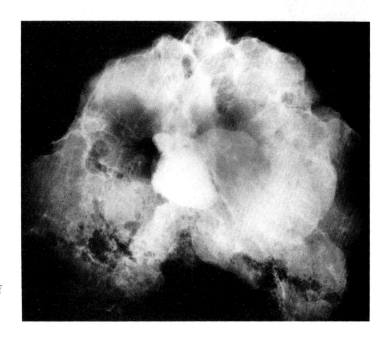

Fig. 3. Radiography of the same specimen as in Fig. 2

The size of the biopsy specimens varied between 5 and 109 g, with an average weight of 40 g. This is related to the variation in the size of the individual breasts, which was not determined beforehand.

One important lesson that our experience has taught us is that the maximum dimensions of the lesions do not always coincide with the apparent maximum dimensions in the mammographic image. Even with a generous excision, the intraductal spread of the cancer

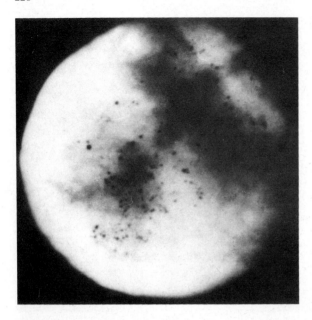

Fig. 4. Fluoroscopic examination of microcalcifications in excised tissue on the image intensifier screen

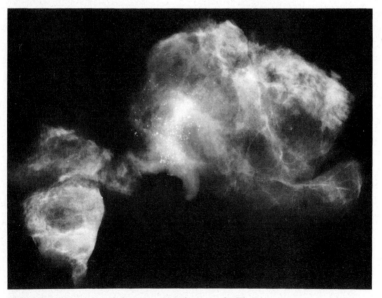

Fig. 5. Radiography of the same specimen as in Fig. 4

Table 1. Indications for 512 excision biopsies

No. of patients	No. of biopsies	Roentgenological indications		Bilateral biopsies
		Micro-calcifications	Occult tumors or opacities	
433	512	357	76	61

Table 2. Reliability of 405 intraoperative biopsies[a] (in 332 patients) alone, without preoperative marking

No. of patients	Percentage		No. of biopsies needed
270	81.3	97.9	Excisions with 1 biopsy
55	16.3		Excisions with 2 biopsies
3	0.9		Excisions with 3 biopsies
4	1.2		Excisions with 4 biospies

[a] Average weight of biopsies 40 g (range 5−109 g)

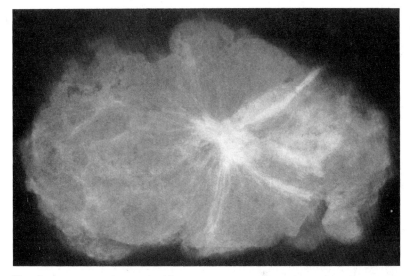

Fig. 6. A generous breast excision

cells still extends beyond the lesion recognizable in the mammogram (Figs. 6 and 7). Anyone who is in the habit of cutting the excised tissue into slices, and subjecting each of these to an x-ray and then to a histological work-up, will know that even in 1-cm-thick slices, cancer having a diameter of up to 15 mm can escape radiologic detection. This point has already been discussed (Tulusan, this volume). Thus, the considerable effort associated with a thorough examination should not be underestimated. It is, perhaps, of considerable importance to note that the most sophisticated euipment for achieving selective removal of tissue must fail if merely a tiny piece of tissue or a few cells are obtained from the center of a scarred area that appears particularly impressive in the mammogram (Fig. 7) while the lesion that is really of importance for the pathologist is located in the immediate vicinity.

The incision for biopsies of the breast should be oriented to the margin of the areola. If the latter is well developed, an incision placed here usually suffices (Fig. 8). In the case of a small areola, it is recommended that the incision be made at the margin of the parenchyma. Sometimes it is also possible, with an incision close to the axilla, where the skin is highly elastic, to combine extensive lymphonodectomy with an excision (Fig. 9).

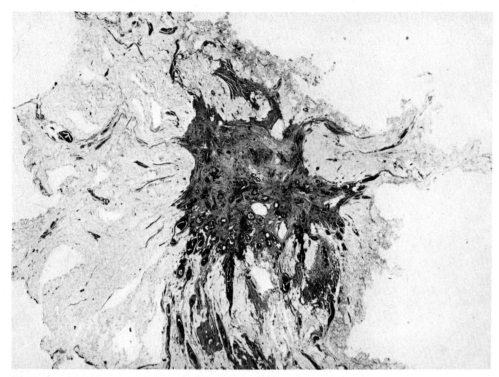

Fig. 7. Histology of the excision tissue from Fig. 6, showing intraductal spread of the cancer extending beyond the recognizable lesion

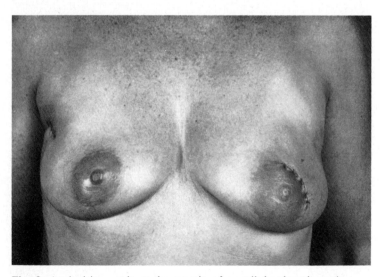

Fig. 8. An incision made at the margin of a well-developed areola

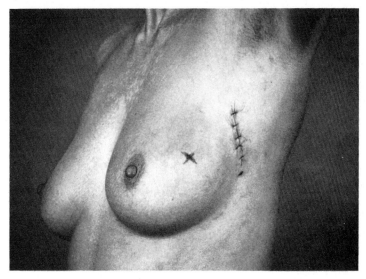

Fig. 9. An incision made at the margin of the parenchyma in the case of a small areola

References

Barth V, Behrends W, Haase W (1977) Methode zur präoperativen Lokalisation nicht palpabler suspekter Mikroverkalkungen im Brustdrüsenkörper (Kugelmarkierung). Radiologe 17: 219–221

Bolmgren J, Jacobson B, Nordenström B (1977) Steriotaxic needle biopsy and preoperative indication of non-palpable mammary lesions. AJR 129: 121–125

Frischbier H, Lobeck J (1973) Frühdiagnostik des Mammakarzinoms. Thieme, Stuttgart

Hoeffken W, Lanyi M (1973) Röntgenuntersuchung der Brust. Thieme, Stuttgart

Kindermann G, Rummel W, Egger H, Weishaar J, Paterok EM, Willgeroth F, Ober KG (1978) Verschiedene Techniken der Brustkrebsfrüherkennung. In: Grundmann E, Beck L (eds) Brustkrebsfrüherkennung. Fischer, Stuttgart, pp 193–197

Nordenström B, Zajicek J (1977) Stereotaxic needle biopsy and preoperative indication of non-palpable mammary lesions. Acta Cytol 21: 350–351

Rummel W, Kindermann G, Egger H, Weishaar J, Müller A, Paterok EM, Willgeroth F (1976) Mikrokalk in der Mammographie, operative Abklärung und histologische Befunde: Geburtshilfe Frauenheilkd 36: 1053–1061

Weishaar J, Paterok EM, Müller A, Rummel W, Willgeroth F (1977) Die Bedeutung der Pneumozystographie in der Abklärung von Mammatumoren. Dtsch Med Wochenschr 102: 958–960

Willgeroth F, Paterok EM (1982) Okkulte Prozesse in der Brust – operatives Management. Schweizer Gesellschaft für Gynäkologie und Geburtshilfe, 25. 6. 1982

Willgeroth F, Rummel W, Säbel M, Kuhn H, Ascherl E (1978) Intraoperativer Nachweis von Mikroverkalkungen der Brust mit einem Durchleuchtungsgerät. Geburtshilfe Frauenheilkd 38: 636–639

Treatment

Conservative Treatment of Potentially Curable Minimal, Occult, and Early Breast Cancer: Experience At Memorial Sloan-Kettering Cancer Center, New York

Jerome A. Urban

Memorial Sloan-Kettering Cancer Institute and Cornell University Medical School,
215 E. 68th St., New York, New York 10021, USA

Conservative Surgery with Radiation Therapy for "Early Breast Cancer

At the Memorial Sloan-Kettering Cancer Center in New York City, we have been careful in adopting this approach to the treatment of early operable breast cancer. It has become obvious from experience in this field that this form of treatment must be guided by careful selection of optimum patient material. Close follow-up must be maintained because of the high incidence of local recurrence and the not infrequent need for salvage surgery. It is also known that these patients must be followed for a long time − a minimum of 10 years, and preferably 15 years.

Between 1980 and 1982, 90 patients were treated by conservative surgery with aggressive radiation therapy at the MSKCC (McCormick B, personal communication). The average tumor size was 1.8 cm, and 43% of patients underwent axillary dissection, 23% showing axillary node involvement. In all cases, complete excision of the tumor with a 2-cm margin about it or a quadrantectomy of the involved portion of the breast was performed. Radiation therapy consisted of the administration of 45−50 Gy electron-beam therapy to the breast and regional nodes, and when indicated, a subsequent 10-Gy boost to the primary site with cobalt-60 therapy, within a 6-week period. More recently, patients have been treated by implantation of radioactive iridium at the primary tumor site following local excision, a tumor dose of approximately 30 Gy being administered to this area by interstitial treatment. This is then followed by 50−60 Gy of external x-radiation treatment using the electron beam applied to the breast, and again to the regional nodes if indicated. Most recently, complete axillary dissection has been added to the conservative treatment protocol. This helps to stage patients accurately and aids in the selection of patients for adjuvant chemotherapy (Table 1).

Preliminary results show good local control considering the short follow-up interval, which ranges between 6 months and 2 years. Three local recurrences have been noted, one in the breast, two in the axilla. In all three cases salvage surgery was performed, and all patients, at present, appear to be free of disease. Distant failures have occurred within the same interval in two patients, one with brain and another with liver metastases (McCormick B, personal communication) (Table 2). It is impossible to draw any valid conclusions from this short presentation of a small group of selected patients, because of the optimal patient material and very short follow-up interval. Close follow-up and long-term follow-up with the use of salvage surgery when indicated must be an integral part of this approach. When dealing with "minimal" early breast cancers − in situ lobular cancer (Rosen et al.

Early Breast Cancer
Edited by J. Zander and J. Baltzer
© Springer-Verlag Berlin Heidelberg 1985

Table 1. Conservative surgery[a] with x-ray therapy[b] for early breast cancer with T1 and small T2 tumors

Year	1980	1981	1982	Total
No. of patients	20	30	40	90
Tumor size	1.8 cm	1.6 cm	1.9 cm	1.8 cm
Axillary. dissection	30%	36%	55%	43%
Positive axilla(e)	2/6; 33%	2/11; 18%	5/22; 23%	9/39; 23%

[a] Complete excision of tumor with 2-cm margin or quadrantectomy
[b] 45−50 Gy to breast and regional nodes with electron beam, plus 10-Gy booster to primary site with Co-60 in weeks

Table 2. Preliminary results obtained with conservative therapy in early breast cancer (follow-up 6 months to 3 years)[a]

Local recurrence (3)		Distant failure (2)		Salvage surgery
				3 (All NED)
Breast	Axilla	Brain	Liver	
1	2	1	1	

[a] Total no. of patients = 90

1978), noninfiltrating intraductal cancer, and infiltrating cancers less than 1 cm in diameter − almost all the residual cancer that may be left behind in the breast following wide local excision of the primary tumor is at the non-infiltrating stage (Rosen et al. 1975) and will not manifest itself as a clinically apparent infiltrating cancer until 9 or 10 years after local excision, even if the breast has not been treated by radiation therapy. When patients with microscopic areas of noninfiltrating intraductal cancer were treated by wide local excision only, clinically apparent infiltrating cancers appeared in 66% of the patients in the same breast, about $9^1/_2$ years after the local excisions (Betsil et al. 1978). No cancers appeared in the opposite breast. Salvage surgery was performed in these patients, usually a radical mastectomy, but 3 years after surgery half these patients, most of whom had nodal metastases, had failed; were living with recurrent disease; or had died of metastatic cancer. The presence of untreated, occult noninfiltrating, intraductal cancer in the breast did not progress into a clinically apparent infiltrating cancer until 9−10 years after the local excision. The survival of the patient was not affected until another 3 years had passed, i.e., 12−13 years after the original local excision. The need for long-term follow-up in evaluating primary therapy of minimal breast cancers is obvious (Rosen et al. 1978).
Some of the factors to be considered in comparing results achieved in different institutions are the degree of selectivity practiced by each group; the proportion of patients considered operable; the number suitable for conservative surgery; the number treated by radical surgery; what was considered to constitute local recurrence; and finally, the clinical staging, which may be quite variable.
Most authors include nodal category N1A (palpable axillary nodes *not* considered to contain cancer) in their stage I cancers (Calle and Pilleron 1979), while some include this finding in their stage II cancer category (Amalric et al. 1982). Thorough evaluation of accurate data, which should include the measured size of the primary tumor, and status of

the axillary nodes by pathological examination, will ultimately help to define any subsets of patients with breast cancer who can be treated equally effectively by conservative surgery plus radiation therapy, while other categories will be managed more effectively by more adequate primary surgery.

In some series of patients treated by conservative surgery and aggressive radiation therapy, anywhere from 20% to 30% (Amalric et al. 1982; Calle and Pilleron 1979) or more of the patients originally seen were not considered suitable for this therapy and underwent primary mastectomy as their initial treatment, being therefore removed from the study group. In our own practice, 97% of patients seen without previous therapy are considered to be operable, and are included in our data. There is some confusion about local recurrence rates. Some individuals consider local recurrence as recurrence adjacent to the local excision area only (Crile et al. 1980). They do not include recurrence in the axilla or recurrence in the remaining breast as evidence of local recurrence. In our own material, local recurrence includes recurrence in the axilla, in the operative area on the chest wall, and in the chest wall itself, especially in the parasternal region.

Treatment of Occult Breast Cancer

The term occult breast cancer is a rather vague one, and is usually applied to patients with cancers detected without definite preoperative diagnosis by physical examination or mammography. We have used the term "occult breast cancer" to define patients with breast cancer whose initial presenting sign consists of a metastatic axillary node and who show no evidence of a primary tumor in the breast at that time (Ashikari et al. 1976; Feuerman et al. 1962). Adult female patients presenting with axillary adenopathy with no obvious inflammatory lesion usually prove to have either malignant lymphoma or metastatic adenocarcinoma in these nodes — the latter almost always secondary to the presence of an occult cancer in the ipsilateral breast. When histopathological examination of an enlarged axillary node has revealed metastatic carcinoma, the breast is the most likely primary source of origin. Lymphoma is next most frequent in this setting. Other sites to be ruled out are melanoma, thyroid, lung, gastrointestinal tract, kidney, and ovary. The help and guidance of a competent, interested pathologist is absolutely essential for satisfactory management of this situation.

Between 1946 and 1975, 42 patients were encountered at the Memorial Sloan Kettering Cancer Institute presenting with an axillary mass that proved to contain metastatic adenocarcinoma, but with no significant clinical finding in the breast (Ashikari et al. 1976). They ranged from 31 to 71 years of age (averaged 51 years). The nodes ranged from 1 to 6 cm in diameter, with an average of 4 cm. Examination of the breast revealed no real clinical findings in 26 patients, and indefinite thickenings in the remaining 16. Mammography was performed in 25 cases, and was reported as negative for any sign of breast cancer in 22, while 3 were highly suggestive of carcinoma.

All patients underwent excisional biopsy of the axillary mass, with careful histopathological examination of these tissues. Frozen sections were not considered adequate — all were examined by the paraffin section technique. All nodes revealed metastatic adenocarcinoma, suggesting a mammary origin. In four cases other primary sources were considered. However, after careful work-up to exclude these other primary sites, all were considered to have metastatic breast cancer in the axillary nodes (Table 3). Four patients refused treatment or were treated elsewhere and were lost to follow-up. All the remaining 38 were

Table 3. Treatment and results[a] in occult breast cancer presenting as node with metastatic adenocarcinoma (Ashikari et al. 1976)

No. of patients	Treatment	Surviving (length of follow-up)	Dead of breast Ca	Dead of other cause	Lost to follow-up
34	Radical mastectomy	26 (6 months to 16 years)	3	4	1
1	Axillary dissection	1 (8 years)			
3	x-Ray therapy	2 (6 months to 4 years)	1		
2	Surgery elsewhere				2
2	Refused treatment				2
42	Overall	29	4	4	5
38	Treated at MSKCC	29	4	4	1

[a] Crude survival 29/38 = 76%; live-table survival 29/33 = 88%

Table 4. Findings and results[a] in 34 cases of occult breast cancer treated by radical mastectomy at MSKCC (Ashikari et al. 1976)

	Findings	No. of patients		No. of patients
Axilla	Positive nodes		Survival, NED	26
Breast	Primary Ca < 1 cm	8	> 5 years	13
	1−2 cm	8	> 10 years	11
	> 2 cm	8	Died of breast Ca	3
	No primary found	10	Died of other cause	4
			Lost to follow-up	1

[a] Crude survival 26/34 = 76%; live-table survival 26/29 = 89%

treated at the Memorial Hospital, 34 by radical mastectomy, 1 by axillary dissection, and 3 by radiation therapy (Table 4).

One of three patients treated by radiation therapy alone died of metastatic breast cancer 20 months after treatment, and the two others are living and free of disease at 6 and 42 months following radiation therapy. One patient treated by axillary dissection was found to be living and free of disease 8 years later. In the remaining patients who were treated by radical mastectomy, 11 of 13 were living and free of disease 10 years after treatment and 2 others had died of other causes. Two of six patients who were followed for 5 years were living and free of disease, while three others had died of breast cancer metastases, and one of other causes while clinically free of disease. Of 15 patients treated within less than a 5-year follow-up 13 were free of disease, 1 died of an advanced cancer of the opposite breast, and the other was lost to follow-up. These data show a surprisingly high survival rate of 29/38 in the overall group treated at Memorial Hospital − 76% crude survival. The actuarial survival was 87%, or 29/33. In only 24 of the 34 patients treated by radical mastectomy was an infiltrating carcinoma found in the breast. Of these, 8 were less than 1 cm in diameter, 8 between 1 and 2 cm, and 8 were slightly over 2 cm in diameter. No evidence of carcinoma was found in the breast from which the mastectomy specimen was taken in 10 patients, despite very detailed examinations with multiple sections and intense examination by our pathologist.

We do not understand why these patients have done so well. None of them received adjuvant chemotherapy, and many of them presented with axillary node disease, which involved anywhere from 1 to 13 nodes. All had relatively small asymptomatic primary lesions in the breast, and in 10 cases the primary lesion was so small that it escaped detection on routine examination. The long-term survival rate in these patients is much better than that usually obtained in patients who have similar nodal involvement in the axilla accompanied by larger primary tumors in the breast. Not infrequently, patients who present with an enlarged node in the axilla are subjected to multitudinous examinations in an effort to find the primary site — usually a fruitless search. These patients should undergo excisional biopsy of the node with careful paraffin section examinations of the node. A competent pathologist can usually determine whether the node is consistent with origin from a breast primary. In this group of patients adequate primary surgical treatment (radical mastectomy) has proved most satisfactory. Although no adjuvant chemotherapy was used following surgery, most of these patients did receive radiation therapy to the peripheral regional nodes (base of the neck, internal mammary area, apex of the axilla) following surgery, receiving a tumor dose of approximately 45 Gy in 5 weeks with cobalt-60 radiation.

Treatment of Minimal Breast Cancer

Until very recently, almost all patients at Memorial Sloan-Kettering Cancer Institute with minimal breast cancer were treated by modified mastectomy (Handley and Thackrey 1969; Wanebo et al. 1974). The phrase "minimal breast cancer" originated with Gallager and Martin (1971), who used it to mean the earliest stage of recognizable breast cancer, including non infiltrating intraductal cancer, in situ lobular cancer, and infiltrating cancers up to 5 mm in diameter when accompanied by clinically negative axillae. In our own approach to this problem, we have expanded the category to include a number of patients with low-grade breast cancers that remain localized to the breast for a relatively long period of time: papillary carcinoma, colloid carcinoma, adenoid cystic carcinoma, early Paget's disease with no gross nodule palpable beneath the nipple, and malignant cystosarcoma phyllodes. We have also included patients with infiltrating lobular and ductal cancers up to 1 cm in diameter when they are not accompanied by suggestive axillary nodes. Between 1955 and 1973, we operated upon 162 patients with minimal breast cancer. Mammography was positive in 60% of these patients. Many of the lesions were detected by contralateral breast biopsy (Urban et al. 1972) at the time of operation for a known cancer in the dominant breast. All patients were treated by modified mastectomy, which included total mastectomy with thorough axillary dissection, at first with preservation of the major and minor pectoral muscles, and more recently with removal of the minor pectoral muscle. Residual carcinoma was found in 52% of the mastectomy specimens following generous excisional biopsies (Wanebo et al. 1974). Among the patients with minimal infiltrating cancers and clinically negative axillae, 16% had micrometastases, i.e., (a) tumor nodule(s) 2 mm or less in diameter, in the axillary nodes. No adjuvant therapy, e.g., x-ray therapy, chemotherapy was administered to these patients, and there were no local recurrences. The crude disease-free survival rate at 10 years in the first 72 patients treated in this fashion is 97% (Table 5) (Wanebo et al. 1974). One patient developed lung metastases 8 years after mastectomy for a noninfiltrating intraductal cancer with negative nodes, and the other

Table 5. Results recorded at 10-year follow-up of 72 patients breated with modified radical mastectomy only for minimal breast cancer (1953–1965)

Pathology	No. of patients	No. of mastectomies	NED
Infiltrating duct Ca	8	9	8
Noninfiltrating duct Ca	27	30	25[a]
In situ lobular Ca	29	37	29
Paget's disease with intraductal Ca	5	5	5
Low-grade Ca	2	2	2
Malignant cystosarcoma	1	1	1
Total	72	82	70 = 97%

[a] One patient died of metastatic carcinoma and one of myocardial infarction

patient with a small infiltrating duct carcinoma died with no evidence of breast cancer from a myocardial infarction. Early in the treatment of this group of patients, when positive nodes were found in the axilla modified mastectomy was replaced by radical mastectomy in 8 patients, to clear the axillae effectively. In none of the 8 cases was any residual carcinoma found, the additional tissue removed by radical mastectomy containing three to four negative nodes in the apex of the axilla.

Modified mastectomy with preservation of the pectoral muscle has proved to be 100% effective in obtaining local control in patients with minimal breast cancer and has yielded an excellent survival rate at 10 years. Other groups have reproduced these results by similar treatment. Of the patients who had undergone wide excisional biopsy of their primary tumors, 52% had residual areas of breast cancer in the mastectomy specimen when examined by conventional postoperative review of the excised tissues. When nodal involvement (Huvos et al. 1971), was found in the axilla it was usually minimal in extent consisting only of micrometastases with lymph nodes containing tumor nodules less than 2 mm in diameter. These optimal results were obtained when adequate primary surgical therapy was applied to a group of patients with a minimal risk of having occult systemic disease at the time of primary treatment.

Primary Treatment of Early Breast Cancer

The great majority of patients with primary breast cancer are still treated according to a selected adequate surgery schedule at the Memorial Hospital in New York City. This involves the use of radical mastectomy, extended radical mastectomy, and modified radical mastectomy, each in the appropriate patients, (Urban 1977, 1978; Urban and Castro 1971) in each instance attempting to obtain maximum local control while preserving the appearance of the patient at an optimal level. None of the patients evaluated in this group received adjuvant chemotherapy. Radiation therapy was administered postoperatively to the adjacent regional nodes in the majority of patients who had positive nodes in the operative specimen, primarily axillary nodes. Our own personal data are representative of the general experience in this hospital. Between 1965 and 1970 we treated 544 patients with

Table 6. Survival in primary operable breast cancer (1965–1970) (Cody et al. 1982)

Type	Mastectomy	No. of patients	5-Year alive	Survival (%) NED	10-Year alive	Survival (%) NED
Infiltrating carcinoma	Radical	351	80	72	70	63
	Extended radical	105	80	69	67	60
	Modified radical	40	92	90	89	86
	Total/mean	496	81	73	71	64
Noninfiltrating carcinoma	Radical	8	(7/8)	(6/8)	(6/8)	(6/8)
	Modified radical	40	100	97	97	97
	Total/mean	48	98	94	94	94
Total/mean for all cases		544	82	75	73	67

Survival calculated by life-table method: complete follow-up on 98% to 5 years and 90% to 10 years

Table 7. Local recurrence rate at 10 years in patients with infiltrating breast cancer (1965–1970) by pathological stage

Pathological stage (AJC/UICC)	No. of patients	Local recurrence as first sign	Local recurrence with or after + systemic disease	Overall local recurrence
I	160	1; 0.6%	0; 0%	1; 0.6%
II	313	13; 4.0%	13; 4.0%	26; 8.0%
III	23	1; 4.0%	2; 9.0%	3; 13.0%
Total	496	15; 3.0%	15; 3.0%	30; 6.0%

primary operable breast cancer, which was infiltrating in 496 cases and noninfiltrating in 48. Of all the patients seen by us at this time with previously untreated breast cancer, 97% were considered to be operable and were included in this series (Cody et al. 1982); 73% of the overall group of patients were alive 10 years later, and 67% were alive and free of disease. Patients with infiltrating breast cancer showed a 10-year survival rate of 71%, while 64% were alive and free of disease at 10 years. Of the patients with noninfiltrating cancer, 94% were alive and free of disease 10 years following treatment (Table 6).

Among the patients with infiltrating breast cancer, 44% had positive axillary nodes. The overall survival of patients with positive axillary nodes was 71% at 5 years, and 58% at 10 years. At 5 years 62% were alive and free of disease, and at 10 years, 50%. When the axillary nodes were negative, patients with infiltrating cancer showed a 5-year survival rate of 88%, while 82% were alive and free of disease. Of these patients, 81% survived 10 years and 75% were alive and free of disease at 10 years (Cody et al. 1982).

Our overall local recurrence rate (recurrences were found in the axilla, parasternal chest wall, and the operative flaps over the chest wall) at 10 years was 6% or 30/496 patients with infiltrating cancer, 2 with recurrence in the parasternal portion of the chest wall, 2 with recurrence in the axilla, and 26 with recurrence in the operative area on the chest wall (Table 7). Only 3% of the overall group showed local recurrence as the first sign of

Table 8. Local recurrence rate at 10 years in patients with breast cancer (1965–1970) by clinical stage

Clinical stage (AJC/UICC)	No. of patients	Local recurrence as first sign	Local recurrence with or after + systemic disease	Overall local recurrence
I	223	2; 0.9%	2; 0,9%	4; 1.8%
II	250	12; 4.8%	11; 4.4%	23; 9.2%
III	23	1; 4.0%	2; 9.0%	3; 13.0%
Total	496	15; 3.0%	15; 3.0%	30[a]; 6.0%

[a] Recurrence in parasternal chest wall in 2 cases; in axilla in 2; and in chest wall flaps in 26

Table 9. Survival following extended radical mastectomy (1965–1970) (Cody et al. 1982)

Nodes	No. of patients	5-Year (%)		10-Year (%)	
		Alive	NED	Alive	NED
All−	54	84	78	78	70
Axillary+/internal mammary−	24	87	75	68	60
Axillary−/internal mammary+	10	68	59	45	45
Axillary +/internal mammary+	17	65	41	47	35
Total	105	80	69	67	60

Survival calculated by life-table method: complete follow-up in 98% (5 years) and 90% (10 years). Of total patients, 39% had positive axillary nodes and 36% received cobalt-60 RT to regional nodes (base of neck)

recurrent cancer. In the remaining 3%, local recurrences appeared concurrently with or subsequent to the appearance of systemic disease (Table 8). None of these patients received adjuvant chemotherapy, but the majority with positive axillary and/or internal mammary nodes received postoperative radiation therapy administered to the regional nodes adjacent to those which were removed surgically: the base of the neck and the internal mammary nodes in patients undergoing radical and modified radical mastectomy; and the base of the neck and apex of the axilla in patients undergoing extended radical mastectomy. Radiation therapy consisted of 45–50 Gy given in divided doses over a 5-week interval in the form of cobalt-60 therapy or electron-beam therapy (Cody et al. 1982).

Patients undergoing extended radical mastectomy (Table 9) had an average tumor size of 3 cm, and most presented with inner or central lesions. In this group 40% showed axillary involvement and 26% had internal mammary involvement (Cody et al. 1982; Lacour et al. 1976; Urban and Casko 1971). At 10 years, 70% of the patients whose axillary and internal mammary nodes were clear were free of disease and well, 45% were free of disease and well when only internal mammary nodes were involved, and 35% were alive and free of disease at 10 years when both axillary and internal mammary nodes were positive. The majority of patients underwent radical mastectomy during this time interval (Table 10). These patients had an average tumor size of 2.4 cm, and 50% had axillary involvement. Of the patients with infiltrating cancer with positive axillary nodes, 70% were alive 5 years

Table 10. Survival following radical mastectomy for infiltrating breast cancer (Cody et al. 1982)

	No. of patients	5-Year (%)		10-Year (%)	
		Alive	NED	Alive	NED
Axilla−	176	89	82	83	75
Level I+	82	79	74	67	61
Level II+	45	69	56	58	40
Level III+	48	54	48	40	33
Axilla+	175	70	62	57	50
Total	351	80	72	70	63

Survival calculated by life-table method: complete follow-up on 98% (5 years) and 90% (10 years) of patients. Of all patients 50% had positive axillary lymph nodes and 47% received cobalt-60 RT to regional nodes

Table 11. Survival with infiltrating breast cancer by stage (1965–1970)

Staging system	Stage	No. of patients	5-Year (%)		10-Year (%)	
			Alive	NED	Alive	NED
Columbia	A	374	88	82	80	74
clinical	B	116	59	47	41	35
	C	6	(4/6)	(3/6)	(3/6)	(2/6)
AJC-UICC	I	223	91	86	85	78
clinical	II	250	73	63	59	52
	III	23	64	55	64	50
AJC-UICC	I	160	92	87	87	82
pathological	II	313	76	67	63	55
	III	23	64	55	64	50
Total		496	81	73	71	64

after radical mastectomy, while 62% were alive and free of disease: 57% survived and 50% were alive and free of disease at 10 years following radical mastectomy. The best survival rate was obtained in the patients in whom the most favorable conditions were present, who underwent modified mastectomy and who usually had minimal infiltrating cancers: a 10-year NED (no evidence of disease) survival rate of 97% for noninfiltrating cancers and a 10-year NED survival rate of 86% for minimal infiltrating cancers (Cody et al. 1982). These excellent survival rates and excellent local recurrence rates, which were attained despite the absence of adjuvant chemotherapy, indicate that most patients with negative nodes and many patients with positive axillary nodes do not have established systemic disease at the time of primary therapy (Table 11). In our own experience the addition of adjuvant chemotherapy has improved the 5-year survival rate of patients with positive axillary nodes by only 5%–10% over that obtained by adequate primary therapy alone in similar patients (Bonnadonna and Valagussa 1981). The current tendency to minimize the importance of adequate primary surgical therapy is without basis (Fisher

1979). Patients with breast cancer will benefit most when adequate primary therapy, which yields excellent local control, is combined with aggressive multidrug adjuvant chemotherapy in appropriate cases.

Although the results of treatment of minimal, occult, and early breast cancer at the Memorial Sloan Kettering Institute do not reflect a wide experience with conservative surgery, the results obtained primarily through radical surgery should serve as a standard against which to compare the results of breast-conserving therapy for operable breast cancer (Calle et al. 1978).

During the last 2 years — 1982 and 1983 — our patient material has improved markedly. The average tumor size is only 1.8 cm, and only about 33% of patients show axillary involvement. The great majority of patients are treated adequately by the Patey-type modified mastectomy, since this procedure is appropriate for these more facorable lesions with a lesser degree and less frequent involvement of axillary nodal disease.

References

Amalric R, Santamaria F, Robert F et al. (1982) Radiation therapy with or without primary limited surgery for primary operable breast cancer: A 20 year experience at the Marseilles Cancer Institute. Cancer 49: 30–34

Ashikari R, Rosen PP, Urban JA, Senoo T (1976) Breast cancer presenting as an axillary mass. Ann Surg 183: 415–417

Betsil WL Jr, Lieberman PH et al. (1978) Intraductal carcinoma: long term follow up after treatment by biopsy alone. JAMA 239: 1863–1867

Bonnadonna G, Valagussa P (1981) Dose response effect of adjuvant chemotherapy in breast cancer. N Engl J Med 304: 10–15

Calle R, Pilleron JP (1979) Radiation therapy with our without lumpectomy for operable breast cancer — 10 year results. Breast 5: 2–6

Calle R, Pilleron JP, Schlinger P et al. (1978) Conservative management of operable breast cancer: 10 year experience at the Foundation Curie. Cancer 42: 2045–2053

Cody HS III, Bretsky SS, Urban JA (1982) The continuing importance of adequate surgery for operable breast cancer: Significant salvage of node positive patients without adjuvant chemotherapy. CA 32: 242–256

Crile G, Cooperman A, Esselstyn CB et al. (1980) Results of partial mastectomy in 173 patients followed from 5 to 10 years. Surg Gynecol Obstet 150: 563–566

Feuerman L, Attie J, Rosenberg B (1962) Carcinoma in axillary lymph nodes as an indicator of breast cancer. Surg Gynecol and Obstet 114: 5

Fisher B (1979) Breast cancer management — alternatives to radical mastectomy. N Engl J Med 301: 326–328

Gallager HS, Martin J (1971) An orientation to the concept of minimal breast cancer. Cancer 28: 1505

Handley RS, Thackrey AC (1969) Conservative radical mastectomy — Patey's operation. Ann Surg 170: 880

Huvos AC, Hutter RVP, Berg JW (1971) Significance of axillary micro and macrometastases in mammary cancer. Ann Surg 173 : 44–46

Lacour J, Buccalossi P, Caceres E et al. (1976) Radical mastectomy versus radical mastectomy plus internal mammary dissection: 5 year results of an international cooperative study. Cancer 37: 206–214

Rosen PP, Fracchia AA, Urban JA et al. (1975) Residual mammary cancer following simulated partial mastectomy. Cancer 35: 739–747

Rosen PP, Lieberman PH, Brun DW, Kosloff C, Adair F (1978) Lobular carcinoma in situ of the breast. Am J Surg Pathol 2: 225–251

Urban JA (1977) Malignant lesions in the breast. In: Hardy JD (ed) Rhodes textbook of surgery. Lippincott, Philadelphia, pp 594−610

Urban JA (1978) Management of operable breast cancer: The surgeon's view. Cancer 42: 2066−2077

Urban JA, Castro EB (1971) Selecting variations in extent of surgical procedure for breast cancer. Cancer 28: 1615−1623

Urban JA, Papachristou D, Taylor J (1977) Bilateral Breast Cancer − Biopsy of the opposite breast. Cancer 40: 1968−1973

Wanebo HJ, Huvos A, Urban JA (1974) Treatment of minimal breast cancer, Cancer 33: 349−357

Conservative Treatment of Potentially Curable Breast Cancer

Experience at the Cleveland Clinic

Robert E. Hermann

Department of General Surgery, Cleveland Clinic Foundation, Cleveland, Ohio, USA

The surgical management of breast cancer changed at the Cleveland Clinic during the mid-1950s from radical operations to conservative operations. This change in our management of breast cancer came about initially through the influence of Dr. George Crile Jr (1956, 1961), and was subsequently taken up by all of the other members of the Department of General Surgery. This report is, therefore, that of our institutional experience.

Our change in the management of breast cancer, from the standard radical mastectomy to conservative operations selected or individualized for each patient, occurred about 10 or 15 years prior to a similar change that has now occurred in the United States. The reasons we changed our management of breast cancer were multiple: (a) we were no longer seeing the large cancers of the breast that we had seen in past years; (b) the importance of a number of prognostic factors (stage of the disease, size of the tumor, histologic type, etc.) other than the type of treatment given was recognized; (c) we were developing an increasing interest in "tumor-host" relationships with regard to regional lymph nodes and humoral factors; (d) breast cancer was being recognized as a potentially systemic disease, and all that could be achieved by operation was local and regional control; and (e) the cosmetic and psychosocial importance of the breast to women was being given increasing importance.

In our opinion, several prognostic factors are more important than the type of treatment when one considers breast cancer. Among these are, most importantly, the stage of the disease when the patient is seen or diagnosed, the histology of the tumor, and the size of the tumor. Other important factors include tumor growth factors such as estrogen and progesterone binding and other immunochemical factors (as yet undiscovered), host-resistance factors, including the immunopathology of regional lymph nodes and the general immune resistance of the patient, the age of the patient, and her menstrual status. Other factors of questionable importance include the location of the tumor in the breast and the duration of symptoms. Finally, treatment factors, the extent of the operative procedure or the use of adjuvant therapy, have been much discussed but are probably of less importance than the stage of the disease, the histology of the tumor, and the size of the primary tumor when diagnosed.

During the past 25 years, we have tried to individualize our treatment of breast cancer depending on tumor size and location as well as clinical stage of the disease (Table 1). We have performed modified radical mastectomy for patients with large tumors (2 cm or larger) or with potentially involved axillary lymph nodes. We have used total mastectomy, with or without axillary exploration and biopsy, for small tumors (2 cm or less) located

Early Breast Cancer
Edited by J. Zander and J. Baltzer
© Springer-Verlag Berlin Heidelberg 1985

Table 1. Surgical management of breast cancer at the Cleveland Clinic

Modified radical mastectomy
  All stage II cancers, stage I < 2 cm

Total mastectomy and axillary biopsy
  Stage I < 2 cm, central lesions

Partial mastectomy and axillary biopsy
  Patient wants breast preserved
  Lesions is peripheral, < 2 cm
  Not lobular or intraductal type

Table 2. Manchester clinical staging of breast cancer

Stage I
  Tumor of any size
  No apparent involvement of lymph nodes
  No distant metastases

Stage II
  Tumor of any size
  Palpable, suggestive axillary lymph nodes
  No distant metastases

Stage III
  Tumor of any size
  Edema of breast, fixation to chest wall
  Ulceration or inflammation
  Large, fixed, or matted lymph nodes
  Supraclavicular nodes
  No distant metastases

Stage IV
  Distant metastases

centrally in the breast or those with a high degree of multicentricity (lobular carcinoma) without apparent clinical involvement of axillary lymph nodes. We have used partial mastectomy, with or without axillary dissection, for small tumors (2 cm or less) located predominantly in the periphery of the breast without apparent axillary lymph node involvement for patients who wish to have the remainder of their breast tissue preserved and reconstructed.

This report analyzes our experience with selective conservative operations for breast cancer in patients primarily treated at the Cleveland Clinic during the years 1955 through 1975. We have used Manchester clinical staging at the Cleveland Clinic for the past 35 years (Table 2). During the 20 years from 1955 through 1975, in all 1,590 patients with breast cancer were seen and received primary treatment at the Cleveland Clinic. Exluded were all patients who had already received primary treated elsewhere, who came to us for follow-up evaluation or for treatment of recurrent disease. We have been able to follow 96% of these patients; 4%, i.e., 61 patients, have been lost to follow-up. Sixty-four percent of the patients were in clinical stage I, 24% in stage II, 6% in stage III, and 5% in stage IV (Table 3).

Our principal operations performed during these years were modified radical mastectomy in 35% total mastectomy in 33%, and partial mastectomy in 18% (Table 4). Radical mastecomy was largely discontinued in 1957; it was performed in only 36 patients − 2%. Biopsy alone and radiation therapy were performed in 10%, and bilateral mastectomy of various types in 2%. Adjuvant radiation therapy was given prophylactically after operation in 14% of the patients in this series. We no longer use prophylactic, postoperative radiation therapy routinely, but use radiation therapy now only with localized recurrences.

Our operative technique is as follows: excision breast biopsy is performed under either local or general anesthesia; local anesthesia is the more common. If a modified radical or total mastectomy is chosen, a transverse incision provides a better cosmetic result. Skin flaps are raised, care being taken to ensure an adequate blood supply and retain

Table 3. Clinical staging[a] of cancer of the breast in 1,590 patients at the Cleveland Clinic (1955–1975)

Stage	No. of patients	Percentage
I	1,025	64%
II	375	24%
III	93	6%
IV	83	5%

[a] Manchester Staging

Table 4. Operations performed for breast cancer in 1590 patients at the Cleveland Clinic (1955–1975)

Radical mastectomy	36 Patients	2%
Modified radical mastectomy	542 Patients	35%
Total mastectomy	520 Patients	33%
Partial mastectomy	289 Patients	18%
Biopsy only	178 Patients	10%
Bilateral mastectomy	25 Patients	2%
Radiation, postoperative	216 Patients	14%

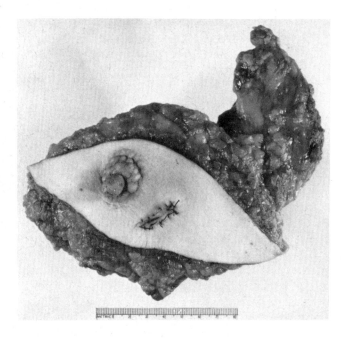

Fig. 1. Operative specimen after modified radical mastectomy

subcutaneous fat. All breast tissue is removed by dissecting in the plane between breast tissue and subcutaneous fat. Both the major and the minor pectoral muscles are preserved, which means that the nerve to the pectoralis major, the long thoracic nerve, and thoracodorsal nerves can be conserved. Suction catheters are placed postoperatively for evacuation of the wound space, and a light dressing is applied for several days. Figure 1 shows a typical operative specimen.

The cosmetic results of modified radical or total mastectomy are equal and can be excellent. With the transverse incision, women can wear low-cut dresses or swimsuits (Figs. 2 and 3), and there is no binding of arm motion. If reconstruction of the breast is desired it can be performed either immediately or 4–6 months postoperatively, including nipple reconstruction if desired by the patient.

Partial mastectomy is performed through the incision depicted in Fig. 4, depending on the location of the tumor. Partial mastectomy should include the skin overlying any previous biopsy site and remove approximately 3–4 cm or normal breast tissue surrounding the previous biopsy site.

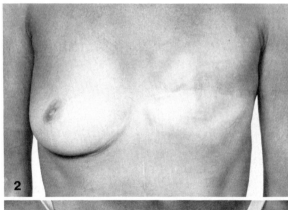

Fig. 2. Cosmetic appearance after left modified radical mastectomy using a transverse incision

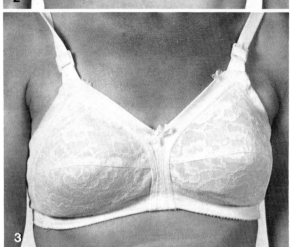

Fig. 3. The same patient wearing a bra with a left breast prosthesis

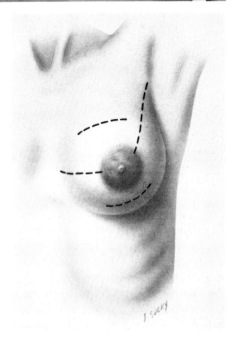

Fig. 4. Incisions used for partial (segmental) mastectomy

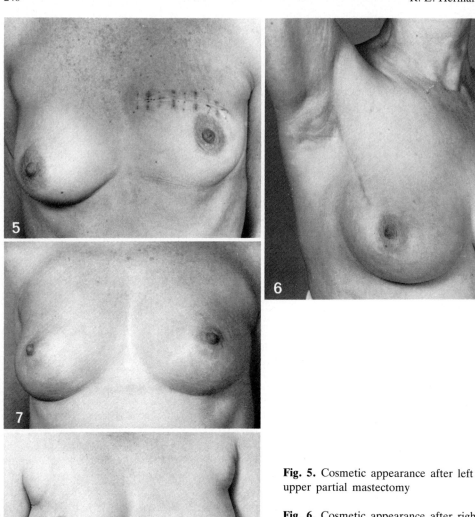

Fig. 5. Cosmetic appearance after left upper partial mastectomy

Fig. 6. Cosmetic appearance after right upper outer partial mastectomy

Fig. 7. Cosmetic appearance after left upper outer partial mastectomy

Fig. 8. Cosmetic appearance after right lateral partial mastectomy

The cosmetic results of partial mastectomy are excellent. Figures 5–8 show patients after partial mastectomy of the left upper central breast, right upper outer quadrant, left upper outer qudrant, and right lateral segment.

One of the controversies about partial mastectomy is the incidence of multicentricity. In the National Surgical Adjuvant Breast Project (NSABP) study, in 904 patients after radical mastectomy the incidence of multicentricity was 13.4% (Table 5) (Fisher et al. 1975b). Noninvasive cancer was more common than invasive cancer. Multicentricity was more

Table 5. Analysis of 904 breast specimens removed because of cancer of the breast (NSABP) (Fisher et al. 1975b)

Incidence of multicentricity	13.4%
Noninvasive cancer	9.3%
Invasive cancer	4.1%
More common with	
Lobular and intraductal types	
Tumors larger than 4.1 cm	
Nipple involvement (11.1%)	
Noncircumscribed primary	

Table 6. Involvement of the nipple and areola in carcinoma of the breast (Smith et al. 1976)

541 Mastectomies:
  66 (12%) Cases of carcinomatous involvement of nipple and areola

Greatest likelihood of involvement:
  Paget's disease or intraductal carcinoma
  Retroareolar location
  Tumor size larger than 2 cm

Least likelihood of involvement:
  Peripheral tumor
  Tumor size 2 cm or smaller

Table 7. Survival rate for breast cancer at the Cleveland Clinic (1955–1975)

Stage	Percentage survival			
	5 Years	10 Years	15 Years	20 Years
Clinical stage I	77	59	45	32
Clinical stage II	54	29	21	16
Clinical stage III	19	4	–	–
Clinical stage IV	13	8	2	2
Clinical stages I and II	71	50	38	27

common with lobular and intraductal types of tumors and tumors larger than 4 cm, and in patients with nipple involvement (intraductal cancer) or noncircumscribed primaries.

Another controversial issue is the incidence of involvement of the nipple and areola in patients with cancer of the breast. At the Mayo Clinic, 541 mastectomy specimens were studied, and carcinomatous involvement of the nipple and areola was found in 12% (Table 6) (Smith et al. 1976). The greatest likelihood of involvement was in patients with Paget's disease, obviously, intraductal carcinoma, a tumor in the retroareolar location, or a tumor larger than 2 cm in size. The least likelihood of involvement was in a patient with a peripheral tumor or a tumor 2 cm in size or smaller.

We have assessed the 5- to 20-year survival of patients operated upon at the Cleveland Clinic during the years 1955 through 1975. Overall survival for all patients and all stages at 5 years was 65%; at 10 years, 46%; at 15 years, 34%; and at 20 years, 27%. The survival of patients in the four clinical stages, stages I through IV, are shown in Table 7. Survival of patients in potentially curable clinical stages I and II are shown at the bottom.

These survival results of our patients in clinical stages I and II have been compared with results published from other centers in the United States during a similar time period for patients with clinical stages I and II disease (Table 8). Results published by the National Cancer Institute Cancer Registry (1982), by the National Surgical Adjuvant Breast Project (Fisher et al. 1975a), by Johns Hopkins Hospital (Lewison and Smith 1963), by Ohio State University Hospital (Minton et al. 1972), and by the Syracuse New York Cancer Registry (Mueller and Jeffries 1975), a total of 21,914 patients, show survival figures at 5 and 10

Table 8. Survival rates at 5 and 10 years for carcinoma of the breast in stage I and II

Study series	Survival	
	5 Years	10 Years
Cleveland Clinic (1955–1975) 1590 patients	71%	50%
NCI Cancer Registry (1955–1965) 14,741 patients	61%	43%
NSABP (1948–1963) 826 patients	64%	46%
Johns Hopkins (1946–1950) 302 patients	52%	33%
Ohio State (1963–1971) 904 patients	62%	48%
Cancer Research Institute USC (1945–1956) 2,038 patients	71%	55%
Syracuse, NY, Cancer Registry (1957–1973) 1,513 patients	58%	38%
Total: 21,914 patients		

Table 9. Survival after various methods of surgical treatment for breast cancer at the Cleveland Clinic (1955–1975)

Surgical treatment	Percentage survival			
	5 Years	10 Years	15 Years	20 Years
Radical mastectomy	61	31	28	16
Modified radical mastectomy	64	44	34	26
Total mastectomy	73	55	40	28
Partial mastectomy	76	57	43	32

years very comparable to those we are reporting with selected conservative operations. Our overall results are, therefore, comparable to or better than those recorded in most other reported series in the United States during these years.

We have been concerned that we might do harm to patients by less extensive or more conservative operative procedures. One of the most interesting facts to come out of our follow-up study is that with partial or total mastectomy patient survival is equal to or better than that with a more radical procedure (Table 9). This, of course, has nothing to do with the operative procedure but represents selection of patients, more favorable patients having lesser operative procedures. It is of interest that of the 289 patients having partial mastectomy, only 18 patients, or 6%, had a new primary cancer develop in the same breast requiring a later complete mastectomy. Survival after this second operative procedure was 79% at 5 years and 47% at 10 years an excellent long-term survival rate.

Table 10. Survival with breast cancer by tumor size at the Cleveland Clinic (1955–1975)

Tumor size	Percentage survival		
	5 Years	10 Years	15 Years
Up to 2 cm (452 patients)	75	57	42
Larger than 2 cm (904 patients)	59	40	29

Table 11. Survival of breast cancer patients by age at the Cleveland Clinic (1955–1975)

	Percentage survival		
	5 Years	10 Years	15 Years
Age − 35 or less	65	53	46
36−65	67	51	40
66 or more	56	29	12
	Determinate survival		
	65	53	46
	71	58	52
	70	55	48

Survival of patients with estrogen-receptor-positive tumors was better than those with estrogen-receptor-negative tumors for both stage I disease and stage II disease.

Survival of patients with small tumors (less than 2 cm) was significantly better than in those with tumors larger than 2 cm (Table 10).

Actual survival figures of patients 35 years of age or younger appeared to be better than those in older groups of patients (Table 11). However, when a determinant survival analysis was made, excluding deaths from other causes and considering only deaths from breast cancer, survival was equal at all ages.

When our three principal operations (modified radical mastectomy, total mastectomy, and partial mastectomy) were analyzed separately in patients with clinical stages I and II, patients having had partial mastectomy did was well as or better than patients having the other operative procedures, at 5 years and up to 20 years of survival (Table 12). In patients with clinical stage II disease, not enough patients had partial mastectomy for 20-year results to be analyzed.

Similarly, when the three principal operations were analyzed in those patients in whom, at histopathological study, all nodes were negative, patients having had partial mastectomy appeared to do better up to 20 years of survival analysis than those patients having had more aggressive operative procedures (Table 13). These results are interesting and require further evaluation for other selection factors not yet identified. When one to three nodes

Table 12. Survival of breast cancer patients by clinical stage and type of mastectomy performed of the Cleveland Clinic (1955–1975)

| | Percentage survival | | | |
	5 Years	10 Years	15 Years	20 Years
Clinical stage I				
Modified radical	73	57	47	33
Total	79	60	43	30
Partial	81	63	48	44
Clinical stage II				
Modified radical	55	30	21	21
Total	51	31	24	20
Partial	60	34	28	–

Table 13. Survival of breast cancer patients by nodal status and type of mastectomy performed of the Cleveland Clinic (1955–1975)

| | Percentage survival | | | |
	5 Years	10 Years	15 Years	20 Years
All nodes negative				
Modified radical	77	60	51	35
Total	83	68	56	32
Partial	95	81	64	53
1–3 Nodes positive				
Modified radical	65	43	35	29
Total	68	26	24	18
Partial	68	45	30	30
4 or more nodes positive				
Modified radical	45	26	12	12
Total	42	24	17	–
Partial	42	17	17	–
No axillary dissection				
Modified radical	–	–	–	–
Total	71	54	37	29
Partial	75	56	42	28

were positive, four or more nodes were positive, or when no axillary dissection was performed, long-term survival results appeared equal.

When the three principal operations are compared in patients with tumors 2 cm or smaller, partial mastectomy appears to have a slight survival advantage (Table 14). In patients with larger tumors, all operations appeared to be equal.

During the past 5 years, we, like groups at many other centers in the United States, have begun to treat many of our patients with local resection of the tumor (tumorectomy), axillary dissection for staging, and radiation therapy to the breast, utilizing the techniques

Table 14. Survival of breast cancer patients by tumor size and type of mastectomy performed of the Cleveland Clinic (1955–1975)

	Percentage survival			
	5 Years	10 Years	15 Years	20 Years
Tumor 2 cm or less				
Modified radical	68	49	41	41
Total	84	72	48	38
Partial	81	57	48	48
Tumor larger than 2 cm				
Modified radical	64	43	32	25
Total	67	45	33	21
Partial	65	54	33	–

advocated by Harris et al. (1978), Almaric et al. (1982), and other radiotherapists throughout the world. Our early experiences with this technique are excellent. The cosmetic results of the treated breast are very good, and the results reported are competitive with those reported by surgeons.

Our experience supports the belief that selective, conservative operative procedures can effectively treat breast cancer by removing local and regional disease, with the same long-term survival rates obtained by radical operations but with improved cosmetic results and function. We believe surgeons can individualize and select the operative procedure for the treatment of breast cancer, depending on the magnitude or extent of the disease. The fact that patients with small, apparently early breast cancers do as well or better after partial mastectomy than after more aggressive operative procedures should be an incentive for women to continue to examine their breasts carefully, so that when a small tumor mass is identified it can be treated promptly by a conservative operative procedure. In the final analysis, earlier diagnosis and treatment may be one of the major benefits of the trend toward more conservative treatment methods.

References

Amalric R, Santamaria F, Robert F, Seigle J, Altschuler C, Kurtz JM, Spitalier JM, Brandone H, Ayme Y, Pollet JF, Burmeister R, Abed R (1982) Radiation therapy with or without primary limited surgery for operable breast cancer. Am Cancer Soc 1: 30–34

Crile G Jr (1956) Cancer of the breast: The surgeon's dilemma. Cleve Clin Q 23: 179

Crile G Jr (1961) Simplified treatment of cancer of the breast. Early results of a clinical study. Ann Surg 153: 1364

Fisher B, Slack N, Katrych D, Wolmark N (1975a) Ten year follow-up results of patients with cancer of the breast in a cooperative clinical trial evaluating surgical adjuvant chemotherapy. Surg Gynecol Obstet 140: 528–534

Fisher ER, Gregorio RM, Fisher B (1975b) The pathology of invasive breast cancer. A syllabus derived from findings of the National Surgical Adjuvant Breast Project. Cancer 36: 1–85

Harris JR, Levene B, Hellman S (1978) The role of radiation therapy in the primary treatment of carcinoma of the breast. Semin Oncol 5: 403

Lewison EF, Smith RT (1963) Results of breast cancer treatment at Johns Hopkins Hospitals, 1946–1950; comparative results and discussion of survival in relation to treatment. Surgery 53:644

Minton JP, Sabback M, Oberle K (1972) Breast cancer survival, the Ohio State University Hospitals. Ohio State Med J 12:1099

Mueller CB, Jeffries W (1975) Cancer of the breast: Its outcome as measured by the rate of dying and causes of death. Ann Surg 182:334

National Cancer Institute (1972) End results in cancer, Report No 4, pp 99–103

Smith S, Payne WS, Carney JA (1976) Involvement of the nipple and areola in cancer of the breast. Surg Gynecol Obstet 143:546

Trials of Wide Excision and Radiation Therapy at the Breast Unit, Guy's Hospital, London

John Hayward

Breast Unit, Guy's Hospital, London, SE1 9RT, England

Introduction

This paper details the results of trials on breast conservation techniques that have been undertaken at Guy's Hospital since 1960. There have been two such trials. In the first one, carried out between 1961 and 1971, 376 patients aged 50 and over with operable breast cancer were assigned by random sample to receive either wide local excision or radical mastectomy, both groups additionally receiving radiotherapy (Atkins et al. 1972). Between 1971 and 1975 a second trial was undertaken in which the same treatments were used, but in this instance only patients with clinically negative axillae were included (Hayward 1977). Patients of all ages were entered into this second series and a further 252 were randomly allocated to either wide excision or radical mastectomy. This paper will describe the results of the first series up to 20 years from the commencement of the trial, in which all patients have been followed-up for a minimum period of 11 years. The second series will be reported up to 11 years from commencement of the trial, and patients have been followed-up here for a minimum period of 7 years. The results of the two series have been reported in more detail elsewhere (Hayward 1983).

Methods

All patients aged 50 and over presenting at the Breast Unit at Guy's Hospital with operable breast cancer were entered into the first series. On confirmation of the diagnosis they were randomly allocated to either wide excision or radical mastectomy. Those receiving wide excision had an excision of the lump together with the surrounding clinically normal breast tissue within 3 cm. The axilla was not disturbed. Postoperatively they received radiotherapy with 38 Gy over 3 weeks by means of a linear accelerator to a glancing field, including the breast and internal mammary chain. Additionally, they received 30 Gy over 2 weeks to the axilla and supraclavicular fossa, using a 300-kV machine. Patients allocated to radical mastectomy received a total mastectomy with full axillary clearance, including removal of the pectoralis minor muscle and that part of the pectoralis major muscle which lay behind the tumour. They received postoperative radiotherapy at a dose of 30 Gy over 3 weeks to the internal mammary, supraclavicular, and axillary fields. This treatment was given by means of a 300-kV machine. In the second series patients of any age with clinically uninvolved axillae were entered, and the surgical and radiotherapeutic treatment options were precisely the same as for patients in series 1.

Early Breast Cancer
Edited by J. Zander and J. Baltzer
© Springer-Verlag Berlin Heidelberg 1985

After treatment, all patients in both series were examined clinically at 3-monthly intervals for the first 3 years after operation, then 6-monthly until 5 years, and subsequently at yearly intervals. No routine investigations were carried out unless demanded by physical signs or symptoms. Nine patients have been lost to follow-up, but data on these have been included in the analysis of results until the time they were last seen. For analysis of the results, all patients have been classified as having either clinical stage I, which is N0 or N1a, or clinical stage II, which is N1b disease. Relapse has been analysed individually for local and distant recurrence. Local recurrence is defined as the development of a lesion within an area bounded by the midline medially, the clavicle superiorly, the posterior axillary line laterally and the costal margin inferiorly. Recurrence in this area may be cutaneous, subcutaneous, nodal or, in the case of patients receiving wide excision, in the retained breast. Additionally, recurrences in nodes in the ipsilateral supraclavicular fossa are categorised as local. Patients are considered to have had a local recurrence even if this is part of disseminated disease. Comparisons of the local and distant recurrence and survival rates have been carried out by the life-table method of analysis, and the significance of differences between curves has been determined by the long-rank method.

Results

In all, 376 patients were entered into the first series, 192 of whom were allocated to radical mastectomy and 184 to wide excision. Figures 1−3 show the life-table comparisons of the local reccurence, distant recurrence and survival rates in patients with stage I disease. Figure 1 shows that patients having a wide excision had a significantly higher incidence of local recurrence than those having a radical mastectomy. Figure 2, however, shows that the curve for distant recurrence was similar for both treatments, and Fig. 3 shows that survival also did not differ between the two groups. Figures 4−6 show the local recurrence, distant recurrence and survival rates for patients with stage II disease. Figure 4, again, demonstrates a significantly higher incidence of local recurrence in patients receiving wide

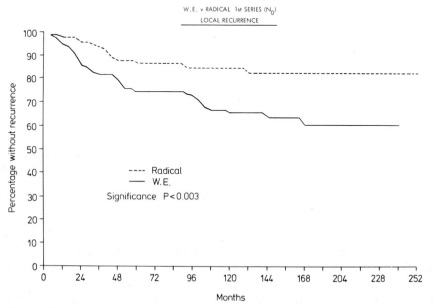

Fig. 1. Comparison of local recurrence rates in patients with stage I disease in the first series

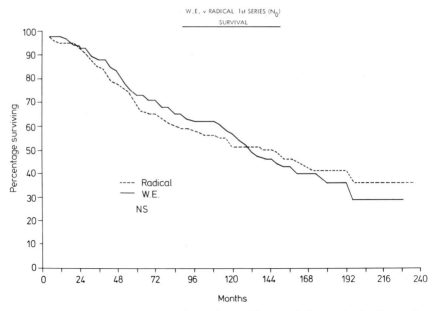

Fig. 2. Comparison of distant recurrence rates in patients with stage I disease in the first series

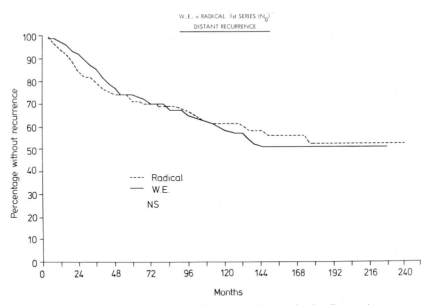

Fig. 3. Comparison of survival rates in patients with stage I disease in the first series

excision. Figure 5, however, shows that distant recurrence was also higher in the wide excision group, although not significantly so, and Fig. 6 shows that survival was significantly worse in the wide excision group.

There were 252 patients in the second series, 130 of whom were allocated to radical mastectomy and 122 to wide excision. Figures 7–9 give the life curves for local recurrence,

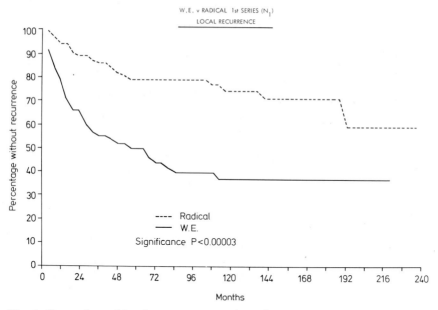

Fig. 4. Comparison of local recurrence rates in patients with stage II disease in the first series

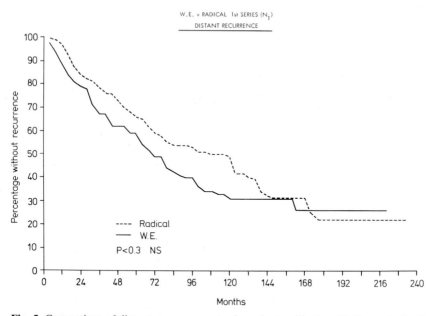

Fig. 5. Comparison of distant recurrence rates in patients with stage II disease in the first series

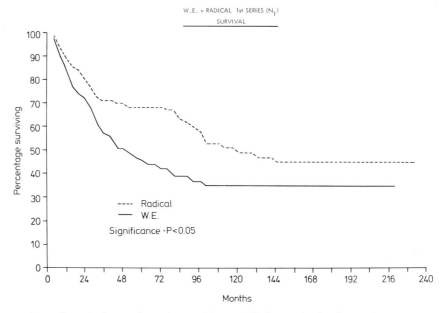

Fig. 6. Comparison of survival rates in patients with stage II disease in the first series

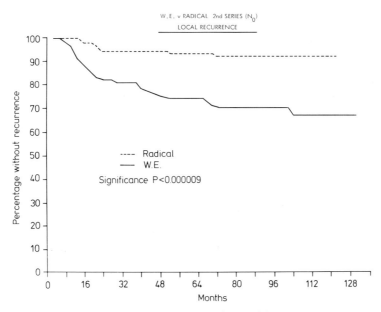

Fig. 7. Comparison of local recurrence rates in patients with stage I diseases in the second series

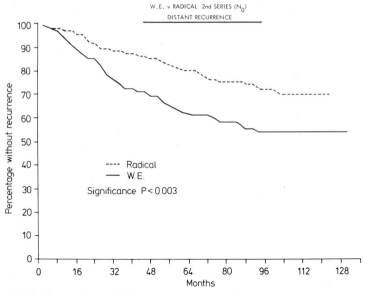

Fig. 8. Comparison of distant recurrence rates in patients with stage I disease in the second series

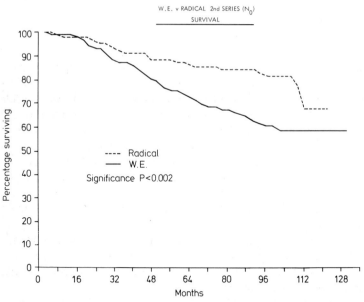

Fig. 9. Comparison of survival rates in patients with stage I disease in the second series

distant recurrence and survival for patients in the two groups. Figure 7 shows that again the local recurrence rate in patients receiving wide excision was significantly higher than in those receiving radical mastectomy. Figure 8, however, shows that unlike the results in stage I disease in the first series, there was a significantly higher incidence of distant recurrence in patients receiving wide excision. Figure 9 shows that in this second series survival was significantly worse in those patients receiving wide excision.

Table 1. Incidence of local recurrence at different sites in patients in both series after wide excision

Site of local recurrence	1st Series		2nd Series N0 (122)
	N1 (63)	N0 (121)	
Skin	11 (17%)	5 (4%)	13 (11%)
Axillary node	13 (21%)	20 (17%)	13 (11%)
Supraclavicular node	1	2	1
Breast	7 (11%)	5 (4%)	5 (4%)
Other	4	6	4
Total	36 (57%)	38 (31%)	36 (30%)

The site of local recurrence in patients receiving wide excision in both series is detailed in Table 1. It can be seen that the major incidence of local recurrence is accounted for by those patients having wide excision who developed metastases in the retained axillary nodes. Recurrence in the retained breast was uncommon, except possibly in those patients with clinically involved axillae, 11% of whom eventually developed a lesion in the ipsilateral breast.

Discussion

In the initial report on the first of these series (Atkins et al. 1972), the results suggested that, with the treatment methods used, wide excision was a safe option for patients with clinical stage I disease, although there was a higher incidence of local recurrence. It was not felt that wide excision was a satisfactory treatment for patients with stage II disease, and because of this such patients were not entered into the second series. It was also thought that the reason for the increased incidence of distant recurrence and diminished survival in patients with stage II disease was the high rate of recurrence observed in the ipsilateral axilla. This high incidence of local axillary recurrence was presumed to be due to the low dose of radiation used. The incidence of local recurrence in patients with stage I disease was apparently not enough to affect distant recurrence rates and survival to any appreciable extent.

In the second series, however, the results of wide excision in patients with stage I disease appear to be much worse than the results obtained with radical mastectomy, and it is interesting to speculate on the reasons for this change compared with patients in the first series, who received precisely the same treatment.

To obtain further information on this point, life curves of patients with stage I disease receiving wide excision in the first series have been compared with similar life curves for patients who received wide excision in the second series. These comparisons are illustrated in Figs. 10–12. Figure 10 compares local recurrence rates, Fig. 11, the distant recurrence rates and Fig. 12, the survival rates. In fact, although there is a slightly higher incidence of distant metastases in patients in the second series, the difference between the curves is marginal, suggesting that the disparity in the results between the two series is not due to the results of wide excision in the second series being worse than in the first. Figures 13–15 give a similar comparison for patients receiving radical mastectomy in tho two series.

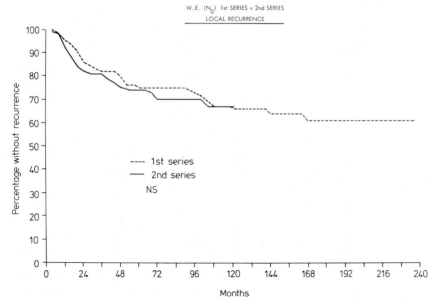

Fig. 10. Comparison of local recurrence rates in patients with stage I disease treated by wide excision in the first and second series

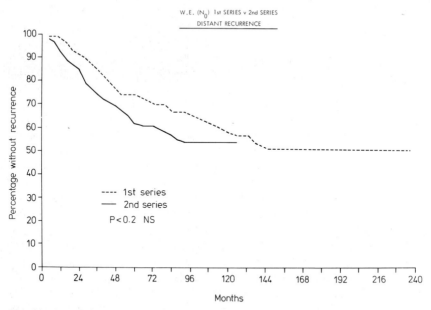

Fig. 11. Comparison of distant recurrence rates in patients with stage I disease treated by wide excision in the first and second series

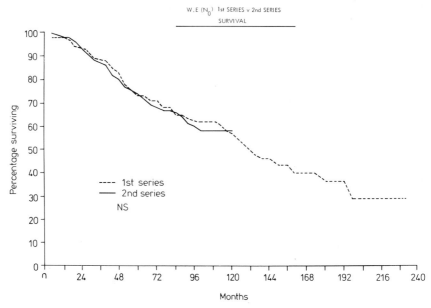

Fig. 12. Comparison of survival rates in patients with stage I disease treated by wide excision in the first and second series

Surprisingly, there is a much greater difference here. Figure 13 shows a comparison of local recurrence and Fig. 14, a comparison of the distant recurrence rate, and it can be seen that these rates are much higher in patients having radical mastectomy in the first series than in the second. Figure 15 compares the survival rate, and here again this is significantly worse in patients having radical mastectomy in the first series than in the second. Admittedly, the follow-up of the second series is not as long as that of the first, but the difference in survival is impressive. It is concluded, therefore, that the reason for the differences in results in the second series is not that patients having a wide excision did materially worse compared with those in the first series, but rather that patients who received a radical mastectomy fared better.

To throw more light on this, the features of the tumours in the two series were compared, to see whether prognostic variables differed to any extent. The pathological stage, histological grade and tumour size were all compared and found not to be significantly different in the two series. There was a slightly lower incidence of local recurrence after radical mastectomy in the second series, which may partly account for the results of the operation being better in that series than in the first.

The principal lesson that can be learned from these series is that local control of disease really is important. It is difficult to attribute the worse prognosis in the wide excision patients to anything other than the high incidence of local recurrence, particularly in the axilla. Additionally, even in the case of radical mastectomy, the incidence of local recurrence may have affected the ultimate result. The series give little information on the safety or otherwise of conservative treatments as such. These were early, relatively unsophisticated trials, and nowadays such low radiation doses to the axilla would not be used. Nevertheless, there is still a considerable number of patients who had their tumour treated by wide excision followed by radiotherapy – albeit at a less than optimum dose – who are still alive, well and free from recurrence today, over 20 years later. What the

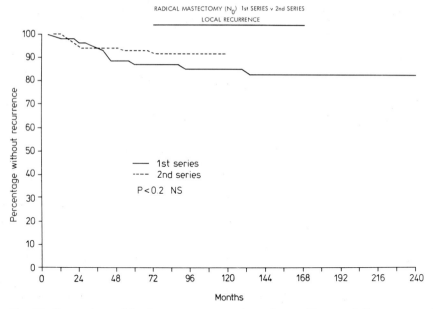

Fig. 13. Comparison of local recurrence rates in patients with stage I disease treated by radical mastectomy in the first and second series

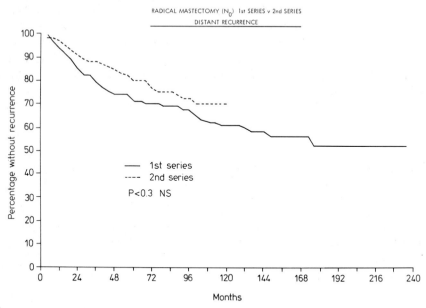

Fig. 14. Comparison of distant recurrence rates in patients with stage I disease treated by radical mastectomy in the first and second series

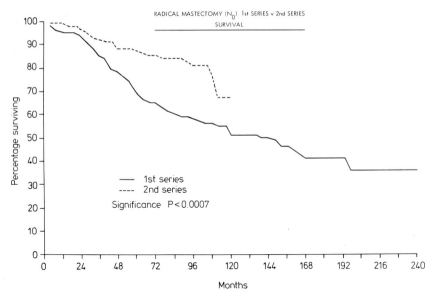

Fig. 15. Comparison of survival rates in patients with stage I disease treated by radical mastectomy in the first and second series

results of these trials do indicate is that any attempt at conservative therapy must entail maximum local control of disease, and that without this the patients' prognosis will be materially worse. What is also demonstrated clearly is the danger of using historical controls. If the radical mastectomy patients who had been used as controls for the first series had also been used as controls for the second, without any subsequent randomisation, the differences between the two treatments shown in the second series would never have been demonstrated.

References

Atkins Sir Hedley, Hayward JL, Klugman DJ, Wayte AB (1972) Treatment of early breast cancer: a report after ten years of a clinical trial. Br Med J II: 423

Hayward JL (1977) The Guy's trial of treatments of "early" breast cancer. World J Surg 1: 314–316

Hayward JL (1983) The Guy's Hospital trials on breast conservation. In: Harris JR, Hellman S, Silen W (eds) Conservative management of breast cancer. Lippincott, Philadelphia

Conservative Treatment of Breast Cancer with the "QU.A.RT." Technique

Umberto Veronesi, Roberto Zucali, Alberto Luini, Filiberto Belli, Sergio Crispino and Mirella Merson

Istituto Nazionale Tumori, Via Venezian 1, 20133 Milano, Italy

Introduction

The vigorous debate over the optimum treatment of breast cancer continues, in particular in countries where more and more cases of breast cancer of limited extent are submitted to primary treatment. There is evidence from many surveys in the United States of America (Scalon 1983; Vana et al. 1981) that the classic radical mastectomy is being abandoned in favor of less mutilating techniques such as the modified radical mastectomy, and in Europe more and more reports show that many centers have adopted a policy of breast-conserving procedures whenever the cases are suitable (Calle et al. 1978; Pierquin et al. 1980; Spitalier et al. 1977). However, the conservative treatments, even for tumors of very limited extent, have not been easily accepted by many surgeons who stress the need for more consistent results from long-term clinical trials to be certain that conservative procedures will give just as good survival rates as the Halsted mastectomy. Unfortunately, the clinical trials comparing the classic extensive mutilating treatments with the conservative ones are few (Hayward 1977; Veronesi et al. 1981; Wolmark and Fisher 1981) and, for various reasons, some of them are not totally acceptable. At the beginning of the seventies we therefore considered it important to design a controlled trial comparing the classic Halsted mastectomy with a conservative procedure that was developed at the Milan Cancer Institute and designated quadrantectomy, axillary dissection, and radiotherapy (QU.A.RT) (Rasponi et al. 1982; Veronesi 1977, 1978).

Patients and Methods

Patients with clinical or mammographic evidence of a breast cancer less than 2 cm in diameter and without palpable lymph nodes (T1 N0) were selected for the trial. If the findings in the excisional biopsy and frozen section were consistent with infiltrating carcinoma measuring up to 2 cm in diameter the patients were randomized to one of the two treatment groups, the first receiving the classic Halsted mastectomy, while the patients in the second group underwent a "quadrantectomy" with simultaneous axillary dissection followed by radiotherapy to the ipsilateral residual mammary tissue. Patients who had had a previous biopsy as outpatients less than 4 weeks before the final surgery were included only after accurate evaluation of the size of the primary tumor. The patients were stratified according to menopausal status. Patients with noninfiltrating carcinoma were excluded as were patients who were older than 70 years or who had had previous malignant disease of any type. Women refusing one treatment procedure or the other and those in whom adequate follow-up was

Early Breast Cancer
Edited by J. Zander and J. Baltzer
© Springer-Verlag Berlin Heidelberg 1985

unlikely because of their geographic location were also excluded from the trial. From 1973 to 1975, patients with histologically proven nodal metastases were further randomized to receive either radiotherapy to the supraclavicular and internal mammary nodes or no further treatment. From 1976 to 1980 the patients with axillary metastases were all submitted to adjuvant chemotherapy (CMF for 1 year).

The patients who were randomized to Halsted mastectomy underwent surgery consisting in an oblique elliptical incision extending to the axillary fossa, complete removal of the minor pectoral muscle, and extensive removal of the major pectoral muscle. All the axillary lymph nodes were removed up to the apex of the axilla. In the last 2 years of the trial the extent of surgery was reduced, with preservation of a large portion of the major pectoral muscle; 54 patients underwent this modified procedure.

Patients randomized to conservative treatment were treated with the quadrantectomy technique, the aim of which is the total removal of the entire quadrant of the breast containing the primary carcinoma, including the overlying skin and the fascia of the major pectoral muscle. The axillary lymph nodes were excised during the quadrantectomy. When the primary cancer was located in one of the upper quadrants the operation was performed en bloc, whereas when the primary site was one of the lower quadrants the axillary dissection was performed separately through a separate incision. All the axillary lymph nodes up to the apex of the axilla were removed, and the minor pectoral muscle was totally removed.

Irradiation of the breast was an integral part of the treatment. A dose of 50 Gy, as calculated at the midplane of the breast, was delivered through two opposing tangential fields with high-energy photons (a cobalt unit or a 6-MeV linear accelerator) and another 10 Gy was given as a booster to the skin surrounding the scar, with orthovoltage radiotherapy. Wedge filters were used if the breast was

Table 1. Menopausal status, size of primary carcinoma, axillary metastases, previous biopsy, and age in patients treated with Halsted radical mastectomy or quadrantectomy

Variable	Treatment	
	Halsted	Quadrantectomy
No. of patients	349	352
Premenopausal (%)	53.9	56.8
Diameter < 1 cm (%)	44.4	46.0
Axillary metastases (%)	24.6	27.0
Previous biopsy (%)	13.7	14.8
Age (years in mean ± SEM)	50.9 ± 0.546	50.1 ± 0.550

Table 2. Distribution of patients by site of primary tumor

Site	Treatment	
	Halsted	Quadrantectomy
	Precentage of patients	
Upper outer quadrant	39.8	44.9
Lower outer quadrant	21.2	14.8
Upper inner quadrant	26.9	27.6
Lower inner quadrant	6.8	9.4
Center	5.7	3.3

Table 3. Frequency of axillary node metastases

Axillary node metastases	Treatment	
	Halsted	Quadrantectomy
	No. of patients (%)	
Absent	263 (75.4)	257 (73.0)
One node	50 (14.3)	50 (14.2)
Two or three nodes	16 (4.6]	27 (7.7)
Four or more nodes	20 (5.7)	18 (5.1)
Total no. of patients	349	352
Total with axillary metastases	86 (24.6)	95 (27)

large and tilted upward. No bolus was used. Radiotherapy was started 15−30 days after surgery and completed within 6 weeks. Until the end of 1975, patients of both groups with positive nodes were randomized to receive adjuvant radiotherapy to supraclavicular and homolateral internal mammary nodes (40−45 Gy) in 4−5 weeks.

Since 1976, all patients with positive nodes were treated with 12 cycles of chemotherapy with the CMF regimen according to the following schedule: cyclophosphamide, 100 mg per m^2 BSA per day for 14 days; and methotrexate, 40 mg per m^2, plus fluorouracil, 600 mg per m^2, on days 1 and 8. Chemotherapy was started 15−30 days after surgery, and in the quadrantectomy group it was begun simultaneously with radiotherapy in most cases. The average quantity of drugs administered was similar in the two treatment groups.

The patients were followed up at quarterly intervals. A chest x-ray examination was requested every 6 months for the first 5 years and then once a year. A complete bone scan or x-ray study was performed every year.

The main data in all patients were recorded and stored in an automated data system after a complete check of the consistency of the data. The data were updated monthly according to the information derived from the follow-up examinations. The calculation of the life-tables was performed by the actuarial method, and the curves were compared by the log-rank test.

From June 1973 to May 1980, in all 701 evaluable patients were entered into the trial; 349 were treated with the Halsted mastectomy and 352 with QU.A.RT. There were no significant differences between the two groups in any of the variables considered, such as age, menopausal status, tumor site by quadrant, dimensions of the primary cancer, incidence of axillary metastases, or previous biopsy (Tables 1 and 2).

The primary cancer measured less than 1 cm in diameter in 44.4% of the patients in the Halsted group and 46.0% in the QU.A.RT group. Microscopical evidence of axillary metastases was found in 24.6% of patients treated with the Halsted mastectomy and in 27.0% of patients treated with the conservative procedure. The breakdown according to the number of lymph nodes involved did not reveal any significant difference between the two treatment groups (Table 3). The two series therefore appeared completely comparable.

Three patients were lost to follow-up; all three were in the Halsted group.

Results

Five patients in the QU.A.RT. group and five in the Halsted group had local recurrences. Moreover, seven patients treated with the conservative technique had a second cancer in the ipsilateral breast 2−5 years after the operation. The diagnosis of a second primary tumor in the ipsilateral breast was recorded after careful clinicopathological evaluation by

Table 4. Local or regional recurrences and second primary breast cancers

Variable	Treatment	
	Halsted	Quadrantectomy
	No. of patients (%)	
Local recurrences	5	5
Second primary tumors		
Ipsilateral breast	–	7
Contralateral breast	12	15

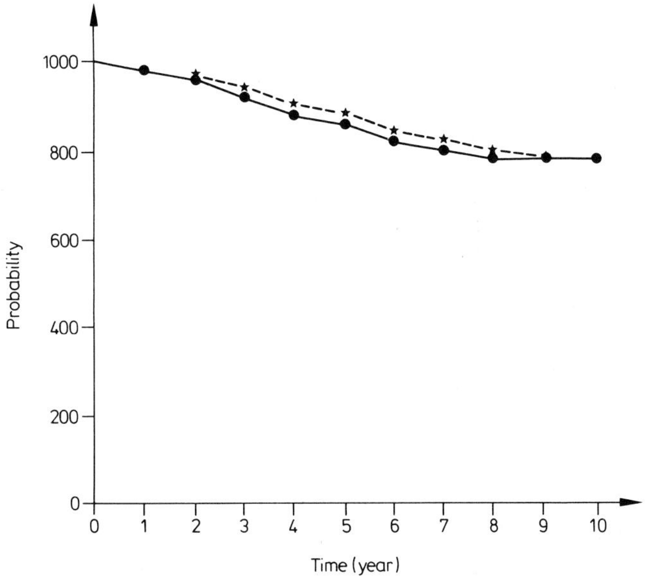

Fig. 1. Actuarial disease-free survival in patients treated with Halsted mastectomy (●———●) or with quadrantectomy axillary dissection, and radiotherapy (✶- - -✶). $n = 701$; $X^2 = 0.69$; $P = 0.40$

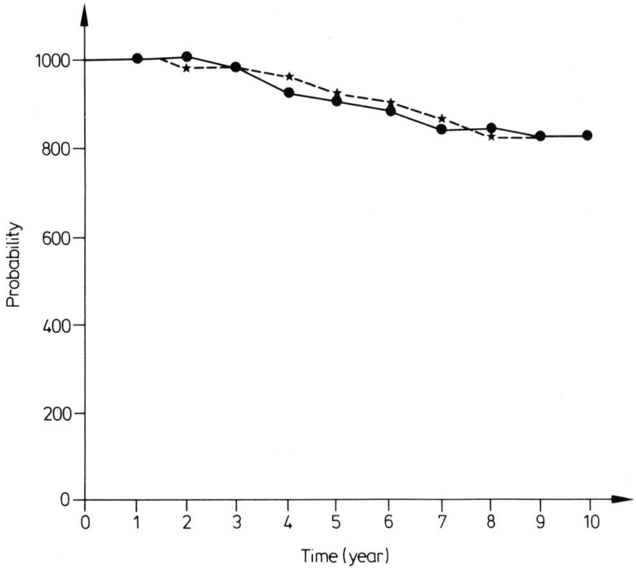

Fig. 2. Actuarial overall survival in patients treated with Halsted mastectomy (●———●) or with quadrantectomy, axillary dissection, and radiotherapy (✶- - -✶). $n = 701$; $X^2 = 0.23$; $P = 0.63$

surgeons, radiologists, and pathologists. Contralateral primary breast cancers numbered 15 in the quadrantectomy group and 12 in the Halsted group (Table 4). By May 1983, there had been 28 deaths from breast cancer in the quadrantectomy group and 28 in the Halsted group.

The data on disease-free and overall survival are shown in Figs. 1 and 2, which do not reveal any difference between the two groups after 3−10 years of follow-up.

Evaluation of disease-free survival by subgroups according to the presence or absence of axillary metastases (Figs. 3 and 4) also did not show differences between the two types of treatment, except an advantage for the patients treated with the conservative procedure in the subgroup of patients with positive axillary nodes. In the first 2 years of the trial, patients

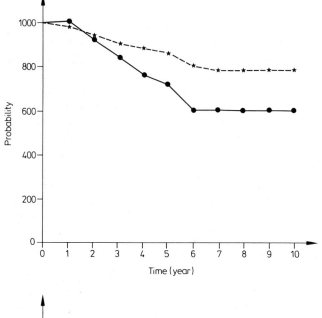

Fig. 3. Actuarial disease-free survival in patients with positive axillary nodes following Halsted mastectomy (●———●) or quadrantectomy, axillary dissection, and radiotherapy (✳- - -✳). $n = 181$; $X^2 = 5.49$; $P = 0.019$

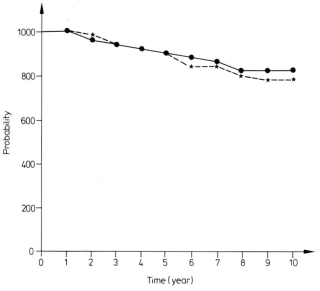

Fig. 4. Actuarial disease-free survival in patients with negative axillary nodes following Halsted mastectomy (●———●) or quadrantectomy, axillary dissection, and radiotherapy (✳- - -✳). $n = 520$; $X^2 = 0.29$; $P = 0.59$

from both groups with positive axillary nodes were further randomized into two different groups; one received no further treatment (23 patients) and the other, additional radiotherapy to regional node stations (33 patients). At 8 years, 18 of 23 patients (78%) without further radiotherapy and 18 of 33 patients (57%) treated with regional radiotherapy were free of disease.

Conclusions

The results presented in this report show that radical mastectomy can be substituted by a less mutilating procedure without any modification of the long-term survival rates or of the rate of local recurrences. Since local recurrence is the main variable in which a difference between the two treatments is expected, there is no reason to expect that the results will be influenced by a longer follow-up period, since most local or regional recurrences generally occur within 3 years of treatment. However, it must be stressed that our data refer to patients with very small breast cancers, their tumors being less than 2 cm in size at the pathological examination.

Whether the procedure can be safely applied to carcinomas more than 2 cm in diameter is at present difficult to say. It is not impossible that extension of the indications for quadrantectomy to include larger tumors might result in a higher rate of local recurrence. Moreover, if the breasts are small a quadrantectomy for a tumor 3 or 4 cm in diameter may give a poor cosmetic result. It is also our opinion that if the QU.A.RT. technique were applied in such cases an increased dosage of the radiation boost over the site of the primary tumor would be necessary. The higher dose could be given either by external radiotherapy or by interstitial implantation of radioactive material. It appears that the planning and implementation of more and more clinical trials of different conservative procedures must go ahead without delay to test the efficacy of the various types of conservative procedures available. The trials will also identify the types of patients who may safely be considered candidates for conservation of the breast.

It is our opinion that with the clinical data now available, it is no longer acceptable for a woman with a small breast carcinoma to be treated with a mutilating operation such as mastectomy when conservative procedures such as QU.A.RT. can provide the same long-term results. In our opinion, it is surprising that the tremendous and successful efforts in the field of diagnostic techniques (which can now detect small carcinomas 5 mm in size) have not been followed by a similar effort to take advantage of these new discoveries in favor of a less traumatic and more humane treatment of the women affected by breast cancer.

References

Calle R, Pilleron JP, Schlieger P, Vilcoq JR (1978) Conservative management of operable breast cancer. Cancer 42: 2045−2053

Hayward JL (1977) The Guy's trial of treatments of early breast cancer. World J Surg 1: 314−316

Pierquin B, Owen R, Maylin C, Otmezguine Y, Raynal M, Mueller W, Hannoun S (1980) Radiation therapy. Int J Radiat Oncol Biol Phys 6: 17−24

Rasponi A, Luini A, Andreoli C, Zucali R (1982) Quadrantectomia più radiotherapia nel carcinoma T$_1$ della mammella. C.E.A., Milano

Scanlon EF (1983) Breast cancer surgery. An overview. In: Feig GA, McLelland R (eds) Breast carcinoma. Masson, New York

Spitalier J, Brandone H, Ayme Y et al. (1977) Cesiumtherapy of breast cancer. A five-year report on 400 consecutive patients. Int J Rad Oncol Biol Phys 2: 231−235

Vana J, Bedwani R, Mettlin C, Murphy GP (1981) Trends in diagnosis and management of breast cancer in the U.S. Cancer 48: 1043−1052

Veronesi U (1977) New trends in the treatment of breast cancer at the Cancer Institute of Milan. AJR 128: 287−289

Veronesi U (1978) Value of limited surgery in breast cancer. Semin Oncol 5: 395−402

Veronesi U, Saccozzi R, Del Vecchio M, Banfi A, Clemente C, De Lena M, Gallus G, Greco M, Luini A, Marubini E, Muscolino G, Rilke F, Salvadori B, Zecchini A, Zucali R (1981) Comparing radical mastectomy with quadrant ectomy, axillary dissection, and radiotherapy in patients with small cancers of the breast. N Engl J Med 305: 6−11

Wolmark N, Fisher B (1981) Surgery in the primary treatment of breast cancer. Brest Cancer Res Treat 1: 339−348

Conservation Therapy of Potentially Curable Breast Cancer: Experience at the Marseilles Cancer Institute

J. M. Spitalier, R. Amalric, H. Brandone, Y. Ayme, and J. M. Kurtz

Institut du Cancer de Marseille, BP 156, 13273 Cedex 09, France

Following the lead of F. Baclesse and his successors at the Curie Institute in Paris, and of other pioneers in Europe and North America, we have used curative radiation therapy in the treatment of 4,160 consecutive operable breast cancers since 1960, with the goal of controlling local-regional disease and avoiding mastectomy.

This presentation deals with 2,321 patients with 5 years' follow-up, 977 with 10 years', and 211 with 15 years': patients lost to follow-up account for 0.01% at 5 years, 0.10% at 10 years, and 0.06% at 15 years. All patients were staged into the operable categories T0−3/n0−1 according to the 1969 UICC TNM system: overed 0.46 were stage I, 0.37 stage II, and 0.17 stage III (Table 1).

Treatment involved curative radiation therapy with or without primary limited surgery; the latter consisted mostly in lumpectomy before 1970; wedge resection after 1972, and wedge resection plus limited axillary dissection after 1975. Excision was performed prior to radiotherapy only in patients with carcinomas less than 5 cm in diameter, having minimal or no adenopathy and no clinical or isolated infrared thermographic indications of rapid

Table 1. Conservative management of operable breast cancer in a consecutive, unselected series of 5-year patients since June 1960 (March 1983)

	T0	T1	T2	T3	
N1	7	128	728	312	1,175
N0	15	397	647	87	1,146
	22	525	1,375	399	2,321

33 Patients lost to follow-up (1.42%) + 62 deaths from other causes (2.67%) = 95 inevaluable patients (4%)
UICC stage I, 1,059/2,321 = 45.63%;
UICC stage II, 863/2,321 = 37.18%
AJC stage I, 412/2,321 = 17.75%;
AJC stage II, 1,510/2,321 = 65.06%
Stage III (T3/N0−1), 399/2,321 = 17.19%
T0 no palpable breast cancer (BC); T1, palpable BC ≤2 cm in diameter; T2, BC > 2 cm ≤ 5 cm in diameter; T3 BC > 5 cm ≤ 8 cm in diamter N0, no palpable axillary node; N1, movable axillary nodes

Early Breast Cancer
Edited by J. Zander and J. Baltzer
© Springer-Verlag Berlin Heidelberg 1985

Table 2. Results[a] of conservative management in a nonselected series of patients with operable breast cancer

	5 Years			10 Years			15 Years		
	A	B	C	A	B	C	A	B	C
T3/N0−1	208	181	125	52	48	25	17	16	8
		385			160			58	
T0−2/N1	641	586	484	161	155	118	27	22	10
		825			264			57	
T0−2/N0	901	856	763	238	232	194	44	40	29
		1,016			325			66	
	1,750	1,623	1,372	451	435	337	88	78	47
		2,226			749			181	

[a] A, alive; B, alive with no evidence of disease; C, alive with no evidence of disease and with breast preservation

growth. All other cancers were irradiated following needle or open biopsy without excision.

The radiation equipment most frequently used was a telecesium unit before 1979, delivering 60 Gy in 6 weeks to the whole breast and axilla, or alterantively 50 Gy in 5 weeks was administered by a telecobalt unit after 1975. Internal mammary and supraclavicular nodes received 40−50 Gy during this period. The tumor received boosters with electron-beam or short-distance cesium, usually to a total of 80 Gy in 8 weeks, reduced to 75 Gy in the event of prior excision. The axilla was received a booster of 70 Gy if clinically or histologically positive.

Following primary treatment patients were followed-up regularly, with mastectomy reserved for apparent local or regional failure. Adjuvant chemo- or hormonotherapy was not routinely given during the period of this study (before 1977).

For our total evaluable unselected series of anatomically operable and conservatively treated consecutive patients, clinical cure rates (survival without evidence of disease) are a function of both initial clinical stage and length of follow-up. They are quite comparable to those seen following primary radical surgery. For all stages taken together the NED survival rates are 73% at 5 years, 58% at 10 years, and 43% at 15 years. These cure rates range from 84% for stage I at 5 years to 28% for stage III at 15 years. The majority of surviving patients have not been required to pay for their cure by loss of the breast (Table 2).

Of particular interest are the relatively favorable group of stages I and II cases who were treated by radiotherapy following primary limited surgery; the crude survival rate is 90% at 5 years 74% at 10 years, and 61% at 15 years; the NED survival rate is 85% at 5 years, 73% at 10 years, and 51% at 15 years, with corresponding breast preservation rates of 95%, 86%, and 70%. These results are particularly good for American Joint Committee stage I (T1/N0).

The series of 10-year patients will be used as the basis for three important analyses: local control rates, results of salvage surgery, and complication rates.

Comparison of our treatment techniques with reference to the control of local and regional manifestations of disease (Tables 3 and 4) in stage I and II patients treated initially with tumor excision, shows that the loco-regional failure rates are similar to those obtained with

Table 3. First clinical recurrences and 10-year isolated loco-regional recurrences[a] following primary limited surgery for operable breast cancer

	Isolated mammary recurrences	Mammary and axillary recurrences	Isolated axillary recurrences	Total loc.-regional recurrences
T2 N1	5/ 69 = 7.25	5/ 69 = 7.25	3/ 69 = 4.35	13/ 69 = 18.84
T2 N0	13/125 = 10.40	2/125 = 1.60	2/125 = 1.60	17/125 = 13.60
T1 N1	2/ 27 = 7.41	1/ 27 = 3.70		3/ 27 = 11.11
T1 N0	11/136 = 8.09	6/136 = 4.41	1/136 = 0.74	18/136 = 13.24
	31/357 = 8.68	14/357 = 3.92	6/357 = 1.68	51/357 = 14.29

All 10-year T'-Mo : 8.68 + 3.92 = 12.60   All 10-year N'-Mo : 3.92 + 1.68 = 5.60

[a] In absence of distant visible disease

Table 4. First clinical recurrences and 10-year isolated loco-regional recurrences[a] following conservative management of operable breast cancer

	Isolated mammary recurrences	Mammary and axillary recurrences	Isolated axillary recurrences	Total loc.-regional recurrences
T3 N1	23/141 = 16.31		5/141 = 3.55	28/141 = 19.86
T3 N0	10/ 41 = 24.39	5/ 41 = 12.20		15/ 41 = 36.59
T2 N1	44/279 = 15.77	35/279 = 12.54	6/279 = 2.15	85/279 = 30.47
T2 N0	34/238 = 14.29	14/238 = 5.88	4/238 = 1.68	52/238 = 21.85
T1 N1	3/ 42 = 7.14	4/ 42 = 9.52	1/ 42 = 2.38	8/ 42 = 19.05
T1 N0	14/158 = 8.86	9/158 = 5.70	1/158 = 0.63	24/158 = 15.19
	128/899 = 14.24	67/899 = 7.45	17/899 = 1.89	212/899 = 23.58

All 10-year T'-Mo : 14.24 + 7.45 = 21.69   All 10-year N'-Mo : 7.45 + 1.89 = 9.34

[a] In absence of visible distant disease

radical primary surgery; with 13% breast failures and 6% axillary failures at 10 years (total: 14%). Mammary recurrence rates were not significantly affected by tumor size below 5 cm (with previous excision), suggesting that surgical removal of the tumor equalizes local recurrence risk.

Only half these local recurrences appear less than 4 years after therapy with 7% of failures occurring after the 10th year. More than 80% of local recurrences are operable (90% in cases of primary limited surgery).

For patients irradiated without previous tumor excision, the local control rates are inferior to those achieved by primary radical surgery, the overall 10-year loco-regional failure rate being 3 out of 10. The value of primary limited surgery is clearly demonstrable for 10-year T2 tumors (36% without and 13% with previous tumorectomy for mammary recurrences).

Among the 5- to 22-year patients 558 salvage operations were performed with mammary and/or axillary residual disease: 24/2,297 = 24% (438 after radiotherapy alone + 120 after

Table 5. 5-year crude survival rates after salvage surgery in 10-year patients (secondary operations with residual disease, performed before January 1977)

	T+ N−	T+ N−	T+ N−	
T3/N0−1	8/16 = 0.50	0/6 = 0.00	6/19 = 0.32	14/41 = 0.34
T1−2/N1	23/31 = 0.74	4/7 = 0.57	7/23 = 0.30	34/61 = 0.56
T1−2/N0	22/31 = 0.71	0/2 = 0.00	5/12 = 0.42	27/45 = 0.60
	53/78 = 0.68	4/5 = 0.27	18/54 = 0.33	75/47 = 0.51

All T+ secondary operations, 57/93 = 61%   All N+ secondary operations, 22/69 = 32%

primary limited surgery). Secondary operations were commonly radical or modified mastectomies. But it is interesting to note that conservative secondary operations were performed in 122/558 (= 22%) of the cases. These conservative operations, reserved for small mammary or axillary recurrences, have become more frequent in recent years, and generally after primary limited surgery (beyond 40%). The results of salvage surgery depend upon both the initial clinical stage and the histological findings in the operative specimen, especially in the axillary dissection. The results are quite acceptable if only the breast is involved: 73% 5-year survival after salvage surgery for initial stages I and II; and 50% of patients surviving after secondary operations for proven loco-regional residual disease (Table 5).

Following axillary dissections we occasionally see transient lymphedema and subacute thrombolymphangitis, and in the long term a few moderately, no disabling, swollen arms. For this reason we advocate restraint in limiting axillary dissection, to obtain 9−12 nodes for adequate staging.

The late sequelae of radiotherapy have been quite acceptable. Fully three-quarters of the patients had minimal or no sequelae, and only 1% had severe complications.

Surgery is the main factor in breast preservation. Although only 40% of the patients were treated by primary limited surgery, two-thirds of the cured patients who have their breasts at 10 years owe this to either primary or secondary conservative surgery.

Our 22-year experience, along with the long-term results from other centers in Europe and North America (Princess Margaret Hospital in Toronto and Fondation Curie in Paris, for instance), has demonstrated that, stage for stage, survival rates are not adversely affected by breast-conserving therapy. Late results are the sole basis of our policies in oncology.

Despite certain objections, we feel strongly that such conservation therapy can be offered with a good conscience to most women with breast cancer that is highly suitable for surgical treatment. But close cooperation between surgeons and radiotherapists is essential. Only the proper use of modern radiation sources will allow maximum sterilization of loco-regional disease with minimal sequelae of radiation.

The best candidates for primary tumor excision are lesions 5 cm or less in size, with minimal or no adenopathy and no skin change and without indications of rapid growth. However, we have recently begun extending the indications of wedge resection to include selected "small" T3 tumors and certain tumors with minimal central skin retraction, removing an ellipsis of skin overlying the cancer. We are also considering the introduction of interstitial iridium implantation.

Along with wedge resection, we feel that the ideal primary conservative operation includes limited dissection of the low and middle axillary levels. Not only does this technique provide all the necessary biologic grading, staging, and binding, but it helps minimize the sequelae of treatment by allowing somewhat less aggressive radiation therapy. Not only can booster doses be reduced, but axillary radiotherapy can be omitted if the axilla is negative on adequate staging.

Although local control is satisfactory following primary limited surgery, patients with larger tumors treated by radiotherapy alone clearly have a higher local recurrence rate than is observed after primary mastectomy. However, this concern about local failure is mitigated somewhat by the good results of salvage surgery. It is clear that local recurrence after conservation therapy must not be viewed in the same pessimistic light as local recurrence following primary radical surgery.

Little by little, the treatment of breast cancer is finally emerging from the constraints of the nineteenth century. Conservation therapy has made its contribution not only in improving the quality of life for many patients, but also in encouraging modern women to seek consultation at an earlier stage of the disease when it is more likely to be curable. In recent years we have seen increasing numbers of small breast cancers with constantly falling numbers of involved nodes: we are seeing a boom of low-failure-risk patients.

Conservative Management of Breast Carcinoma*

The Créteil Experience

B. Pierquin, Y. Otmezguine, and P. A. Lobo

Département de Carcinologie, Hôpital Henri Mondor, 94010 Créteil, France

Introduction

More than 900 patients with breast carcinoma have received conservative treatment during the past 21 years. The aim was to give the patient with breast malignancy a treatment preserving the breast malignancy a treatment preserving the breast and thus avoiding the psychologic trauma that follows a mastectomy, at the same time guaranteeing the patient loco-regional control equivalent to that obtained by radical treatment methods which result in loss of the breast. The survival, local recurrence, cosmetic appearance, and iatrogenically induced complications are now reported. Tumorectomy before or after radiation therapy will also be discussed.

Methods

The following criteria were used to select the patients for conservative treatment: (a) Not previously treated for breast malignancy; (b) absence of distant metastasis at the time of presentation; (c) absence of other primary lesions in the contralateral breast or other locations; (d) all patients with T1, T2, or T3 lesions less than 7 cm who refused surgery; and (e) all N0, N1a and N1b lesions less than 2 cm.

The majority of the patients with T1 lesions (80%) were initially treated with tumorectomy without axillary lymph node dissection (except certain N1b). This was followed by preliminary external irradiation with telecobalt delivered to the breast and underlying chest wall by tangential beams and to the axillary, supra- and subclavicular, and internal mammary lymph nodes by a direct field technique, up to a dose of 45 Gy. Electron boosts (10–13 MeV) were given to the internal mammary lymph node chain (15 Gy) and to axillary lymph nodes (24 Gy). On completion of the electron boosts iridium was implanted in the breat in the area containing the residual tumor (boost dose 37 Gy) or that from which the tumor had been excised (boost dose 25 Gy). For T2 lesions the same method was applied, but the proportions of tumorectomies performed before and after irradiation were reversed (20% before). For T3 lesions the treatment was mostly nonconservative, consisting in preliminary external irradiation with telecobalt up to a dose of 45 Gy followed by radical surgery (Patey type mastectomy with axillary dissection). Patients who refused surgery received radical irradiation similar to that given for the T1 and T2 lesions (boost dose 37 Gy).

---

* First published in: Acta Radiologica Oncology 22 (1983)

Early Breast Cancer
Edited by J. Zander and J. Baltzer
© Springer-Verlag Berlin Heidelberg 1985

Results

The survival is presented in Table 1 after a minimum follow-up of 5, 7, and 10 years for T1, T2, and T3 lesions. The incidence of N1b is low for T1 (4%) and T2 (12%) lesions, but much higher (35%) for T3 lesions. Even though the survival rates are different at 5 years between the T1 (84% NED), T2 (75% NED), and T3 lesions (65% NED, Table 2), it is interesting to note the equalization of the rates at 10 years between the uncorrected and NED survivals, on the one hand, and between the survival of patients with T1 and T2 lesions on the other. It seems there is no further new manifestation of the disease after about 10 years for T1, T2, or T3 lesions, and the long-term prognosis for T1 and T2 lesions seems to be identical once the maximum risk for development of metastases has passed during the first few years. At the same time it is worth noting the identical rate (27%) of distant metastasis at 10 years for T1 and T2 lesions (Table 3).

After 5 years, the rate of local recurrence in the breast or peripheral lymph nodes rapidly reaches a plateau of less than 10% for T1 and T2 and less than 20% for T3 lesions (Table 4). The recurrence rate at 10 years is almost identical for T1 and T2 lesions (T1 8%, T2 9%). It is to be noted that the proportion of breasts preserved amongst the NED patients at 5, 7, and 10 years remains high and unchanged. Of the 39 local recurrences detected clinically during the last 10 years of observation, the majority (32/39) were found in the breast itself, half of these being localed at a distance from the initial site of involvement (19/39). No

Table 1. Distribution of patients by classification and follow-up (5, 7, and 10 years). The percentage is of N1b is shown for each T category

	5 years			7 years	10 years
	No. of cases	%	% N1b		
T1	99	24	4	66	26
T2	235	58	12	145	67
T3	74	18	35	57	33
Total	408			268	126

Table 2. Uncorrected and NED survivals at 5, 7, and 10 years for T1, T2, and T3 lesions. Percent in parentheses

	T1			T2			T3		
	No. of cases	Alive	Alive NED	No. of cases	Alive	Alive NED	No. of cases	Alive	Alive NED
5 years	99/408	89/99 (90)	83/99 (84)	235/408	192/235 (82)	177/235 (75)	74/408	51/74 (69)	48/74 (65)
7 years	66/268	54/66 (82)	50/66 (76)	145/268	114/145 (79)	103/145 (71)	57/268	37/57 (65)	29/57 (51)
10 years	26/126	17/26 (65)	17/26 (65)	67/126	46/67 (68)	43/67 (64)	33/126	15/33 (45)	15/33 (45)

Table 3. Distribution of distant metastases at 5, 7, and 10 years. Percent in parentheses

	T1	T2	T3
5 years	14/99 (14)	49/235 (21)	23/74 (31)
7 years	13/66 (20)	35/145 (24)	23/57 (40)
10 years	7/26 (27)	18/67 (27)	15/33 (45)

Table 4. Local recurrence rate for T1, T2 and T3 lesions. Proportions of breasts preserved among NED patients. Percent in parentheses

	T1		T2		T3	
	No. of cases	Breast/ NED	No. of cases	Breast/ NED	No. of cases	Breast/ NED
5 years	3/99 (3)	82/83 (99)	15/235 (6)	169/177 (95)	12/74 (16)	41/48 (85)
7 years	3/66 (5)	48/50 (96)	13/145 (9)	98/103 (95)	10/57 (17)	25/29 (86)
10 years	2/26 (8)	16/17 (94)	6/67 (9)	40/43 (93)	5/33 (15)	12/15 (80)

Table 5. Distribution of clinically detected local recurrences

	No. of cases	T	N	T & N	Total
T1	99	3	0	1	4
T2	235	19	0	2	21
T3	74	10	2	2	14
Total	408	32	2	5	39

isolated lymph node recurrences were observed for T1 and T2, and such recurrences were infrequent for the T3 lesions (2/74). Local recurrences in the breast occurring at the same time as lymph node metastases detected clinically remain rare for T1 and T2 (3/334) as well as for T3 lesions (2/74; Table 5). Surgical cure by mastectomy and axillary dissection (according to Patey or Halsted) was possible in most cases (33/39). Four cases needed skin grafts (2 T2 and 2 T3; Table 6). Overall, the proportion of local recurrences with lymph node metastases remains low; only 5 (1.5%) lymph node recurrences confirmed microscopically were observed during 10 years (Table 7).

The cosmetic results stabilize around 3 years after treatment. The physical appearance of the breast is classified according to three categories: (a) Very good, for those without sequelae or with only a discrete change not apparent at first glance; (b) quite good, for those developing obvious sequelae such as telangiectasia or alteration of breast contour but acceptable in preference to mastectomy; and (c) poor, when the cosmetic results are such that initial surgery would have been preferable. The observations at 5, 7, and 10 years are

Table 6. Surgical control of loco-regional recurrences

	Radical surgery	Uncontrolled	Total
T1	4	0	4
T2	20[a]	1	21
T3	9[a]	5	14
Total	33	6	39

[a] Two T2 and two T3 with graft

Table 7. Histopathologic information regarding T and N for 33 patients operated upon with radical surgery for local recurrences

	T+N−	T+N−	T−N+	Total
T1	3	1	0	4
T2	16	4	0	20
T3	3	4	2	9
Total	22	9	2	33

Table 8. Assessment of cosmetic results for patients with local control at 5, 7, and 10 years. Percent in parentheses

	Years	Very good	Quite good	Poor	Total	
T1	5	32	4	0	36	
	7	34	3	0	37	
	10	12	4	1	17	
Total		78 (87)	11 (12)	1		90
T2	5	33	23	5	61	
	7	39	28	4	71	
	10	21	16	4	41	
Total		99 (54)	67 (39)	13 (7)		173
T3	5	3	4	3	10	
	7	9	9	1	19	
	10	4	5	2	11	
Total		16 (40)	18 (45)	6 (15)		40

summarized in Table 8: 87% very good for T1 lesions, 54% for T2, and 40% for T3 lesions. The poor results are 1% for T1, 7% for T2, and 15% for T3 lesions. In assessing the cosmetic results for patients subjected to tumorectomy it must be emphasized that only the tumor bed was excised and the boost dose was relatively moderate (25 Gy instead of 37 Gy). Very good cosmetic results were obtained in 90% of the T1 patients in whom tumorectomy was performed, versus 72% in those without tumorectomy. For the T2 lesions, the results were less spectacular (65% versus 51%). A comparison between the patients operated upon at this hospital and at another hospital before referral reveals that

Table 9. Cosmetic results in relation to tumorectomy. Very good results at 5 years and more. Percent in parentheses

	Tumorectomy		No tumorectomy	Total
T1	65/72 (90)		13/18 (72)	78/90 (87)
T2	24/37 (65)		69/136 (51)	93/173 (54)
	Inner	Outer		
	15/18 (83)	9/19 (47)		
T3				16/40 (40)

the very good results are as high as 83% at this hospital, compared with a much lower rate (47%) for those operated upon in another hospital (Table 9).

Iatrogenic complications other than those affecting the cosmetic appearance of the breast are relatively unimportant. Therefore, only those of a definite and lasting nature will be considered. Minor pains were observed in the breast or scapular region in less than 5% of cases. Amongst the NED patients, up to the present time no case of severe neuritis involving the brachial plexus has been observed. The same applies to paresis or paralysis of the nerve roots. Minor limitations of shoulder movements were observed in 5%−10% of the cases, probably due to radiation-induced sclerosis of the pectoralis major muscle. No case of severe impairment of shoulder movement has been observed. Lymphedema of the upper extremity was rare (less than 5% of cases) and of a limited degree when present. Only one case of radiation-induced breast necrosis was observed which necessitated mastectomy (T2, boost dose 37 Gy) (Calitchi et al. 1984).

Discussion

Patients with carcinoma of the breast have been treated since 1961 with the aim of conservative management if possible.

The results at 10 years compared with the results at 5 (Pierquin et al. 1980) and 7 years have demonstrated a plateau in survival. This probably indicates that the potential for the development of late local recurrence or distant metastasis is extremely low, and if metastases appear they have a very slow progression (Clark et al. 1982).

These results are comparable to those obtained with surgery or combined radiation therapy and surgery (Hannoun 1978). However, it must be kept in mind that these comparisons are made in nonrandomized series.

The only randomized trial was published by Veronesi et al. (1981), in which the conservative (quadrantectomy and radiation therapy) and nonconservative techniques (Halsted type operation) were shown to produce identical survival rates at 5 years (Table 10). This trend was confirmed at the 7-year follow-up (Veronesi 1982).

The low rate of local recurrence in the present series (less than 10% at 10 years for T1 and T2 lesions) is in accordance with experience at the Curie Institute (Calle et al. 1978; Calle 1982) for T1 and T2 lesions subjected to tumorectomy, but differs for T2 and T3 lesions not operated upon; the incidence of local recurrence is higher at the Curie Institute (Table 11). Overall, the proportion of breasts preserved at 10 years is identical at the two centers for T1 and T2 lesions subjected to tumorectomy and is in the order of 95% for the NED patients. On the other hand, this proportion remains high for patients with T2 and T3 lesions not

Table 10. Survival at 5 years following Halstedtype operation or quadrantectomy and radiation therapy at Istituto Nazionale Tumore, Milan 1981 (percentages)

	Halsted ($n = 349$)	Quadrantectomy + radiation therapy ($n = 352$)
N−	75	73
Local recurrences	0.8 ·	0.2
Distant metastases	8	6
Overall survivals	90	90
NED survivals	83	84

Table 11. Percentage of breasts preserved (T1−T2, alive NED) at Institut Curie and Hôpital Henri Mondor (Créteil)

	Tumorectomy + radiation therapy	Radiation therapy alone
5 years		
Curie	95	47
Créteil	97	96
10 years		
Curie	88	53
Créteil	95	95

undergoing tumorectomy treated at this hospital (95% for T2, 80% for T3), while it is around 50% for patients treated at the Curie Institut. This may be due to the technique of dose delivery. After tumorectomy it is sufficient to give a boost of 20−25 Gy to the original tumor area, which is easily done with external irradiation (telecobalt or electrons), or by interstitial therapy (^{192}Ir). When tumorectomy has not been performed it is necessary to deliver a higher boost, in the order of 35−40 Gy, to the residual tumor to obtain an overall rate of control equivalent to that obtained when a tumorectomy has been performed. The total dose delivered locally exceeds 90 Gy (50 Gy for a reference isodose of 45 Gy − preliminary irradiation, plus > 40 Gy for a reference isodose of 37 Gy − boost irradiation), which is achieved by means interstitial therapy. Due to the limiting factor of the skin tolerance, the boost delivered by external irradiation should not exceed 25 Gy (total dose should not exceed 80 Gy). This fact should be modified, as at the Curie Institute a large number of the patients irradiated without tumorectomy are not given a full tumor dose if the tumor regression is insufficient after 50−55 Gy. These patients are then operated upon with a modified radical mastectomy with axillary dissection. These failures of radical irradiation cannot be considered in the same light as failures of irradiation taken to full tumor doses.

The survival, local recurrence, or distant metastases at 10 years are nearly identical for T1 and T2 lesions. Therefore, conservative management appears possible for all tumors of 1−5 cm (Harris and Hellman 1982). The same does not apply to the T3 lesions, as the survival of these patients at 10 years, though stable, is clearly very low with a high rate of local recurrence. It is worth noting that conservative management was used in selected T3 lesions only if three conditions were fulfilled: (a) the primary tumor less than 7 cm; (b) appreciable tumor reduction (50%) after preliminary external irradiation; and (c) if the

Table 12. Incidence of second primary in contralateral breast at 5, 7, and 10 years. Percent in parentheses

	5 years	7 years	10 years
T1	6/99 (6)	6/66 (9)	2/26 (8)
T2	4/235 (2)	6/145 (4)	3/67 (4)
T3	5/74 (7)	6/57 (10)	3/33 (9)
Total	15/408 (3.6)	12/268 (6.7)	8/126 (6.3)

patient expressed a strong desire to keep her breast, understanding and acceptance of the increased risk of local failure or poor cosmetic result. On the whole, the results for T3 lesions treated conservatively after proper selection are relatively satisfactory and worthy of consideration.

The cosmetic results are clearly related to the total dose delivered to the tumor bed in the breast. The best results were obtained (90% very good) when a tumorectomy could be performed, thus permitting a reduction of the boost dose. The poor cosmetic results (retraction, telengiectasia) were as a rule limited to the area which received the boost dose. The breast usually retains a near-normal appearance if the dose of external irradiation does not exceed 50 Gy. How the tumorectomy is performed also plays an essential role in the final cosmetic result. Large excisions, particularly if deep, may cause retraction from scar tissue, which is further aggravated by radiation-induced fibrosis. It is therefore important that this combined treatment with irradiation and surgery be carried out by members of an oncology team working closely together. It should be noted that any assessment of cosmetic results can only be made after a relatively long period of observation (3 years after treatment) (Table 9).

Local pains of a minor nature and slight limitation of shoulder joint movements are infrequent. This is valid for up to 10 years of observation. It is too early to make any prediction about the remaining life span of the patients.

The incidence of a second primary in the contralateral breast continues to remain low. On average it does not exceed 6% at 10 years, with a plateau being reached at 7 years (Table 12).

In the light of the present satisfactory results the treatment protocol has been modified in an attempt to further refine the indications for tumorectomy (with or without axillary lymph node dissection of limited extent). Tumorectomy before irradiation of T1 lesions is recommended. For T2 lesions tumorectomy before irradiation is also recommended if it is felt that the excision will not adversely affect, the cosmetic result tumors up to 3 cm in size. For larger lesions (over 3 cm) the indications for tumorectomy are extended by delivering a preliminary course of external irradiation (45 Gy) and closely monitoring the reduction in tumor size in the hope that the size will decrease to less than 3 cm. The outcome of this preliminary radiation determines the subsequent treatment: (a) If no tumor reduction is noted it is preferable to perform radical surgery or deliver the maximum permissible boost dose of 37 Gy by interstitial therapy; (b) with complete tumor regression as determined clinically and radiologically a boost dose of 25 Gy to the tumor bed by interstitial therapy is adequate; (c) with reduction of tumor size to below 3 cm but without complete regression a simple tumorectomy is recommended followed by a boost of 15 Gy by [192]Ir (Fig. 1).

The role of axillary dissection limited to the lymph nodes in the inferior portion of the axilla remains to be defined. It may provide information of prognostic importance in predicting

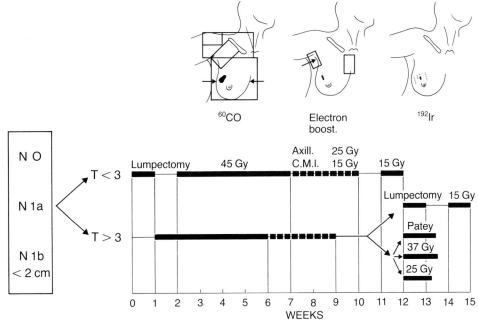

Fig. 1. New treatment protocol for breast carcinoma

the risk of developing distant metastases and in deciding what adjuvant therapy is indicated (hormonal or chemotherapy). However, it has no influence on the local control of lymph node metastasis; only 1.5% microscopically proven recurrences were detected at 10 years after irradiation alone (T1 and T2). Therefore, it can be stated that radiation therapy alone is capable of controlling nearly al micrometastases in the lymph nodes in the case of T1 and T2 lesions classified as NO and N1a, and even in the N1b lesions provided they are less than 2 cm in size.

Summary

The results obtained with conservative management of breast carcinoma are presented. The disease-free survival for patients with T1 lesions was 84% at 5 years, 76% at 7 years, and 65% at 10 years; the corresponding figures for patients with T2 lesions were 75%, 71%, and 64%; and those for patients with T3 lesions, 65%, 51%, and 45%. Among the patients who were free of disease at 10 years, the affected breast had been preserved in 94% with T1 lesions, 93% with T2 lesions, and 80% with T3 lesions. The cosmetic results were very good in the case of T1 lesions, good in the case of T2 lesions, and quite good in the case of T3 lesions. Up to 1981 simple tumorectomy was performed for most T1 lesions and some T2 lesions, followed by radical radiation. Most of the T2 and T3 lesions were treated exclusively with radical irradiation. In an attempt to improve the cosmetic results, since 1981 the indications for tumorectomy have been extended to include some of the T2 lesions and, whenever possible, some of the T3 lesions. In these cases tumorectomy with limited axillary dissection is performed either before or after irradiation.

Acknowledgements. The authors wish to thank the entire staff of the Department of Oncology at Hôpital Henri Mondor, particularly the surgical group − A. Germain, M. Julien, A. Bisson, S. Hanoun, J. Lange, C. Thomsen − and the radiotherapy group − F. Baillet, J. P. le Bourgeois, M. Raynal, C. Maylin, M. Salle, J. J. Mazeron, E. Calitchi, M. Martin − and G. Marinello, PhD.

References

Calitchi E, Cheula JM, Otmezguine Y. Roucayrol AM, Mazeron JJ, Le Bourgeois JP, Pierquin B. (1984). Analyse retrospective á 10 ans des séquelles du Tradement loco-regional des cancers du sein. Bull. Cancer. 71 : 100

Calle R (1982) Breast carcinoma local treatment − place of conservative surgery and irradiation exclusively for early breast cancer. International Conference on the Use of Conservative Surgery and Radiation Therapy in the Treatment of Early Breast Carcinoma, Cambridge, Mass

Calle R, Pilleron JP, Schlienger P, Vilcoq JR (1978) Conservative management of operable breast cancer. Ten years experience at the Foundation Curie. Cancer 42: 2045

Clark RM, Wilkinson RH, Mahoney LJ, Reid JG, MacDonald WD (1982) Breast cancer. A 21 year experience with conservative surgery and radiation. Int J Radiat Oncol Biol Phys 8: 967

Hannoun S (1978) Cancers du sein classés T1, T2. Etude comparative à propos de 387 cas répartis en 2 séries traités respectivement par chirurgie mutilante (128 cases) ou radiothérapie (259 cases): MD Thesis, University of Paris

Harris JR, Hellman S (1982) Primary radiation therapy for early breast cancer: the experience at the Joint Center for Radiation Therapy. Internationl Conference on the Use of Conservative Surgery and Radiation Therapy in the Treatment of Early Breast Carcinoma, Cambridge. Mass

Pierquin B, Owen R, Maylin C, Otmezguine Y, Raynal M, Mueller W, Hannoun S (1980) Radical radiation therapy of breast cancer. Int J Radiat Oncol Biol Phys 6: 17

Veronesi U (1982) Conservative treatment of early breast cancer at the Istituto Nazionale. International Conference on the Use of Conservative Surgery and Radiation Therapy in the Treatment of Early Breast Carcinoma, Cambridge, Mass

Veronesi U, Saccozi R, Del Vecchio M, Banfi A, Clemente C, De Lena M, Gallus G, Greco M, Luini A, Marubini E, Muscolino G, Rilke F, Salvadori B, Zecchini A, Zucali R (1981) Comparing radical mastectomy with quandrantectomy, axillary dissection and radiotherapy in patients with small cancers of the breast. N Engl J Med 305: 6

Conservative Treatment of Potentially Curable Minimal, Occult, and Early Breast Cancer: Experience at the Universitäts-Frauenklinik Hamburg

K. Thomsen

Universitäts-Frauenklinik Hamburg-Eppendorf,
Martinistrasse 52, 2000 Hamburg 20, Federal Republic of Germany

I would like to give a brief description of our Hamburg trial of conservative treatment of T1 tumors of the breast; our patient sample is small compared with that in the Milan study and the NSABP program. But first let me say something in review about our motivation. Long ago we had the impression that the fate of patients suffering from breast cancer depended more on other conditions than on the extent of operation. At the Congress on Conservative Treatment of Breast Cancer in Strasbourg 1972, I was deeply impressed with the 5- and 10-year survival rates following wide excision and irradiation. These results were obtained without public discussion as is usual nowadays. Many doctors now feel they are being progressive when they perform a breast-preserving operation even without having the necessary personal experience and technical conditions. In addition, they do not like to be involved in a controlled study. For the patient this is a risk trend, which could also discredit the trials under way.

Table 1 recapitulates some of the data presented in Strasbourg in 1972. Due to the different classifications (i.e., TNM system, Columbia, or Manchester classification) only a restricted comparison is possible. Nevertheless it can be stated that the 5- and 10-year survival rates for cases in stage T1 are comparable, with those after radical operation. The results in stage T2 are demonstrably worse than those after radical surgery. Hayward found the same in a randomized trial of patients over 50 years of age. After 5 years there was no significant difference between the results of conservative and radical treatment of stage T1, but worse results were seen in stage T2 after conservative treatment (see results of Schlienger, Rissanen, and Hayward (Table 1). In the group of conservatively treated patients the number of local recurrences was twice as high as with radical treatment.

In Germany there are no institutions like that in Milan with more than 1,000 cases of primary breast cancer to be treated yearly. A cooperation of different institutions in a protocol like in the National Surgical Adjuvant Breast Program could not be realized in Hamburg or even in all West Germany. Actually such a cooperative randomized trial is no longer necessary, as the main problems under discussion today in Munich are being investigated in current randomized trials.

Therefore, in 1972 we started a controlled but not randomized trial of T1N0M0 breast cancer to be treated with *wide excision and irradiation*.

According to the findings of Shah and Rosen and others, limited, breast-preserving operation modalities must be expected to be an insufficient therapy for stage T1 cases. In the prospective study of Rosen, in which partial mastectomy was simulated at the time of radical mastectomy for known breast cancer, 56% of the patients had a primary tumor less

Early Breast Cancer
Edited by J. Zander and J. Baltzer
© Springer-Verlag Berlin Heidelberg 1985

Table 1. Results of conservative treatment in the form of wide excision and irradiation

Author	Stage	No. of cases	Survival rate 5 years	10 years
Spitalier	T1 + T2 N0 M0	38	97%	
Mustakallio	T1 + T2	702	90% 83%	81% 58%
Schlienger	T1 N0 M0 T2 N0 M0	64	90% 60%	
Delouche	T1 N0 M0 T2 N0 M0	92	88% 77%	
Rissanen	T1 N0 M0 T2 N0 M0	150 189		73% 49%
Birkner	?	110	63%	
Peters	I and II	124	76%	45%
Wise	?	96	95%	62%
Atkins	T1/T2 N0	70	56%	
Hayward	T1 N0 T2 N0	182 188	78% 56%	
Papillon	T1/T2 N0	127 62	69%	66%
Svoboda	T1/T2 N0	83	67.9%	
Prosnitz et al.	I II	49 101	91%[a] 60%[a]	

[a] Recurrence-free

Table 2. Factors requiring exclusion from conservative treatment

Tumor over 2 cm in diameter
Poorly bounded tumors with high capability to spread
Lymphangiosis in tissue surrounding the tumor
Incomplete removal of a tumor
Removal of a tumor with too small a margin of uninvolved tissue
Concomitant preinvasive carcinoma

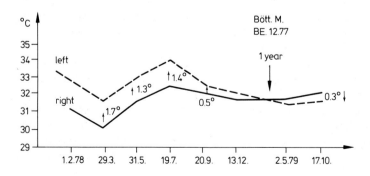

Fig. 1. The treated left breast became isothermic with the right breast after 1 year

Table 3. Local recurences and distant metastases by group

Group	No. of patients	Local recurrence	Distant metastases	Second carcinoma
I	84	4	1	–
II	50	4	1	1
	134	8	2	1

Table 4. Five-year survival following conservative management of breast cancer

Group	No. of patients	Disease-free	Local recurrence	Metastases
I	35	32	3	
II	17	14	2	1
	52	46	5	1

than 2 cm in diameter. In 22% non infiltrating carcinoma were found in the residual three quadrants, but 11% showed residual areas with infiltrating cancer. These findings negated the concept of unicentricity, even for such small lesions. If such patients are treated by surgery alone the need for total mastectomy for optimal control ist evident. If they are treated by breast-perserving surgical modalities additional x-ray treatment to the remaining breast and the regional lymph node areas is necessary.

Our trial was terminated at the end of 1981 after 10 years. Due to the restriction of selection only 25% of our patients with T1 stage, disease, i.e., 134 cases, could be included in this study. The conditions requiring exclusion from this type of conservative management are summarized in Table 2.

For the wide excision, needle localization with x-ray control is necessary, since most of these small tumors are not palpable. The excised specimen is examined by specimen *radiography* and by *step sections*. If the above-mentioned conditions are confirmed, telecobalt irradiation is started 10 days after the operation. The breast is exposed to a tissue dose of 60 Gy, and the lymph nodes, including the parasternal chain, to a dose of 55 Gy.

The patients are followed-up at frequent intervals by the same team as is responsible for the primary therapy. In follow-up, thermography plays a dominant role. After irradiation the temperature of the treated breast exceeds that of the untreated breast by 1.5 to 2.5 deg C. After 1 year both breasts should be isothermic, as demonstrated in Fig. 1.

So far we have treated 134 patients with wide excision and x-ray therapy without excavation of the axilla. When we started this program little was known about the significance of adjuvant chemotherapy in patients with lymph node involvement. In group I all the above-mentioned conditions were present. In this group we observed 4 cases with local recurrence and 1 case with distant metastases. In group II, of 50 cases there were 4 with local recurrences, 1 with distant metastases, and 1 with a cancer in the contralateral breast (Table 3).

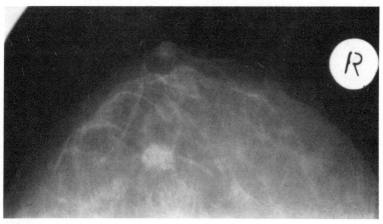

Fig. 2. A 35-year-old patient with a small tumor 1 cm in diameter diagnosed only by mammography

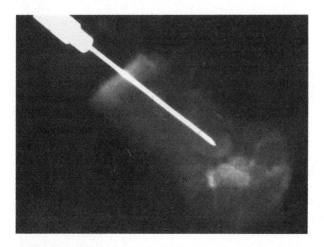

Fig. 3. The specimen radiogram after needle localization

In group II not all of the above-mentioned conditions were present, for example a poorly bounded tumor. The results in this group are clearly worse, which means that this modality of management of stage T1 breast tumors should be applied *only* when all the above-mentioned conditions are present, i.e., under ideal conditions.

Table 4 shows our 5-year survival rates: almost 90% of the patients are disease-free after 5 years. According to other trials this figure is expected to drop in the next 5 years. Figures 2–7 show a representative case.

The conditions necessary for conservative treatment in this trial are summarized in Table 5.

This is a preliminary report of a controlled but nonrandomized trial. Our patients are too few and the follow-up too short to allow a final conclusion.

After termination of this study we started a new trial including all stage T1 cases without special selection. The maximum diameter of the cancer will be measured by radiography and by our pathologist in the specimen. The operation is done by segmental resection with removal of the underlying fascia and excavation of the axilla.

If there is no node involvement only the preserved breast is subjected to an x-ray treatment with 60 Gy. If the lymph nodes are involved chemotherapy is applied for six cycles

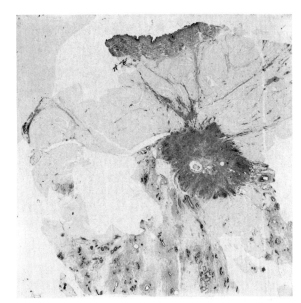

Fig. 4. A giant section of the tumor

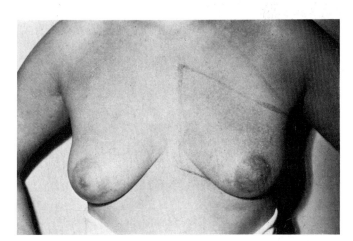

Fig. 5. The patient after x-ray therapy

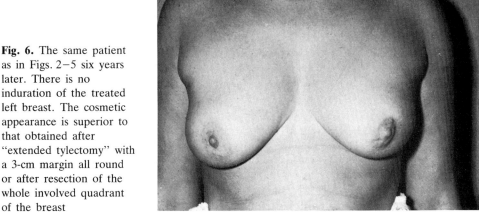

Fig. 6. The same patient as in Figs. 2–5 six years later. There is no induration of the treated left breast. The cosmetic appearance is superior to that obtained after "extended tylectomy" with a 3-cm margin all round or after resection of the whole involved quadrant of the breast

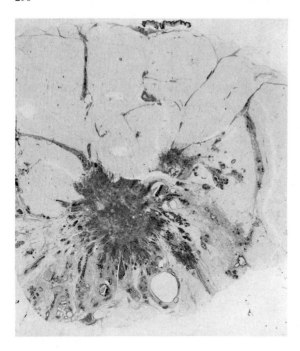

Fig. 7. A giant section from a tumor 1.5 cm in diameter but with a satellite tumor excluded from our trial

Table 5. Necessary conditions for conservative treatment

1 Close cooperation between surgeon, radiologist, and pathologist, who *share* responsibility for deciding on and carrying treatment and for follow-up at frequent intervals

2 Stage T1 N0 M0
   Tumor should be sharply outlined and surrounded by sufficient uninvolved tissue (min. 1 cm). Measurement of tumor, step sections

3 Irradiation of breast and regional lymph nodes with 60 Gy

4 Follow-up with mammography and thermography; modified radical mastectomy if tumor not sterilized

Table 6. Conservative procedures applied in breast cancer patients staged T1 N0 M0

Procedure	No. of patients
Wide excision + radiation	134
Segmental excision + axillary excavation + radiation	35 (5)[a]
	169

[a] Five with lymph node involvement

according to the CMF protocol used in Milan. We have treated 35 cases in this way so far. Of these, 5 had lymph node involvement. We hope to achieve results as good as those in Milan.

So far we have treated 169 cases conservatively (Table 6). Worldwide experience with conservative treatment modalities for early breast cancer provides no evidence that radical surgery gives better results than conservative procedures. If no difference in long-term survival can be stated than conservative breast-preserving operations have the advantage of providing *better cosmetic and functional results and an improvement in the quality of life.* The knowledge that the breast can often be saved in selected cases that are diagnosed early, should stimulate women to examine their own breasts, to have periodic mammograms, and to contact their physician at the first suspicion of breast disease. This may decrease the incidence of death from breast cancer.

The patient suffering from breast cancer needs an individualized therapy adapted to the individual situation. But this can only be realized on the basis of 10- and 15-year results of the main randomized trials under way today.

Conservative Treatment of Potentially Curable, Minimal, Occult, and Early Breast Cancer

K. G. Ober

Universitäts-Frauenklinik, Universitätsstrasse 21/23, 8520 Erlangen,
Federal Republic of Germany

Only someone who is perfectly aware that he does not know enough about the matter could include such differing terms as "potentially curable", "minimal", "occult" and "early cancer" in the same title. For, in the last resort, these terms have not yet been defined, and I cannot imagine how they could be defined with any accuracy within the next 10 years.

Gynecologists have gained experience with cancer of the cervix. Although, here, the conditions are considerably more favorable, we must still expect to encounter great problems of communication even in this area.

The fashionable solution of the programmed, prospective randomized study is in my view to be rejected. There has been a great deal of discussion on this, and international opinion varies conderably. Anyway, we shall find no answer here.

An alternative would be accurate documentation, which, however, would involve a considerable amount of work. Again, comparison with carcinoma of the cervix suggests itself, in which this procedure has yielded the only really useful results to date. Professor Zander presented a report on this in 1980. In the case of the breast, a great deal more time will be needed, since this disease requires longer observation periods and, in addition, accurate documentation of disease is very much more difficult in a paired organ with eight quadrants than in the case of the uterine cervix, which can after all become pathologic only in a region the size of the first joint of the thumb. We have already heard some facts and figures on this from my co-workers (Egger et al., this volume). Serious discussions require measurements. Assessments based on the sensitivity of the fingertips are just as ineffectual in our times as the midwife's stethoscope as a means of monitoring a high-risk birth.

My own approach the the choice of treatment involves personal talks with the patient, whom I observe very closely. Occasionally, I experience something of a conflict within me, but, as a rule, I answer my own question, namely: How would you choose if the patient were a member of your own family?

We have carried out tumor excision and quadrantectomy both for palliative and, after long and careful consideration, for specifically therapeutic reasons. The indications for subcutaneous mastectomy are based on very stringent and strictly applied criteria. Basically, this is a non-classic operation, which really ought to be the final step in the diagnostic work-up rather than a form of primary treatment.

At present, our sample is small; Tables 1−4 show the results we have achieved to date. Of special interest is the fact that each case is particularly thoroughly and accurately documented. Perhaps the results can be evaluated in 10−15 years' time. We have gained similar experience in the case of cancer of the cervix.

Early Breast Cancer
Edited by J. Zander and J. Baltzer
© Springer-Verlag Berlin Heidelberg 1985

Table 1. Observations in patients receiving palliative surgery

Case no.	Patients	Age (years)	Tumor diameter	LN	RAD	CHT	Follow-up
1	H. H.	83	> 80	Ø	−	−	† 1 year
2	D. B.	75	18	Ø	−	−	† 2 years
3	W. A.	42	99	++	+	+	† 3 years
4	B. R.	34	99	++	+	+	NR − 10 years
5	D. A.	61	> 35	−	−	−	Recurrence − 1 year
6	S. U.	36	Right 18 Left 12	++	+	+	NR − 7 years
7	H. M.	67	99	−	−	+	Recurrence-3.5 years
8	K. K.	32	20	+	+	+	† 1 year
9	Sch. A.	72	99	++	−	+	† 1 year
10	E. O.	59	10	−	−	−	NR − 3 years
11	A. A.	61	20	Ø	−	−	† 1 year
12	M. A.	67	29	−	−	−	NR − 2 years
13	K. M.	69	18	+	−	−	NR − 1 year
14	H. H.	46	18 + 11	+	−	+	Dec. 1982 Status quo
15	B. U.	63	> 30	+	−	+	NR − 1 year

LN, lymph node status; RAD, adjuvant radiation therapy; CHT, adjuvant chemotherapy; 99, tumor diameter not precisely measurable because of multiple invasion; ø not done

Table 2. Observations in patients receiving lumpectomy

Case no.	Patients	Age (years)	Tumor diameter	LN	RAD	CHT	Follow-up
1	St. D.	50	13	Ø	+	−	NR − 9 years
2	Sch. H.	50	10	−	−	−	Recurrence − 1 year
3	St. E.	57	20	−	−	−	NR − 5.5 years
4	Sch. R.	29	50	−	+	−	† 2 years
5	A. H.	60	24	−	−	−	NR − 4 years
6	W. M.	39	20	+	+	+	NR − 4 years
7	H. H.	40	9	−	−	−	NR − 2 years
8	C. L.	55	23	−	−	+	NR − 2 years
9	F. M.	27	99	−	−	−	NR − 2 years
10	F. T.	71	15	++	−	+	NR − 2 years
11	M. M.	50	15	(−) Sinus-meta	−	+	NR − 2 years
12	E. K.	71	15	Ø	−	−	NR − 1 year
13	R. C.	30	22	+	−	+	NR − 1 year
14	R. E.	34	14	−	−	+	NR − 1 year

Abbreviations as in Table 1

Table 3. Observations in patients subjected to quadrantectomy

Case no.	Patients	Age (years)	Tumor diameter	LN	RAD	CHT	Follow-up
1	W.P.	51	10	−	−	−	NR − 10 years
2	K. J.	65	30	−	−	−	Recurrence − 8.5 years
3	St. E.	36	10	−	+	−	NR − 5.5 years
4	L. E.	62	99	+	+	+	NR − 5 years
5	H. G.	41	15	−	+	−	Recurrence − 2 years
6	B. U.	35	16	++	+	+	† 1 year
7	B. G.	50	11	−	+	−	NR − 5.5 years
8	H. K.	58	12	−	+	−	NR − 6 years
9	U. E.	81	20	+	−	−	NR − 1 year †
10	St. E.	56	25	−	+	−	NR − 3 years
11	K. S.	37	22	+	+	+	Recurrence − 2 years † 3 years
12	U. M.	68	17	+	+	+	NR − 3.5 years
13	G. A.	73	8	Ø	−	−	NR − 3.5 years
14	E. H.	68	17	−	+	−	NR − 3.5 years
15	G. M.	42	99	−	+	+	Recurrence − 2.5 years
16	A. A.	77	25	−	+	−	NR − 2 years
17	St. E.	49	13	(+) Micro-meta	+	−	NR − 2.5 years
18	L. A.	70	99	−	−	−	NR − 2 years
19	R. G.	32	20	−	−	−	NR − 2 years
20	L. M.	41	15	−	−	+ Nissen-Meyer	Recurrence − 2 years
21	Sch. E.	41	26	+	−	+	NR − 1 year
22	G. B.	74	15	−	−	−	NR − 1 year

Abbreviations as in Table 1

Table 4. Observations in patients subjected to subcutaneous mastectomy

Case no.	Patients	Age (years)	Tumor diameter	LN	RAD	CHT	Follow-up
1	G. E.	46	2	Ø	−	−	NR − 10.5 years
2	P. H.	40	2	−	−	−	NR − 7.5 years
3	K. V.	48	2	Ø	−	−	NR − 5 years
4	K. W.	49	4	Ø	−	−	NR − 4 years
5	H. L.	46	2	Ø	−	−	NR − 4 years
6	T. K.	31	1−22	Ø	−	−	NR − 4 years
7	K. H.	46	10	Ø	−	−	NR − 4 years
8	H. C.	44	3	Ø	−	−	NR − 4 years
9	K. E.	51	2	Ø	−	−	1 year
10	M. G.	48	5 + 2	Ø	−	−	6 months

Abbreviations as in Table 1

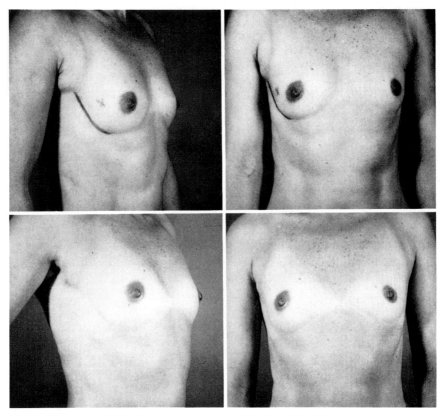

Fig. 1. Appearance following quadrantectomy with a lateral incision

Over the last $2^1/_2$ years, we have frequently carried out the so-called quadrant resection with a lateral incision. Experience shows that from the aspect of the number of lymph nodes removed, lymphonodectomy is just as possible as is Patey's operation, but the cosmetic results are better (Fig. 1).

References

Zander J, Baltzer J, Lohe KJ, Ober KG, Kaufmann C (1981) Carcinoma of the cervix: An attempt to individualize treatment. Am J Obstet Gynecol 139: 752–759

Subcutaneous Mastectomy with Lymphadenectomy and Irradiation for Primary Treatment of Breast Cancer

F. K. Beller and E. H. Schmidt

Frauenklinik der Westfälischen Wilhelms-Universität,
4400 Münster/Westfalen, Federal Republic of Germany

Introduction

The trend towards replacing radical procedures for the primary treatment of breast cancer by conservative operations is obvious from the literature. In 1970 more than 75% of American surgeons preferred Halsted's radical procedure. Only a few surgeons were beginning to apply less radical operations. Data have become available indicating that in most patients breast cancer is already a systemic disease at the time of diagnosis. Any type of operation can achieve only local cancer control at best.

There has been a long list of surgeons performing limited operations with subsequent irradiation for local cancer control. The results of tylectomy (lymphectomy) and wedge resection (quadrant resection), with or without axillary node dissection, will be discussed at this meeting. The German, Hirsch, used primary irradiation in 1928 and the attempts of French radiologists to perfect the radiation techniques are well known.

The "modified radical procedure" is a technical term that has been used by various surgeons in different ways. In any event, the transverse (Stewart) incision replaced the longitudinal (Halsted) incision, and the pectoralis major muscle was left intact. This type of operation is often historically, although not quite correctly, associated with the name of Patey as the originator. This type of surgery has reversed the radical situation of surgical procedures, since in 1979 less than 25% of surgeons preferred Halsted's procedure for the primary operation.

A variety of randomized studies comparing ultraradical with radical, and radical with modified radical techniques, gave to better results than the conservative operations such as wedge resection or tylectomy (Fig. 1). Annual mortality figures have not changed during the last 6 decades, which is another indication that the type of operative procedure is of minor or no significance (Vorherr 1981).

It is rather remarkable that surgeons place so much emphasis on the removal of large portions of skin even when data are lacking to indicate skin involvement. Skin metastasis is a pathophysiologic type of development, which is not related to skin involvement of the primary tumor. This is also indicated by the fact that more skin is removed by Halsted's procedure than by the modified radical mastectomy, but local recurrence rates are identical (Fig. 2). An even more perplexing situation concerns involvement of the areola and nipple. Lack of technical standards and criteria resulted in wide variations ranging from 2% to 20% in stage 1 disease. This explains attempts to transplant the areola into the groin or store it in the refrigerator to re-implant it later. The cosmetic results were poor, either because the

Early Breast Cancer
Edited by J. Zander and J. Baltzer
© Springer-Verlag Berlin Heidelberg 1985

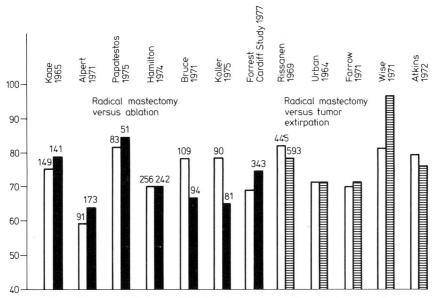

Fig. 1. Various "early" trials reveal 75% survival after 5 years regardless of the type of surgery. (Beller and Möhlen 1978)

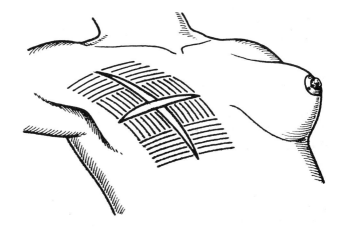

Fig. 2. Areas of skin resected during Halsted's operation and the modified radical procedure. Although less skin is resected during the latter, the local recurrence rate is not increased

transplanted areola failed to take or because the implanted areola lost its natural color.

It remains puzzling why the modified radical procedure was not replaced by a subcutaneous mastectomy with subsequent immediate or delayed augmentation. The areola and the nipple, rather than breast size, are the accepted marks of femininity in the western world. Could it be that surgeons felt they were being "radical" by removing the areola in an otherwise "modified radical" procedure? Such a thought may be substantiated when surgeons leave the skin overlapping the tumor intact but remove the nipple in small tumors far distant from the areola. Only Freeman (1973) in the USA and Gynning et al. (1975) in Sydney used subcutaneous mastectomy in very small tumors.

In any event, the quality of life is better with less radical operations (Fig. 3). After consideration of the pertinent literature, in 1974 we started to perform subcutaneous

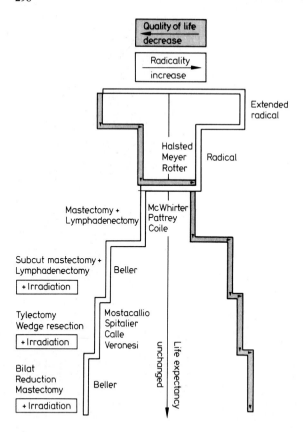

Fig. 3. Quality of life increases with reduced operations, though life expectancy remains unchanged

mastectomy and lymphadenectomy, followed by irradiation, in patients with stage T1 breast cancer (Beller and Schnepper 1976). Initially, we restricted this technique to patients with a tumor located at least 3 cm away from the areola area. After 18 months we abandoned this restriction because the areola and nipple were routinely biopsied and areolar involvement was found only in 4% (Fig. 4).

This operation is termed "extended subcutaneous mastectomy" (Table 1). If cancer was found in the areola or nipple, they were excised. In patients with large breasts weighing 500 g or more, after subcutaneous mastectomy the excessive skin mantle was reduced. We regard it as important to leave the skin sheet containing the areola flat without wrinkles. In regard to the lymphadenectomy technique, perivascular connective tissue of the axillary vein was left intact to prevent lymphedema. Enlarged lymph nodes above the axillary vein were removed bluntly by means of a thread-glove. Complete lymph node dissection was not performed, since this procedure does not seem to be curative.

Irradiation was felt to be necessary in all conservative surgery (tylectomy, quadrant resection), and therefore also to be required subsequent to subcutaneous mastectomy (Fig. 5).

At this time, the indications for adjuvant chemotherapy are not well defined and the ultimate benefits to the patient have not been determined. Because only 15%−25% of breast cancer patients with positive axillary nodes have recurrent disease within the first 2 years following primary therapy, 75%−85% of patients received adjuvant chemotherapy at a time when systemically disseminated cancer cells were dormant or their proliferation

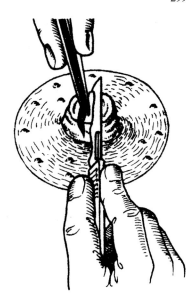

Fig. 4. Frozen section of nipple and areola base allows
this important area to be left intact

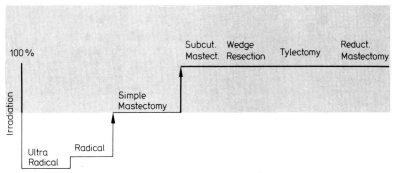

Fig. 5. Necessity for irradiation in relation to surgical procedures. Ultraradical and radical operations
do not need irradiation, and the necessity after simple mastectomy is debatable. With reduced surgery
irradiation is part of the primary treatment

Table 1. Procedure adopted at the University Hospital for Women, Münster,
for extended subcutaneous mastectomy (Beller and Schnepper)

1	Resection of glandular tissue by approx. 95%
2	Frozen section of both areola and mamilla
3	Lymphadenectomy
4	Irradiation, + adjuvant chemotherapy in stage N1

minimal and chemotherapy therefore not effective (Vorherr 1981). Accordingly, it is
imperative to strive for identification of patients in whom subclinical cancer growth most
probably exists at the time of primary therapy. In such patients adjuvant chemotherapy
may be successful in delaying recurrent disease.

Adjuvant chemotherapy was administered to node-positive patients as shown in Table 2.
There is still no general agreement on the optimum duration of adjuvant chemotherapy.

Table 2. Adjuvant treatment of breast cancer

Cyclophosphamide	600 mg/m²
5-Fluorouracil	500 mg/m²
Vincristine	1 mg/m²
Methotrexate	300 mg/m²

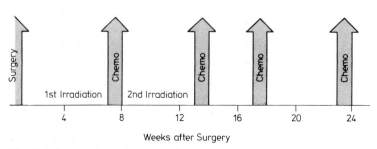

Fig. 6. Adjuvant chemotherapy regimen

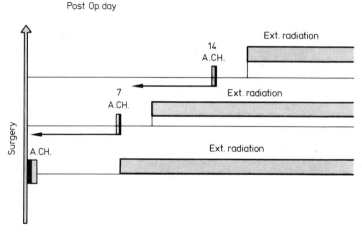

Fig. 7. Predating of the adjuvant chemotherapy (*A. CH.*) The first infusion is now given in the recovery room since it has become obvious that wound healing is not influenced

According to Bonadonna et al. (1981), adjuvant chemotherapy for 6 months is as effective as a 12-months regimen. We have given four cycles of high-dose infusions within 6 months (Fig. 6). The adjuvant chemotherapy was predated when it was realized that it did not interfere with wound healing. At present the first treatment cycle is administered immediately after surgery when the frozen section has revealed positive nodes (Fig. 7).

Breast reconstruction by silicon implant was done after the irradiated skin had become soft again; this was usually the case within 6–12 months.

In view of the risk of synchronous and metachronous contralateral and ipsilateral breast cancer in 10%–20% of all patients, we recommended bilateral subcutaneous mastectomy, especially in high-risk patients (10%–30%) with (1) unilateral premenopausal breast

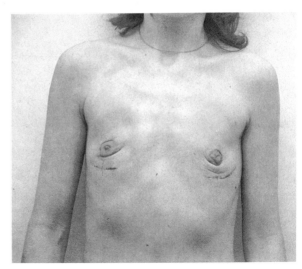

Fig. 8. Situs after bilateral subcutaneous mastectomy with reduction of skin. Note the absence of wrinkles

cancer and a positive family history; (2) multicentric cancer; (3) unilateral cancer and contralateral precancerosis (atypical proliferation); (4) unilateral lobular or tubular carcinoma; and (5) unilateral cancer and suggestive contralateral mammogram with dysplasia, microcalcification, and abnormal tissue structure. Surprisingly, only 25% of these patients followed our advice. In contrast, almost all patients with a precancerous conditions (severe dysplasia and cellular atypia) agreed to have a bilateral operation, for both prophylactic and cosmetic reasons. This discrepancy in acceptance of bilateral surgery between cancer patients and women with premalignant lesions is most probably due to the enormous psychoemotional strain on the cancer patient, connecting bilateral surgery with increased fear and seriousness of her problem. It also astonished us that only 25% of patients desired breast reconstruction. After our unilateral or bilateral surgery the majority of patients indicated that they did not feel mutilated (Fig. 8). Thus, it appears that when areola and nipple are left intact the patients do not feel mutilated, and that the size of the breast is of secondary importance.

Treatment Results

We have previously reported results after 8 years by single case analysis (Beller and Schnepper 1981). Mean while all cases have been computerized and life-table analysis has been performed according to Chiang.

The results of all stage I tumors, including T0N1, are presented in Fig. 9. They do not differ from those obtained in patients treated by a modified radical mastectomy, but we must point out that this was not a randomized study.

The disease-free survival time is also comparable between the two groups (Fig. 10). This result is not surprising since subcutaneous mastectomy differs from modified mastectomy only in the retention of skin, areola, and nipple.

In view of tumor pathobiology and the effectiveness of postoperative irradiation, I find it difficult to accept that healthy-looking skin should be resected, even though lymphatic connections between tumor and skin may exist.

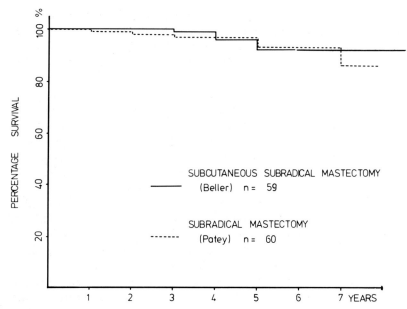

Fig. 9. Percentage survival after subcutaneous mastectomy compared with modified mastectomy (Patey) both with irradiation and lymphadenectomy

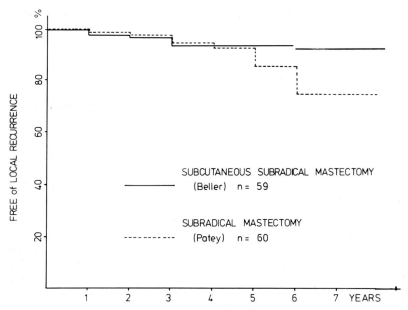

Fig. 10. Time lapse between primary treatment and local recurrence or metastatic growth, also in comparison with subcutaneous mastectomy and modified radical mastectomy (Patey)

In summing up our experience, subcutaneous mastectomy, lymphadenectomy, and post-operative irradiation provide equally effective therapeutic alternatives for primary breast cancer as treatment by lumpectomy or quadrantectomy followed by radiotherapy. However, none of the presently applied treatment modalities solve the problem of the "other breast".

Whereas by virtue of the specific pathobiology of breast cancer no significant differences in long-term survival rates can be expected, it was astonishing to realize that in patients with lumpectomy [Spitalier et al. 1973 (Toulouse); Calle and Pilleron 1982 (Paris)] and quadrantectomy [Veronesi et al. 1981 (Milan)] second cancers have rarely developed from remaining breast tissue. It must be remembered that breast cancer is multifocal (multicentric) in 25%−40% of patients. Accordingly, one may project that in up to 25%−40% of postlumpectomy breast cancer patients a second breast cancer will eventually be diagnosed. However, this was not the case. We concluded, therefore, that irradiation following lumpectomy or quadrantectomy effectively destroys multifocal lesions or prevents them from progressing to cancer. As a consequence, one is tempted to simply remove the malignant tumor and irradiate the remaining breast tissue. In patients with a high risk of bilaterality the contralateral breast can also be irradiated.

According to results derived from our work and literature data, the conclusion seems to be obvious that meticulous removal of glandular tissue is not necessary, especially since in plastic surgery it has often been held preferable to resect only 85% instead of 95% of the glandular body, to improve the cosmetic result. In light of the effectiveness of radiotherapy, the amount of glandular tissue left behind seems of little importance. It seems to be important (a) that the malignant tumor has been removed within healthy tissues (as determined by multiple frozen sections), and (b) that the remaining breast tissue is irradiated (not less than 40 Gy).

Surgical Technique Presently Applied

Since January 1982 we have removed the tumor and the bulk of the glandular body. Glandular tissues with connective tissue septa (Cooper's ligaments), which are close to and run into the panniculus adiposus and overlying breast skin, remain in situ. Thus the glandular, connective, and adipose tissue left behind is used to construct a smaller breast by a technique slightly modified from the reduction mammaplasty we described earlier (Beller and Wagner 1974). The preoperative marking of the breast skin is accomplished by a modified Strömbeck pattern and the entire figure is de-epithelialized. Subsequently, the glandular body is separated from the underlying pectoral fascia in the caudocranial direction, and the pectoral fascia is removed. The lateral Biesenberger figure is then performed. The healthy tissue plate underneath the areola is turned up (Figs. 11 and 12). The malignant tumor is removed within healthy tissue, as determined by multiple (up to 10) frozen sections of samples taken from the surrounding tissue of the tumor bed. Subsequently, the axilla is opened for lymph node dissection up to the axillary vein. Reconstruction of the breast is depicted in Figs. 13 and 14. When the frozen sections reveal positive nodes, adjuvant chemotherapy is administered before the patient awakes from general anesthesia in the recovery room.

When, after paraffin embedding and serial sections, lymph node metastasis is diagnosed, adjuvant chemotherapy is instituted on the 7th postoperative day. If the biopsy from nipple and areola base shows carcinoma in the frozen section, areola and nipple are resected.

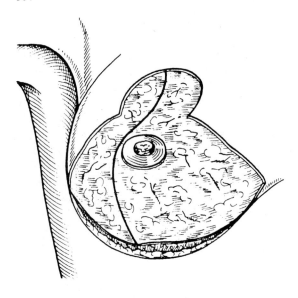

Fig. 11. Surgical technique (Beller). After de-epithelialization, Biesenberger incision is indicated. (Beller 1985)

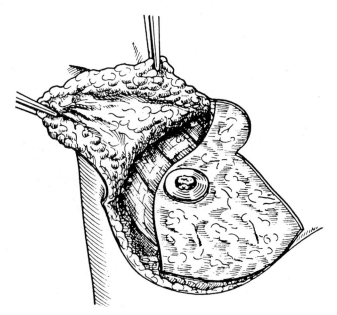

Fig. 12. Surgical technique: After mobilization of the breast from the pectoralis fascia and incision the two segments can be turned around, to allow removal of the tumor and the bulky breast tissue. (Beller 1985)

This procedure is called a "partial subcutaneous mastectomy with lymphadenectomy and simultaneous mammaplasty" (Table 3). The glandular tissue is also removed below the areola [where it is mostly left because of fear of tissue sloughing (Fig. 15)].

Since January 1982, 150 patients with breast cancer and 50 women with severe cellular atypia have undergone this type of surgery. In all but two patients bilateral reduction mastectomy was performed. Patients with cellular atypica did not undergo lymphadenectomy and irradiation. In patients with unilateral breast cancer the noninvolved breast was reduced but lymphadenectomy and irradiation were not performed. *There was no local recurrence or skin metastasis.*

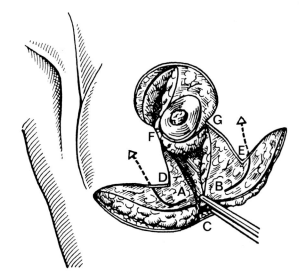

Fig. 13. Surgical technique: After removal of the glandular part a breast is formed from the remaining fat. Points *F* to *G* are sutured together, and *D/E*, to *C*. The tissue *A* and *B* is introverted. (Beller 1985)

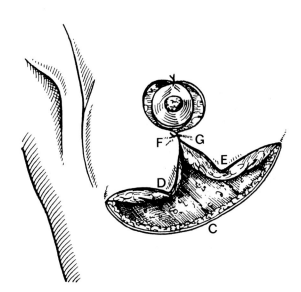

Fig. 14. Surgical technique: Situs after relocation of the areola. Corner *F* is sutured to *G,* and *D* and *E* will be sutured to *C*. (Beller 1985)

Table 3. Advantages of bilateral partial subcutaneous mastectomy as performed by Beller with lymphadenectomy and irradiation

1	A plastic procedure (reduction and lifting) replaces a radical procedure
2	Bilaterality solves the problem of the contralateral breast
3	No multilation
4	No lymphedema
5	Mammography without foreign body

Secondary mastectomy in case of recurrence

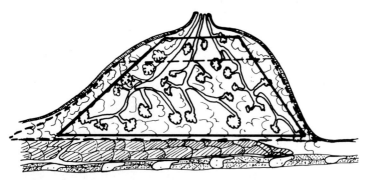

Fig. 15. Schematic showing surgical technique. *Black lines* indicate the area of glandular tissue removed. Note that reduced subcutaneous mastectomy frequently means removal of gland and fat while leaving tissue below the areola for fear of slough. This is different from our technique

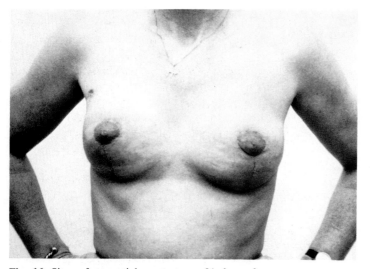

Fig. 16. Situs after partial mastectomy 21 days after surgery

Table 4. Partial subcutaneous mastectomy with lymphadenectomy. (Beller 1982)

---

1   Reduction of the bulky glandular part, leaving fat from which the new breast is formed
2   Bilateral performance of the operation (two teams)
3   Lymphadenectomy of the cancer site
4   Irradiation of cancer site and ipsilateral breast when histology reveals a secondary primary

---

We believe that this operation largely solves the problem of the other breast (Table 4). The cosmetic results are also very satisfactory (Fig. 16 and Table 4). Prophylactic contra-lateral subcutaneous or simple mastectomy are procedures that are too extensive to be justifiable, especially when a silicon implant, with its high complication rate, is desired.

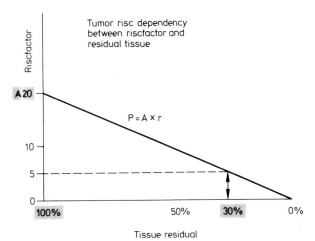

Fig. 17. Tumor risk after bilateral partial mastectomy, which is calculated to be less than 5%

However, the reduced subcutaneous mastectomy with subsequent augmentation without silicon seems acceptable.

Because our surgical technique leaves approximately 30% of the glandular tissue behind, some may consider this as an inadequate therapy. However, in patients with lumpectomy and quadrantectomy larger glandular portions remain, yet due to irradiation survival rates are equal to those patients who have had radical surgery. Nonetheless, theoretical considerations also support the technique of a reduced subcutaneous mastectomy. Atypical epithelial proliferation is considered to be a precancerous condition. Not less than 20%–30% of these patients will eventually develop cancer.

Assuming this is correct (some authors dissent), for a patient in whom 30% of glandular tissue is left the chance of developing malignancy is less than 5%, i.e., a risk similar to that of the average postmenopausal woman (Fig. 17). Moreover, since both breasts are reconstructed from remaining breast tissues, and the breasts are smaller, clinical examination, mammography, and sonography of these small breasts are diagnostically more effective. In view of these deductions, the calculated risk appears to be acceptable. In our 150 patients with breast cancer no local recurrence has been observed so far.

Finally, I would like to express my views on the treatment of patients with tumors larger than stage T1, i.e., carcinomas more than 2 cm in diameter. The general tenor of contemporary publications on breast cancer therapy emphasizes tumor stage-related surgery, which calls for a small operation in patients with a small tumor and for extended surgery in patients with a larger tumor. However, it is common experience that patients with a large tumor have more extensive local and systemic spread, curtailing their survival. Thus the patient's fate is not decided by the cancerous breast, but by distant metastases to lung, bone, liver, brain, and other organs.

In these patients the lethal outcome is predetermined long before the breast is operated on. Therefore, we do not endorse this commonly accepted concept of tumor stage-related surgery, whereby patients are mutilated with a reduced life expectancy. Therefore, the approach to tumor stage-related surgery has been reversed. The 8-year survival results in T2 tumors (Fig. 18) and the data on freedom from local recurrence (Fig. 19) do not differ from the figures obtained with modified mastectomy.

A patient with a large tumor and positive axillary (parasternal) nodes should have the most conservative treatment. We include these patients in the group for reduced subcutaneous

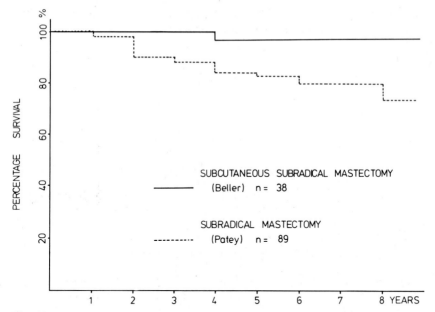

Fig. 18. Percent survival after subcutaneous mastectomy compared with modified radical mastectomy in T2 cancers

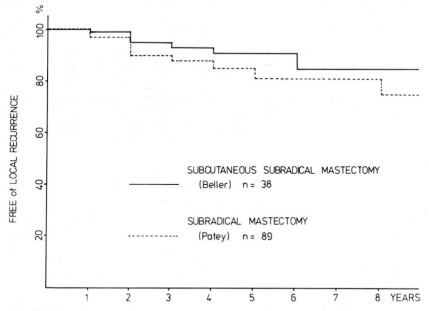

Fig. 19. Free of metastatic growth or local recurrence in T2 tumors

mastectomy. Despite the poor prognosis the quality of life is improved and an optimistic outlook on life preserved. Based on our treatment results and on survival rates reported in the literature, we are convinced that our patients are not at a disadvantage in regard to length of survival.

References

Beller FK, Bohmert H (1984) Atlas der Operationen an der weiblichen Brust. Schattauer, Stuttgart

Beller FK, Möhlen KH (1978) Operative Behandlung des Mammakarzinoms, heutiger Stand und Problematik. Med Welt 29: 77

Beller FK, Schnepper E (1976) Die mamillenerhaltende Operation zur Behandlung kleiner Mammakarzinome. Senologia 3: 27

Beller FK, Schnepper E (1981) Konservative Primäroperation des Mammakarzinoms. Dtsch Med Wochenschr 106: 329

Beller FK, Wagner H (1978) Die Technik einer Reduktionsplastik der weiblichen Brust. Zentralbl Gynakol 100: 1599

Bonadonna C, Rossi A, Tancini C, Brambilla C; Marchini S, Valagussa P, Veronesi U (1982) Multimodal therapy with CMF in resectable breast cancer with positive axillary nodes. Recent Results Cancer Res 80: 149

Calle P, Pilleron JP (1982) Nichtverstümmelnde Behandlungsverfahren beim operablen Brustkrebs. In: Frischbier HJ (ed) Die Erkrankungen der weiblichen Brustdrüse. Thieme, Stuttgart, p 207

Freeman OS (1973) Subcutaneous mastectomy for central tumors of the breast with immediate reconstruction. Past Reconstr Surg 51: 263

Gynning J, Jacobson S, Linell F, Rothmann V, Östberg G (1975) Subcutaneous mastectomy in 80 patients with breast tumors. Acta Chir Scand 141: 488

Hirsch J (1927) Radiomchirurgie des Brustkrebses. Dtsch Med Wochenschr 53: 1419

Spitalier JM, Robert F, Seigles J, Almaric R (1973) Césium therapy curative des cancers du sein de petite taille. Nouv Presse Med 4: 2249

Veronesi J, Saccozzi R, del Veccio M, Baufi A et al. (1981) Comparing radical mastectomy with quadrantectomy, axillary dissection, and radiotherapy in patients. N Engl J Med 305: 6

Vorherr H (1981) Pathobiology of breast cancer: hypothesis of biological predetermination and long-term survival. Klin Wochenschr 59: 819

Our Experiences in Setting Up the BMFT*-Multicenter Trial: Therapy of Small Breast Cancer

H. Rauschecker[1], R. Sauer[2], A. Schauer[3], H. Scheurlen[4], and H.-J. Peiper[1]

[1] Chirurgische Universitätsklinik, Robert-Koch-Strasse 40, 3400 Göttingen,
  Federal Republic of Germany
[2] Strahlentherapeutische Klinik der Universität,
  Krankenhausstrasse 12, 8520 Erlangen, Federal Republic of Germany
[3] Pathologisches Institut der Universität,
  Robert-Koch-Strasse 40, 3400 Göttingen, Federal Republic of Germany
[4] Zentrum für die Methodische Betreuung von Therapiestudien der Universität,
  Landfriedstrasse 12, 6900 Heidelberg, Federal Republic of Germany

"The medical community in the Federal Republic is obviously unable to design an interdisciplinary therapeutic concept for cancer diseases to be realized on a broad basis. With its program on the promotion of research and development for the benefit of health, the Federal Government created the organizational and financial basis for cooperative study groups and the structural requirements for the realization of multicenter therapeutic trials."

This statement was made in June 1978 at Schloss Reisensburg by the representative of the Federal Ministry of Research and Technology. By invitation of the Ministry, oncologists from all over the Federal Republic met there to work out strategic concepts for the activation of clinical trials. In a first step, an inquiry to estimate the demand for cancer trials was initiated at every university and major community hospital troughout the country. The result indicated that breast cancer was among these malignant diseases that deserved priority. In February 1979 representatives of those institutions interested in a cooperative breast preservation study commissioned us to coordinate this project and finally, in July 1983, the Ministry gave us the permission to activate this trial.

The cartoon by B. Fisher demonstrates impressively the influences we have been confronted with while planning the study over the past 4 years (Fig. 1).

First of all, the study design had to be set up. A planning committee of 12 specialists from the fields of surgery, gynecology, pathology, radiotherapy, and statistics decided on the protocol outline. As we have learned from this symposium, opinions on tumor extent in conservative breast surgery are rather controversial. We decided on a tumor stage T1N0M0 according to pathohistological criteria, differing in this respect from other study groups but being aware that this made the practical side of the study even more complicated.

The major objectives behind this decision were
1) Clear definition of the patient selection criteria.
2) Avoidance of objections to the study on the grounds of too generous patient selection criteria.

It was our goal to have as many institutions as possible participating in the study to meet the requirements of the Ministry by realizing new therapeutic concepts on a broad basis. This is only possible if the technical, apparative, and timing requirements of the protocol can be realized not only by specialists working in university institutions, but also in medium-sized

---

* BMFT = Bundesministerium für Forschung und Technologie (Federal Ministry of Research and Technology)

Early Breast Cancer
Edited by J. Zander and J. Baltzer
© Springer-Verlag Berlin Heidelberg 1985

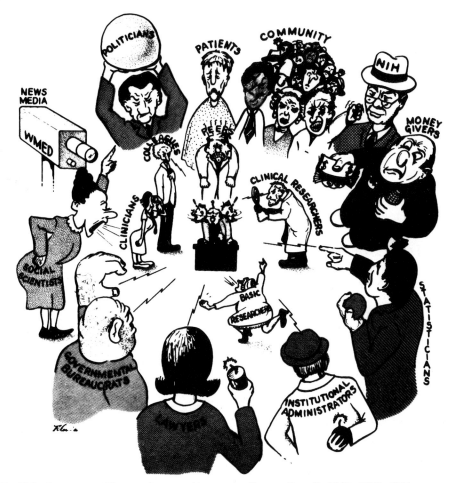

Fig. 1. B. Fisher's cartoon: The maelstrom of research. Cancer Res 40: 3863–3874, 1980

hospitals. Quality control is guaranteed by the reference centers for surgery, pathology, and radiotherapy together with the statistics center.

Figure 2 is the scheme of the study design: a patient qualifies for the study if – after routine examinations – a pathohistological tumor stage T1N0M0 is established. The patient will then be randomized to one of the two treatment modalities: (a) mastectomy or (b) radiotherapy. In case of medial tumor location additional irradiation of the regional (parasternal, supra- and infraclavicular) lymph nodes will be performed.

Parallel with the set-up of the protocol went the recruitment of trialists. At first, there was great enthusiasm due to the prospects of governmental funding for personnel and apparatus. As a consequence of the governmental money shortage the promised structural improvements were cut back to a relatively modest sum for each case entered. This caused a sudden decline of interest in multicenter trials, since most of our colleagues thought the financial support offered was an inadequate compensation for the additional effort needed to treat and monitor each patient in such a way as to meet protocol and documentation requirements.

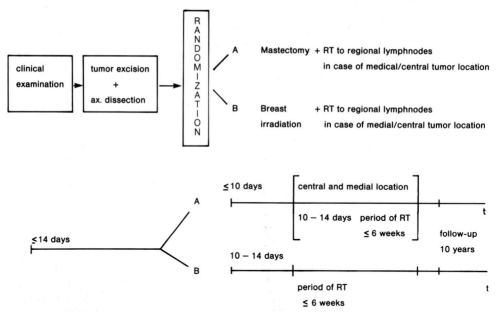

Fig. 2. Study design of the BMFT Multicenter Trial: Therapy of Small Breast Cancer

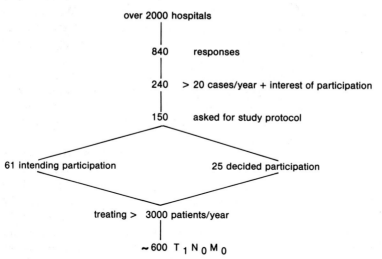

Fig. 3. Breast cancer inquiry regarding interest in participation in the study

In late 1980, we asked more than 2,000 hospitals in our country whether there was still interest in the study and whether the number of patients mandatory for a valid result could be entered. Replies were received from 840 institutions, and 230 treating 20 breast cancer patients or more showed interest. Of 150 requesting the protocol, 61 are willing to cooperate and 25 institutions have already definitely decided to participate. These 86 institutions treat about 3,000 breast cancer patients a year. Estimating stage T1N0M0 to account for 20% of all cases, in theory 600 patients per year could be entered (Fig. 3).

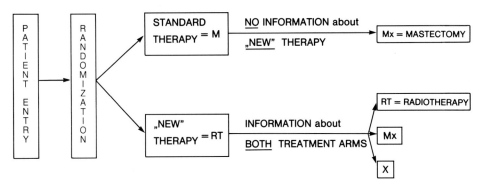

Fig. 4. Zelen's modification of the randomization procedure. N Engl J Med 300: 1242–1245, 1988

To answer the question as to whether, in breast cancer of the pathohistological stage T1N0M0, a breast-preserving therapy is as good as mastectomy with respect to the further course of disease, the statistical center estimated that 400 randomized patients per treatment modality are required within 3 years. This confronts us with the big question mark – randomization: will the number of patients willing to undergo randomization be sufficient for a statistically significant evaluation? At this point, a discussion would be speculative. In the United States of America, apparently up to 90% of all patients give informed consent to randomization to the different treatment modalities. We will know later whether this is also possible in our country. At present, experience with this problem is lacking not only among doctors, but also among patients, legal experts, and governmental agencies.

The matter of informed consent requires enormous effort, especially in the area of guidance and psychological understanding of each patient. No information scheme exists that can equally well be applied to each patient. We believe that if there is optimum individual patient information (which is rather time-consuming) the often cited doctor-patient relationship will not be disturbed.

There are several ways to avoid informed consent: Marvin Zelen developed a randomization modus which we also discussed for our study (Fig. 4). Patients randomized to breast preservation, i.e., the "new" therapeutic modality, also had to be informed about mastectomy, whereas patients randomized to standard therapy, i.e., mastectomy, were given no information about the new therapy. The benefit of this modus is that there will be enough patients in the mastectomy arm. On the other hand, it implies that the randomization is done before the patients receive any information. Thus the doctor knows what treatment arm the patient is randomized to and can influence the patient according to his point of view. This is not only unfair towards the patient, but is also statistically and legally debatable.

In this context, we might comment on something mentioned earlier, the lack of experience of legal experts with clinical studies. This study was the first one being legally evaluated. It took 9 months before we received the lawyer's reply. During that period the experts' opinion on Zelen's randomization modus had swung from agreement to a strict rejection, and we therefore returned to the randomization form with "fully informed consent." After full information, it is left to each individual patient to undergo randomization or choose the treatment herself (Fig. 5).

What happens to those patients who are not willing to undergo randomization?

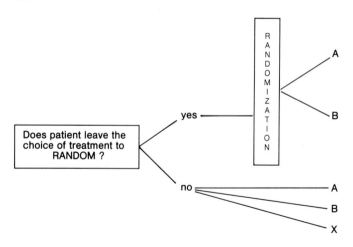

Fig. 5. Randomization procedure applied in the study

As shown in Fig. 6, the postoperative care will be the same as for randomized patients, provided that entry criteria are fullfilled. In this way, we collect information on how many and which kind of patients (regarding age, educational, and social status) decide on which treatment modality and what role the so-called hospital factor (role of the hospital personnel involved) will play. Furthermore, the study should yield information about possible connections between the self-selection of treatment, survival time, and quality of life. With the assistance of Peter McGuire in Manchester (England), who is an expert in the field of oncological psychiatry, a patient questionnaire has been prepared, from which we hope to derive details about the psychological effects of the two treatment modalities.

These additional endeavours should not diminish efforts to obtain informed consent to randomization from as many patients as possible. A drop out rate of only 10% (as is reported from the United States of America) seems unachievable in Germany. Due to the general lack of public information on the value of clinical trials, consent to randomization will depend ultimately on the commitment of the informing doctor and whether he has a positive attitude to this project. Dr. van Dongen, who is coordinating the EORTC breast preservation study imparts the relevant information to all patients who undergo breast surgery in his hospital himself, and very few refuse randomization.

Finally, another problem should be mentioned, namely the two-stage procedure necessary for patients randomized to mastectomy. This was thoroughly discussed with study participants, legal experts, and representatives of the government agencies. Tumorectomy and associated lower axillary dissection are part of the diagnostic procedure. Randomization takes place after pathohistological diagnosis of the primary tumor and the axillary lymph nodes. Women agreeing to randomization have to undergo a second operation about 10 days later if they are randomized to mastectomy.

This two-stage procedure can be avoided by

1) Changing the patient entry criteria, i.e., disregarding the pathohistological status of the lymph nodes.
2) Informing the patient before the diagnostic operation.
3) Altering the mode of randomization.

We have already discussed the last possibility. The point mentioned first is applied in almost all other breast cancer studies. In the United States of America tumorectomy with local anesthesia is becoming increasingly a routine practice. As soon as the surgeon is notified of the final pathohistological diagnosis (on average 5 days later) the patient is informed of the histological tumor diagnosis and − if she has clinically negative axillary

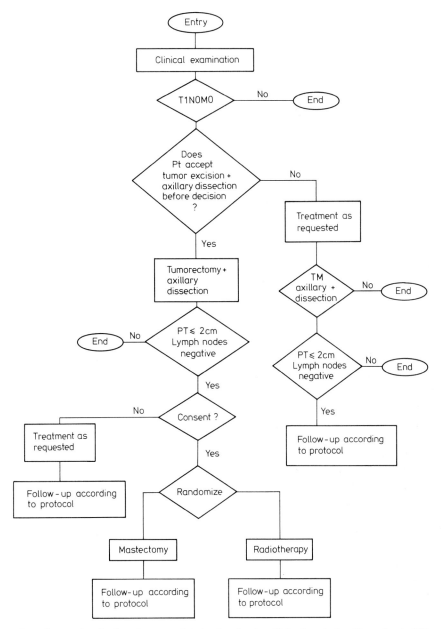

Fig. 6. Flow chart for randomized and nonrandomized patients within the study. *Pt,* patient; *PT,* primary tumor; *TM,* tumorectomy

lymph nodes − of the study and the treatment arms being investigated. If the patient consents to participate in the study she is then randomized and treated accordingly. If positive axillary lymph nodes are revealed on pathohistological examination an adjuvant radiation or systemic therapy follows after wound healing. The majority of our trialists decided to keep the pathohistological staging of the axillary lymph nodes as a study entry criterion. It is only possible to bring forward patient information without changing entry

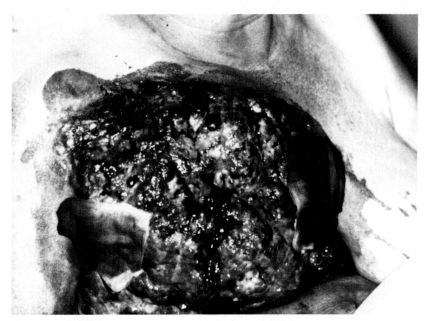

Fig. 7. Inoperable metastatic breast cancer in a 60-year-old patient

criteria if the lymph node diagnosis is also established by frozen section. This kind of lymph node work-up is painstaking and can only be performed at institutions that have the necessary manpower.

Patient information before the diagnostic operation has the disadvantage of leaving too many questions open. After extensive and strenuous discussions the following compromise was achieved: Before the diagnostic procedure, i.e., tumorectomy, the patient will be informed of the ongoing study and its therapeutic modalities, and then she decides whether to participate or to choose between the two therapeutic options. If she selects mastectomy the operation can be performed as soon as the frozen section diagnosis of the primary tumor is made. For patients participating in the study the two-stage procedure is mandatory.

The aforementioned comments touch only on some difficulties we have faced while setting up the study over the past 4 years. At times they endangered the entire project, but this learning process was necessary at times for the benefit of the study. However, considerable delay was caused by factors depicted in Fisher's cartoon (Fig. 1).

In breast cancer, *mastectomy* is still the *standard procedure* and breast preservation an experimental treatment modality which should only be offered to patients under study conditions. This implies that cancer patients in whom the breast is preserved must be absolutely certain that a high therapeutic standard is guaranteed and particular care taken with follow-up. Also, we hope to make a valid contribution towards answering the question as to whether conservative treatment is equivalent to mastectomy with regard to the further course of the disease, as reported by other study groups from the data of uncontrolled trials. There are still patients who do not see the doctor in time because they are so afraid of losing their breast that they wait until they are inoperable, like the patient whose lesion is shown in Fig. 7. She came to us with intolerable dyspnea due to pulmonary metastases.

With our trial we want to relieve women of the anguish of losing a part of their femininity and to encourage them to undergo early screening for their own benefit.

Subject Index

Adjuvant Chemotherapy of Breast Cancer

Editor: **H.-J.Senn**
1984. 98 figures, 91 tables. XIII, 243 pages. (Recent Results in Cancer Research, Volume 96). ISBN 3-540-13738-6

Clinical Interest of Steroid Hormone Receptors in Breast Cancer

Editors: **G.Leclercq, S.Toma, R.Paridaens, J.C.Heuson**
1984. 74 figures, 122 tables. XIV, 351 pages. (Recent Results in Cancer Research, Volume 91). ISBN 3-540-13042-X

Early Detection of Breast Cancer

Editors: **S.Brünner, B.Langfeldt, P.E.Andersen**
1984. 94 figures, 91 tables. XI, 214 pages. (Recent Results in Cancer Research, Volume 90). ISBN 3-540-12348-2

N.Becker, R.Frentzel-Beyme, G.Wagner

Atlas of Cancer Mortality in the Federal Republic of Germany

2nd edition. 1984. 44 coloured maps, 178 graphics.
VI, 383 pages in German and English. ISBN 3-540-13413-1

Manual of Clinical Oncology

Edited under the auspices of the International Union Against Cancer
3rd fully revised edition. 1982. 44 figures. XV, 346 pages
ISBN 3-540-11746-6

UICC
International Union Against Cancer
Union Internationale Contre le Cancer

TNM-Atlas

Illustrated Guide to the TNM/p TNM Classification of Malignant Tumors
Illustrations by U.Kerl
Editors: **B.Spiessl, P.Hermanek, O.Scheibe, G.Wagner**
2nd edition. 1985. 323 figures. Approx. 280 pages
ISBN 3-540-13443-3

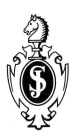

Springer-Verlag
Berlin
Heidelberg
NewYork
Tokyo